Research on Cognition Disorders

Benito Damasceno

Research on Cognition Disorders

Theoretical and Methodological Issues

Springer

Benito Damasceno
Department of Neurology
State University of Campinas (UNICAMP)
Campinas, São Paulo, Brazil

ISBN 978-3-030-57265-5 ISBN 978-3-030-57267-9 (eBook)
https://doi.org/10.1007/978-3-030-57267-9

This Springer imprint is published by the registered company Springer Nature Switzerland AG
The registered company address is: Gewerbestrasse 11, 6330 Cham, Switzerland

To my wife Dione, my sons Eduardo and Alfredo, and my uncle Eduardo who raised me with love and wisdom.

Preface

This book is addressed to all those interested in studying the human mind, especially in doing research on disorders of cognition, being intended for graduate and postgraduate students (in projects of scientific initiation, master's and PhD theses) as well as for postdoctoral researchers in the areas of neurology, cognitive neuroscience, psychology, neuropsychology, psychiatry, education, and linguistics. It is the result of my theoretical and practical experience in teaching and researching in neurology, neuropsychology, and cognitive neuroscience at the State University of Campinas (UNICAMP, Brazil) since 1986. The focus is on theoretical-methodological issues, controversies, and limitations of current studies in cognition disorders.

Part I is about cognitive functions and their interrelationships. Functions such as perception, attention, visuospatial-motor abilities, memory, language, and intellectual reasoning are conceived, not as isolated mental "faculties," a priori existing, or as "modules" located in restricted brain center, but as complex functional systems which represent the world by means of signs (mainly those of language), result from the appropriation (internalization) of external actions and relations of the individual with other persons and things, and have a cerebral organization distributed in various interconnected regions. Theoretically, several studies conceive the cognitive functions as neurofunctional networks, but in the methodological implementation of their research they do not consider them as functional systems, with each function being reciprocally influenced by others, particularly by those most relevant for the execution of the proposed test or task.

Part II deals with the historical-cultural origin of cognition, presenting its phylogenetic and ontogenetic development, from perception to theory of mind, social cognition, language, and intellectual reasoning. A problem with various studies is their exclusively biological or computational approach to the human mind. Obviously, our mind is the product of a long biological evolution, besides being mediated by biological, neurophysiological, and neurochemical processes. Computations also underlie the mental functioning and have even been implemented in electronic neural networks, helping us to better understand, for example, visual perception. Notwithstanding, the human mind is an emergent property of these processes and cannot be reduced to them; it is the interface between the organism and the world, being mediated by signs, particularly those of language, and therefore by internalized social-cultural elements acquired in joint social practice, and whose lack or deprivation in the critical periods of the mental-cerebral development impairs the acquisition of a normal mind. In addition to the biological and computational processes, the mental act of the human being also involves subjectivity, free will, and the social regulation of attitudes and decision making.

Part III addresses methodological issues of the neuropsychological investigation of patients with brain disease, focusing on brain-behavior correlations, especially on detection of impaired basic mental mechanisms or operations and, in this way, drawing inferences about the regional distribution of the brain lesion or dysfunction. Based on the systemic approach, the neuropsychological battery has to include appropriate tests for the function being studied, including control tests (counter-proofs) and control conditions, particularly the comparison with healthy matched subjects. For example, performance in a test of learning and delayed recall of a list of words may be affected by impairment of other functions such as attention, verbal fluency, motivation (apathy), and humor state (depression). Thus, for knowing whether the low scores in this test are due to a primary impairment of episodic memory (and, by inference, to a hippocampal lesion) or due to a disturbance of other mental functions (e.g., attention, verbal fluency, humor state), we need control tests (counter-proofs) for these other functions. The influence of these variables (mainly subject variables such as age and education) should be foreseen in the planning phase of the project, or should be verified after data collection by means of a multivariate analysis. So, it is emphasized to use appropriate study designs as well as randomization and matching for controlling subject variables which could, otherwise, confound the results of the investigation.

Part IV presents the fundamentals of descriptive and inferential statistics applied to biomedical and psychological research. The four chapters in this part cover definitions of basic concepts, elements of statistical analysis, hypothesis testing, and choice of tests. The intention is to make the science of statistics more interesting and easier to be understood even by graduate students. With this purpose, practical illustrations are given about how to calculate Z score, effect size, chi-squared (χ^2) test, t-test, Pearson´s correlation coefficient (r), and simple linear regression. Obviously, these tests can be immediately run by online calculators of free software programs, but the idea here is to teach the student the rationale behind such tests.

Part V deals with methodological issues in cognition research on three selected conditions: multiple sclerosis, temporal lobe epilepsy, and Alzheimer's dementia. Why these conditions and not others? I chose them because they have been the objects of my neurological practice, teachings, and researches, including clinical trials, since I started as professor at the Department of Neurology, UNICAMP, decades ago, and even before, under my medical residency and specialization in Neurology at Sahlgrenska University Hospital (Gothenburg, Sweden). The problems and limitations of researches on these conditions are critically discussed from the point of view of a systemic and interfunctional approach of cognition, as thoroughly presented in Parts I and III.

With this kind of approach, by showing the complexity of the human mind, I hope this book will be useful to all those who are interested in doing research on cognition disorders.

Campinas, São Paulo, Brazil Benito Damasceno

Acknowledgments

I am deeply grateful to all patients and colleagues of the Department of Neurology, UNICAMP Medical School and Clinics Hospital (Brazil), for giving me the opportunity to work together and better understand the human mind and treat its disorders. I am indebted particularly to those colleagues with whom I researched together, namely, Fernando Cendes and Andrea Allesio in the area of epilepsy; Márcio Balthazar, in dementia; Alfredo Damasceno and Leonilda Santos, in multiple sclerosis and neuroimmunology; and Edwiges Morato and Maria Irma Coudry, in neurolinguistics (UNICAMP Aphasia Centre). Special thanks to Alfredo Damasceno for reviewing and suggesting improvements to the manuscript. I am also thankful for the invaluable support and grants given by CNPq (National Council for Scientific and Technological Development, Brazil) and especially by FAPESP (São Paulo Research Foundation, Brazil) all these years. And I cannot forget those colleagues at Sahlgrenska University Hospital (Gothenburg, Sweden), who taught me neurology (particularly Lorenz Bergmann), the fundamentals of neuropsychology (Peter Borenstein), and neurophysiology (Gaby Bader) as part of my medical residency and specialization in neurology.

Contents

Abbreviations

AD	Alzheimer´s disease
ADNI	Alzheimer´s Disease Neuroimaging Initiative
ADRDA	Alzheimer´s Disease and Related Disorders Association
AMPA	α-amino-3-hydroxy-5-methyl-4-isoxazolepropionic acid
ANCOVA	analysis of covariance
ANOVA	analysis of variance
APOE	apolipoprotein E
APP	amyloid precursor protein
BDI	Beck Depression Inventory
BDNF	brain-derived neurotrophic factor
BICAMS	Brief International Cognitive Assessment for Multiple Sclerosis
BNT	Boston Naming Test
BRB-N	Brief Repeatable Battery of Neuropsychological Tests
BVMT	Brief Visuospatial Memory Test
CDR	Clinical Dementia Rating
CSF	cerebrospinal fluid
COWAT	Controlled Oral Word Association Test
CVD	cerebrovascular disease
CVLT	California Verbal Learning Test
D-KEFS	Delis-Kaplan Executive Function System
DMN	default mode network
DSM	Diagnostic and Statistical Manual of Mental Disorders
EDSS	Expanded Disability Status Scale
EEG	electroencephalography
FAQ	Functional Assessment Questionnaire
FCSRT	Free and Cued Selective Reminding Test
FDG	fluorodeoxyglucose
FSMC	Fatigue Scale for Motor and Cognitive Functions
FSS	Fatigue Severity Scale
FTD	frontotemporal degeneration
FTDP-17	Frontotemporal dementia and parkinsonism linked to chromosome 17

GM	gray matter
IADL	instrumental activities of daily life
ICD-10	International Statistical Classification of Diseases and Related Health Problems – 10th Revision
ILAE	International League Against Epilepsy
IWG	International Working Group
LNI	Luria´s Neuropsychological Investigation
MACFIMS	Minimal Assessment of Cognitive Function in Multiple Sclerosis
MCI	mild cognitive impairment
MADRS	Montgomery-Åsberg Depression Rating Scale
MFIS	Modified Fatigue Impact Scale
MMSE	Mini-Mental State Examination
MRI	magnetic resonance imaging
MS	multiple sclerosis
MSFC	MS Functional Composite
MTLE	medial temporal lobe epilepsy
NFT	neurofibrillary tangle
NIA-AA	National Institute on Aging – Alzheimer's Association
NINCDS	National Institute of Neurological and Communicative Disorders and Stroke
NMDA	N-methyl-D-aspartate
PASAT	Paced Auditory Serial Addition Test
PET	positron emission tomography
PFC	prefrontal cortex
PiB	Pittsburgh compound B
PM	prospective memory
PSEN	presenilin
RAVLT	Rey Auditory Verbal Learning Test
SDMT	Symbol Digit Modalities Test
SPART	10/36 Spatial Recall Test
SPECT	single photon emission computerized tomography
SRT-DR	Selective Reminding Test – Delayed Recall
ToM	theory of mind
WAIS-R	Wechsler Adult Intelligence Scale – Revised
WLG	Word List Generation
WM	working memory
WMS	Wechsler Memory Scale

Chapter 1
Introduction

1.1 Theoretical Approach

1.1.1 Introduction

Cognition is a set of processes by which knowledge is acquired, stored, and manipulated in the mind. These processes start with sensation and comprise other interrelated mental actions involved in perception, attention, visual-spatial-motor abilities, memory, language, and intellectual reasoning. As a component of the mind, cognition has reciprocal relationships with other noncognitive functions, such as emotion, volition, and self. Cognitive functions are not isolated or a priori existing "faculties" located in circumscribed brain center, but complex, distributed, and dynamic functional systems, which represent the natural and social world by means of signs (this is their mediated, semiotic nature) and results from the internalization or appropriation by the individual of external actions and relations with things and persons (their social-historical-cultural origin) [1, 2].

1.1.2 Cognition as a Dynamic Functional System

As a functional system, mind and cognition comprise a network of various basic mental operations (processes) organized in a set of interconnected brain regions, each region contributing with its specific operation to the functioning of the system as a whole. This concept of functional system can be illustrated with the way we solve a problem given orally, e.g., "John has 10 apples and Joe has 3 apples less than John. How many apples do they have?" or "A man needed to cross a river using a very small canoe. He had to bring three things across the river: a hen, a basket of corn, and a fox. Because of the size of the canoe, he could only cross with one thing at a time. If he crossed with the fox first, the hen would stay behind with the corn

B. Damasceno, *Research on Cognition Disorders*,
https://doi.org/10.1007/978-3-030-57267-9_1

and eat it. If he took the basket of corn first, the fox would stay behind with the hen and eat it. What would he have to do to get all three things across the river?". The solution requires an ensemble of various crucial mental operations and their corresponding brain regions or networks, such as (1) phonemic analysis and synthesis for understanding words (left superior-posterior temporal gyrus and neighboring associative cortex); (2) semantic analysis of sentences and the text as a whole as well as interpretation of the logico-grammatical relationship expressed by the phrase "less than," plus symbolic-spatial reasoning involved in the subtraction 10 minus 3 (mainly left inferior parietal and neighboring lateral temporal associative cortex); (3) memory processes for maintaining online in the focus of consciousness, both short-term, new incoming information (sensory-perceptive, spatial, verbal-phonological) and long-term, old information, collected from episodic, semantic, and procedural memory (prefrontal in connection with temporal regions); and (4) hypothesis testing, establishment of a goal and plan of solution, monitoring the execution of the plan, and lastly verifying whether the result obtained is according to the final question and to the data and constraints of the problem (prefrontal regions).

Another characteristic of the mind's functional system is its dynamic structure, that is, the composition of the whole set of mental operations and brain regions' changes from moment to moment insofar as each task consecutively switches from one to the other. At each moment, each intermediary task requires a different ensemble of cognitive operations suitable to achieve the main objective (i.e., to achieve the goal or to answer to the final question of a problem). Besides these cognitive operations, an adequate level of motivation, volition, and affective state is critical. So, the final objective of the activity as a whole remains constant, but the methods and cognitive operations involved can vary [3].

This conception of the mind represents a great theoretical-methodological contribution to basic and clinical scientific research on mental-cognitive issues, since it takes into account relationships and reciprocal influences between task-relevant psychological variables, whose unique (independent) contribution to the fulfillment of the task can be controlled beforehand (when planning the study) or can be determined by multivariable statistical analysis after data collection. Based on this conception, a clinical neuropsychological research has also to take into consideration the influences exerted by symptoms or syndromes on each other, for example, the interplay between depression, apathy, fatigue, sleep disturbance, psychosocial stress, and side effect of drugs. In clinical practice, a thorough anamnesis with detailed analysis of each of these accompanying disorders or comorbidities may disclose which of them is the main or primary contributor to the cognitive impairment.

As regards the mediated character of cognition, it is given by the fact that the individual relates himself with other things and persons not directly, but by means of the signals and signs (mediators) which represent these things, persons, their properties, and behaviors. Sensations are the first step to getting knowledge about the outside world. The physical, chemical, and spatial-temporal properties of external things and phenomena stimulate the sensory cells' receptors, where these properties are transduced and converted into trains of action potentials along the sensory cells' axons, whose frequency and rhythm codify (as neural codes) the information about those external things. From the most primitive and simple signals (as those of conditioned reflexes) to the signs of human language (e.g., words), the meaning of the mediators becomes more generalized and abstract [4].

1.1.3 Historical-Cultural Origin of Cognition

The historical-social-cultural origin of cognition is based on the appropriation (internalization) by the individual of external, practical relationships, and interactions with other people and objects. These interactions, particularly those of cooperative labor activities, are mediated by two kinds of instruments: material (tools, artifacts) and psychological (signs, words), the first ones for acting on nature and the second ones, on other people [5]. The appropriation process, firstly by imitation learning and then through the subsequent mastery of these instruments, particularly the signs of language (words), enables the individual to construct his/her internal language, ideal actions, and thought as action, which will precede any external activity [6, 7]. For this reason, cognition may be conceived as a kind of internal (mental and cerebral) version of the external, vitally, and socially relevant activity, as we have seen in problem-solving. The joint social practice with other people is a sine qua non condition for the acquisition of a normal healthy human mind. The lack or deprivation of adequate sensory, linguistic, and socioemotional interaction in critical periods of the mental-cerebral development can lead to serious cognitive and behavioral consequences, as found in orphaned and abandoned children raised in institutions [8, 9]. According to observational and interventional case-control studies in these children, intellectual-executive and memory functions are the most impaired, accompanied by psychiatric disturbances ranging from autistic-like to inattentive, hyperactive, and aggressive behavior [10–12]. In children with early psychosocial deprivation, neuroimaging studies have shown structural abnormalities predominantly in prefrontal and medial temporal regions, with reduced connectivity in frontal, temporal, and parietal white matter, including components of both uncinate (amygdala-frontal connection) and superior longitudinal fasciculi (parietal-temporal-occipital connection to frontal regions), which are respectively involved in emotional control and higher psychological functions. These white matter abnormalities have been correlated to duration of time in the orphanage and to scores of inattention and hyperactivity [13].

1.2 Methodological Issues

Research on cognitive disorders may have as objectives (1) to detect which basic mechanism or mental operation is impaired as well as which symptom or syndrome is primary or secondary and, in this way, to diagnose the regional distribution of the brain lesion or dysfunction, yielding valuable information for establishing an appropriate rehabilitation program; (2) to provide a baseline and profile of neuropsychological impairment for future comparisons; and (3) to predict the patient's behavior in real-world settings on the basis of his/her performance on neuropsychological tests. The first and third objectives are particularly challenging due to the complex, interrelated, and dynamic nature of our mental functions.

1.2.1 Neuropsychological Diagnosis of the Impaired Basic Mental Mechanisms and Lesion Localization

Modern techniques as magnetic resonance imaging (MRI) can localize the brain damage with high accuracy, but an MRI may not show signs of lesion where the neuropsychological evaluation indicates there is a dysfunction, as in patients examined 2 h after an acute ischemic stroke manifested exclusively as Wernicke-like aphasia or in the early phase of Alzheimer's disease presenting solely with episodic memory impairment (amnesia). Neuropsychological evaluation takes into account the following principles proposed by Luria [2] and Mesulam [14]:

1. Some brain regions, especially those of so-called convergence-divergence zones or hubs (e.g., left temporal-parietal junction), process some basic mental operations (e.g., spatial reasoning) needed for performing different complex tasks (e.g., construction of a model using multicolored Kohs cubes, chess game, left-right orientation, subtraction 51–17, and understanding of relational expressions as "the father's brother"). Therefore, a lesion in such a region (e.g., left inferior parietal) will produce not an isolated symptom but a whole syndrome comprising, e.g., constructional apraxia, acalculia, spatial disorientation, and aphasic difficulties – also known as Gerstmann syndrome. As a corollary, the finding of such a syndrome obtained by means of a comprehensive neuropsychological assessment strongly suggests a lesion in that brain region.
2. The various basic operations required to fulfill a complex task can be impaired by damage to a brain region (or interconnecting pathways) that processes any of them. For instance, incapacity to solve a problem may be due to lesion in any brain region that process some of the basic operations needed for resolving it. So, it may result from a working memory and/or intellectual-executive dysfunction (prefrontal lesion), aphasia (left temporal cortex), or acalculia (left inferior parietal region).

Therefore, to disclose the impaired basic mental operation and, by inference, the corresponding brain region that is damaged, we need a comprehensive battery of appropriate tests, including control tests (counterproofs) and control conditions. One crucial control condition is the comparison of the patient's test performance with that of healthy subjects matched to the patient as regards variables that can influence performance, such as age, sex, and educational level. This comparison is necessary for ascribing the patient's inferior performance to his brain lesion.

The selection of the tests is based on their accuracy to detect and measure those basic mental operations hypothetically required for executing the complex task in which the subject is disabled. This can be illustrated with the neuropsychological investigation of patients with medial temporal lobe epilepsy (MTLE), the most common epilepsy type in adults, frequently associated with medial temporal lesions and memory decline, but presenting good outcome after resection of the epileptogenic focus. The best surgical outcomes are obtained when the results of neuropsychological, electroencephalographic (video-EEG-telemetry), and neuroimaging (e.g., MRI, SPECT, PET) are concordant, each one independently indicating the same side and local of the brain dysfunction. In MTLE cases, the main challenge to the neuropsychologist is to localize the brain dysfunction without knowing or being influenced by the EEG and neuroimaging data. For attaining this goal, the neuropsychological investigation has to satisfy the following conditions:

1. As regards memory, the test battery has to take into account the existence of its different subtypes (episodic, semantic, working memory) as well as the putative functional differences between the left and right temporal lobes concerning representation of verbal and visual-spatial memory. According to the so-called material specific memory model (MSMM) [15, 16], the left temporal lobe is dominant for mediating memory for verbal material (e.g., list of abstract words) and the right one, for nonverbal material (e.g., abstract designs). This material-specific lateralization has been confirmed strongly as regards the relation between left temporal epileptogenic focus (or lesion) and verbal memory [17–21] but weakly as concerns right-sided focus (lesion) and nonverbal (visual, spatial) memory deficits, probably due to the verbalizability of the visual material employed or because visual-spatial memory has a more diffuse or bilateral brain representation. Moreover, there is "paradoxical" evidence of impairment of nonverbal (visual, spatial) memory in cases with left hippocampal sclerosis or left anterior temporal resection [22], as well as of verbal memory after right temporal resection [23].
2. Another problem is that the patient's inferior performance on a memory (learning) task may be caused not by a primary disorder of episodic memory (or medial temporal lesion) but by impairment of another cognitive function that is crucial for executing that task (e.g., auditory or visual perception, attention, verbal fluency), or it may also be due to a more widespread or diffuse disturbance (e.g., depression, fatigue, drowsiness, side effect of drugs) whose influence should have been controlled, minimized, or removed. For this reason, all these variables (i.e., other non-memory cognitive functions or diffuse disturbances) that can

influence the execution of a memory task have to be assessed by means of appropriate control tests (counterproofs), for example, examining visual perception with Poppelreuter's overlapping figures [2] or form discrimination [24]; attention with "A" Random Letter Test [25] or WAIS-R digit span [26]; verbal fluency with category (animals) or FAS [27]; mood with the seven items of Beck's Depression Inventory Fast Screen (BDI-FS) [28]; and fatigue with the Modified Fatigue Impact Scale (MFIS) [29, 30]; or the Fatigue Scale for Motor and Cognitive Functions (FSMC) [31]. An issue here is that depression and fatigue are subjective overlapping syndromes, with fatigue being a component of the DSM-5 diagnostic criteria for depression [32], but the differentiation between both may be achieved by employing the BDI-FS plus MFIS or FSMC. BDI-FS prioritizes depressive thought content (e.g., feelings of worthlessness or inappropriate guilt) and mood (e.g., dysphoria, anhedonia) and excludes items in which depression is confounded with fatigue or cognitive impairment; and the MFIS or FSMC measures specifically fatigue (both physical and cognitive, psychosocial fatigue).

1.2.2 Brain-Behavior Correlations

1.2.2.1 Control of Influential Variables: Study Design

The relationship between a patient's brain disease or lesion A (e.g., hippocampal atrophy) and his/her cognitive-behavioral syndrome B (e.g., amnesia) or performance on neuropsychological tests is not straightforward or linear, but mediated by extraneous influential variables other than the lesion itself, e.g., age, education, mood state, psychosocial stress, cognitive and brain reserve, and comorbidities (Fig. 1.1).

Variable is any characteristic of persons, things, or phenomena, which can vary, presenting different types, levels, or values. A variable is called *independent* (IV; e.g., age) when it can affect another one, called *dependent* variable (DV; e.g., logical

Fig. 1.1 Multiple factors (*C*, *D*, *E*, *F*, *G*, *H*) that can influence (modify) the relationship between a brain lesion (*A*) and a cognitive syndrome (*B*).

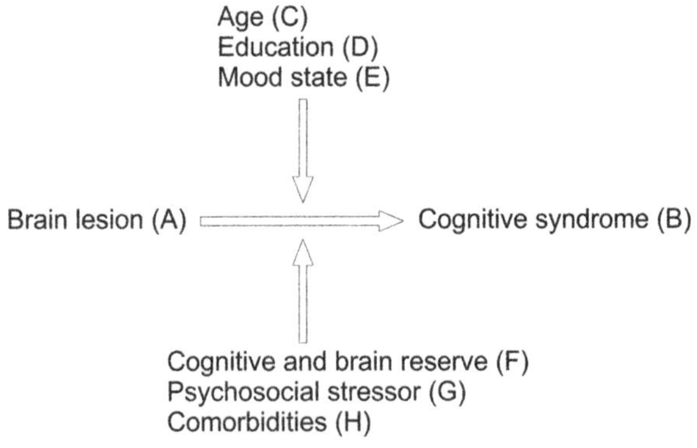

reasoning). In research on cognition, the investigator manipulates an IV and looks for changes in a DV. The power of such a research is given by its ability to ensure that only the IV is permitted to vary across the conditions of the testing. So, the investigator has to control (remove) the influence of any variable (other than the IV being studied) which could have an effect on the DV; otherwise, the results of the investigation may be difficult to be interpreted and inconclusive. These extraneous variables are called *covariates*. A covariate is called *confounder* (e.g., age, in the example of Fig. 1.1) when it influences both the IV that is being studied (e.g., hippocampal atrophy) and the DV or outcome (amnestic syndrome or memory performance), since it is known that aging leads to both increasing hippocampal atrophy and memory impairment. Another kind of covariate is the *mediator*, which occurs, for example, when an IV (e.g., temporal-limbic encephalitis) can lead to change in a covariate, e.g., mood state (manifested as an asthenoemotional syndrome), which in its turn leads to change in a DV, e.g., performance on memory tests. In this case, the covariate "mood state" is a *mediator*.

Test performance may be influenced by variables related to the subject, to the test (e.g., type of stimulus, psychometric and metacognitive characteristics, previous instructions), or to the testing situation (e.g., local with bothersome light, temperature, or noise; the experimenter's strange or exaggerated appearance, attitude, and behavior). Among subject variables, age and education are the most important, but cognitive performance may also be influenced by sex, handedness, intelligence level, motivation, humor state, variations of the individual's circadian rhythm, side effect of drugs, polyglotism, and previous experience with the proposed tasks.

In research in the fields of neuropsychology, behavioral neurology, and cognitive neuroscience, control of variables is achieved by means of an *experiment*, which is a procedure carried out under controlled conditions, consisting in intervening, manipulating, and altering the state of the participants. An experiment is, for this reason, the best method for testing hypothesis and verifying cause-and-effect relationships or, at least, associations between events. An experimental design may be "cross-sectional," by collecting data from different subjects that belong to two or more groups at a single point in time, or "longitudinal," or "prospective," by gathering data from the same sample of subjects on two or more occasions. The longitudinal design has higher probability to provide evidence supporting cause-and-effect relationships.

The influence of subject variables can be removed or minimized by means of group studies, which can adopt (1) a "within-subject" (also called "repeated measures") design, using the same subjects in each of the experimental conditions and testing sessions, or (2) a "between-subjects" or "between-groups" design, allocating different subjects in each experimental group by means of randomization and matching.

In *randomization*, each subject gets a number or code which has equal probability as all other subject numbers and codes for being randomly chosen and allocated in each subgroup. Randomization does not eliminate interindividual differences (subject variables) but reduces their effect on the performance of each subgroup. Another way to reduce the influence of subject variables is by increasing sample size. Nevertheless, randomization alone cannot increase the sensitivity of an experiment in detecting a small effect of an IV on a DV, but this deficiency is overcome by *matching*, that is, by selecting pairs of subjects with similar characteristics (age, sex, education, intelligence) which can influence test performance and have an effect on the DV and then allocating randomly each subject of the pair in each subgroup. In summary, influential variables should be controlled or maintained the same between testing sessions of the same individual or between groups of individuals being compared. In case-control group studies, confounders should be assigned equally to both groups.

Nowadays, grant-giving institutions require that the project present, already in its planning phase, before data collection, a detailed description of study design, methods for controlling influential variables (especially confounders), and type of statistical analysis of the data. For this purpose, the investigator has to know beforehand which covariates would be the most influential in the relationship between the IV and the DV (outcome) to be studied. If these requirements were not fulfilled beforehand, then, after the data have been collected, a multivariate statistical analysis may disclose that, after adjusting for the most relevant covariates, a brain lesion or dysfunction (e.g., hippocampal atrophy or epileptogenic focus) has an independent percentage of contribution to the low memory scores of the patients. In such a situation, by using a multivariate analysis (such as backward stepwise regression or ANCOVA), we can demonstrate a primary, memory-specific impairment associated with that brain dysfunction.

As compared to case studies, group studies are more complex, require large enough sample sizes, take longer time due to rigorous inclusion criteria, but are the best method for balancing interindividual variations in biological, sociocultural, and psychological characteristics, as well as for increasing intragroup homogeneity and for gathering more reliable data in clinical trials and brain-behavior correlation studies.

The within-subject design has the advantages of maximally removing the influence of interindividual variability and of requiring fewer participants, since the subjects performing in later repeated testings are controls for themselves performing in former ones (e.g., in the baseline evaluation). In spite of the advantages of the within-subject design, two problems may arise with it: (1) the *order effect*, with the subject's performance on the second testing being influenced by his/her performance on the first one due to practice or fatigue (this effect may be overcome by randomizing the order of the tests among all subjects of the group, with half the subjects following the order A → B and the other half the inverse order B → A), and (2) the *carryover effect*, with the subjects remembering some items (e.g., words) of the first testing and intrusively introducing them in the second or third testing, even when tested with different items (e.g., another list of words).

The between-groups design is often used in case-control clinical trials comprising a subgroup of *cases* that receive the new intervention or treatment being tested (e.g., a new drug, surgical procedure, or rehabilitation method) and the *controls*, which do not get the new treatment but instead are given a placebo, a traditional treatment, or no treatment at all. A condition for gathering reliable data and detecting even small treatment effects in clinical trials, besides a large enough sample size, is *double-blinding*, that is, neither the participant subjects nor the investigators know the kind of treatment the participants are receiving.

1.2.2.2 Issues Related to Lesion Analysis

As regards the lesion, a cognitive-behavioral syndrome cannot be explained exclusively by the loss of function supposedly performed by the damaged brain region [33], since the syndrome results from the combination of other factors, which may be (1) psychological (motivation, humor state), (2) neuropsychological (systemic and dynamic character of mental functions, type and severity of the cognitive disorder), and (3) dysfunction of other intact brain structures interconnected to the damaged one, since lesion in one region causes change of neurotransmission, excitation-inhibition balance, and blood flow in other neighboring and distant brain regions. Some of these regions that normally were activated or inhibited by the damaged one become denervated and consequently hypo- or hyperactive, in this way also producing symptoms and contributing to the syndrome as a whole. In addition, there is a continuous postlesional transformation of the syndrome (Leischner's "syndromenwandel") [34] due to an interplay between secondary axonal degeneration, functional reorganization, and recovery (plasticity). A typical example is the case of an acute ischemic stroke causing initially a global aphasia, which evolves after months to a Broca's aphasia. For all these reasons, to localize a lesion even with high-resolution MRI does not imply in localizing in the same region the whole syndrome.

On the other hand, the image of a lesion seen on MRI may not correspond to the real degree of nervous tissue (cells and axons) destroyed, as happens in cases of space-occupying lesions (e.g., parenchymal hematoma or infiltrating neoplastic tumor), in which the abnormal imaging area does contain functionally competent neurons and fibers. For this reason, for valid brain-behavior correlations in studies of groups of patients, Damasio and Damasio [35, 36] suggested to include preferentially ischemic stroke (infarction) in its chronic phase, more than 3 months old, when the abnormal MRI image will correspond to actual (complete or partial) brain parenchyma destroyed and the resultant syndrome will be in stable phase, thus allowing safer brain-behavior correlations. As regards such correlations, structural MRI also has other limitations: (1) its modularity assumption that cognitive functions are mapped in functional modules which would have the same location in different individuals, not taking into account individual variations in neural-cognitive organization nor considering that natural lesions (diseases) may be spread beyond the limits of such functional modules [37], and (2) its low temporal resolution as regards detection of functional changes that occur in other brain regions following the acute phase of a focal lesion. The combination of structural and perfusion imaging [38] as well as of functional MRI (fMRI) has partly overcome this last limitation. In fMRI, stimuli or tasks are presented to the subject, leading to increase in blood flow and ratio of oxygenated to deoxygenated hemoglobin, which creates the BOLD (blood oxygenation level dependent) signal needed to image construction. Indeed, fMRI determines the brain regions involved with a task, but it does not reveal which structures are necessary or critical for performing the task, besides having other limitations, such as its time resolution (the cognitive processing of a stimulus takes only tens of milliseconds, while the first hemodynamic changes are observable 1–2 s later), and its susceptibility to artifacts, particularly in frontal and medial temporal lobes [37, 39]. These authors call attention to the complementary information that these neuroimaging methods can give, and, therefore, they propose to combine brain activation (such as fMRI) with brain disruption techniques (such as lesion-behavior mapping), since there may be theoretical questions or brain functions that cannot be solved or determined only by means of the lesion method or the functional neuroimaging alone.

1.3 Conclusion

Cognitive functions as memory, language, attention, and intellectual reasoning depend on each other and are also influenced by changes of motivation and humor, such as apathy, depression, fatigue, and sleep disturbance, which require a detailed anamnesis for disclosing the most influential. The aims of a neuropsychological evaluation may be (1) to analyze the syndrome as a whole attempting to detect the impaired basic mental operations, in this way contributing to diagnose the regional distribution of the brain lesions; (2) to establish an appropriate rehabilitation program; (3) to provide a baseline of cognitive deficits for future comparisons; or (4) to predict the patient's behavior in real-world settings. With the first aim, the researcher has to conceive the mental functions, not as isolated "faculties" or "modules" located in circumscribed brain center, but as complex neurofunctional systems and networks. For example, assessment of episodic memory using a word list learning task has to consider other subtypes of memory as well as the influence of other mental functions needed for performing the task. Inferior performance in such a task may be caused not by a primary disorder of episodic memory but by impairment of other required cognitive functions (e.g., attention, perception, verbal fluency), or by a diffuse disturbance (depression, fatigue), or even by age and educational level. So, the neuropsychological assessment has to include appropriate control tests (counterproofs) for perception, attention, and verbal fluency, as well as scales for depression and fatigue. The influence of other variables (covariates) can be minimized by adopting a group study, be it with a "within-subject" ("repeated measures") design, using the same subjects in each group, or with a "between-subjects" ("between-groups") design, allocating the subjects in each group by means of randomization and matching.

As regards clinicopathologic correlations, the problem is that a cognitive-behavioral syndrome cannot be explained exclusively by the loss of function of a damaged region. Even when the MRI lesion is well delimited, its image may not indicate the real degree of nervous tissue destroyed, besides other interconnected intact brain structures becoming dysfunctional, hypo- or hyperactive, in this way also contributing to the syndrome. For such correlations, it is suggested to give preference to cases with brain infarction in chronic phase and to combine brain activation (e.g., fMRI) with brain disruption techniques (lesion-behavior mapping).

References

1. Vygotsky LS (1934/1982) Psychology and the theory of localization of psychic functions. In Vygotsky LS (ed) Sobranie sochinenij. Tom 1. Voprosy teorii i istorii psikhologii. Pedagogika, Moscow (in Russian)
2. Luria AR (1966/1980) Higher cortical functions in man, 2nd edn. Basic Books, New York
3. Luria AR (1973) The working brain: an introduction to neuropsychology. Basic Books, New York
4. Rubinstein SL (1972) Princípios de Psicologia Geral, 2nd edn. Estampa Editorial, Lisbon (translated from the original title in Russian: Osnovy Obschei Psijologuii)
5. Vygotsky LS (1978) Mind in society: the development of higher psychological processes. Harvard University Press, Cambridge
6. Galperin PY (1976) An introduction to psychology. Moscow University Press, Moscow. (in Russian)
7. Wertsch JV (1998) Mind as action. Oxford University Press, New York
8. Spitz RA, Wolf K (1946) Anaclitic depression. Psychoanal Stud Child 2:313
9. Nelson CA III, Bos K, Gunnar MR, Sonuga-Barke EJS (2011) The neurobiological toll of early human deprivation. Monogr Soc Res Child Dev 76(4):127–146. https://doi.org/10.1111/j.1540-5834.2011.00630.x
10. Rutter M, Andersen-Wood L, Beckett C et al (1999) Quasi-autistic patterns following severe early global privation. J Child Psychol Psychiatry 40(4):537–549
11. Tizard B, Rees J (1974) A comparison of the effects of adoption, restoration to the natural mother, and continued institutionalization on the cognitive development of four-year-old children. Child Dev 45(1):92–99
12. Nelson III CA, Zeanah CH, Fox NA (2019) How early experience shapes human development: The case of psychosocial deprivation. Neural Plasticity 1676285, 12 p. https://doi.org/10.1155/2019/1676285
13. Govindan RM, Behen ME, Helder E, Makki MI, Chugani HT (2010) Altered water diffusivity in cortical association tracts in children with early deprivation identified with tract-based spatial statistics (TBSS). Cereb Cortex 20(3):561–569. https://doi.org/10.1093/cercor/bhp122
14. Mesulam MM (1990) Large-scale neurocognitive networks and distributed processing for attention, language, and memory. Ann Neurol 28:597–613
15. Milner B (1972) Disorders of learning and memory after temporal lobe lesions in man. Clin Neurosurg 19:421–446
16. Jones-Gotman M (1996) Psychological evaluation for epilepsy surgery. In: Shorvon S, Dreifuss F, Fish D, Thomas D (eds) The treatment of epilepsy. Blackwell Science, Oxford, pp 621–630
17. Hermann BP, Seidenberg M, Schoenfeld J, Davies K (1997) Neuropsychological characteristics of the syndrome of mesial temporal lobe epilepsy. Arch Neurol 54:369–376
18. Baxendale SA, Thompson PJ, van Paesschen W (1998) A test of spatial memory and its clinical utility in the pre-surgical investigation of temporal lobe epilepspy patients. Neuropsychologia 36:591–602
19. Jones-Gotman M, Harnadek MCS, Kubu CS (2000) Neuropsychological assessment for temporal lobe epilepsy surgery. Can J Neurol Sci 27(Suppl 1):S39–S43
20. Leone AA, Damasceno BP, Cendes F, Guerreiro CAM (2001) Memory deficits in patients with temporal lobe epilepsy. J Int Neuropsychol Soc 7:429

21. Alessio A, Pereira FR, Sercheli MS, Rondina JM, Ozelo HB, Bilevicius E, Pedro T, Covolan RJ, Damasceno BP, Cendes F (2013) Brain plasticity for verbal and visual memories in patients with mesial temporal lobe epilepsy and hippocampal sclerosis: a fMRI study. Hum Brain Mapp 34(1):186–199
22. Glikmann-Johnston Y, Saling MM, Chen J, Cooper KA, Beare RJ, Reutens DC (2008) Structural and functional correlates of unilateral mesial temporal lobe spatial memory impairment. Brain 131(Pt 11):3006–3018. https://doi.org/10.1093/brain/awn213
23. Gleissner U, Helmstaedter C, Schramm J, Elger CE (2002) Memory outcome after selective amygdalo-hippocampectomy: a study in 140 patients with temporal lobe epilepsy. Epilepsia 43:87–95
24. Benton AL, Hamsher K, Varney NR, Spreen O (1983) Contributions to neuropsychological assessment. Oxford University Press, New York
25. Strub RL, Black FW (2000) The mental status examination in neurology, 4th edn. F.A. Davis Company, Philadelphia
26. Wechsler D (1981) Wechsler adult intelligence scale – revised. Psychological Corporation, New York
27. Lezak MD (1995) Neuropsychological assessment, 3rd edn. Oxford University Press, New York
28. Beck AT, Steer RA, Brown GK (2000) BDI-fast screen for medical patients: manual. Psychological Corporation, San Antonio
29. Fisk JD, Pontefract A, Ritvo PG, Archibald CJ, Murray TJ (1994) The impact of fatigue on patients with multiple sclerosis. Can J Neurol Sci 21(1):9–14
30. Téllez N, Rio J, Tintoré M, Nos C, Galán I, Montalban X (2005) Does the modified fatigue impact scale offer a more comprehensive assessment of fatigue in MS? Mult Scler 11(2):198–202
31. Penner IK, Raselli C, Stöcklin M, Opwis K, Kappos L, Calabrese P (2009) The fatigue scale for motor and cognitive functions (FSMC): validation of a new instrument to assess multiple sclerosis-related fatigue. Mult Scler 15(12):1509–1517
32. American Psychiatric Association (2013) Diagnostic and statistical manual of mental disorders, 5th edn. Author, Washington, DC
33. Fuster JM (1989) The prefrontal cortex: anatomy, physiology, and neuropsychology of the frontal lobe, 2nd edn. Raven Press, New York
34. Leischner A (1972) Über den Verlauf und die Einteilung der aphasichen Syndrome. Archiv für Psychiatrie and Nervenkrankheiten 216:219–231
35. Damasio H, Damasio AR (1989) Lesion analysis in neuropsychology. Oxford University Press, New York
36. Damasio H, Damasio AR (1997) Chapter 5: The lesion method in behavioral neurology and neuropsychology. In: Feinberg TE, Farah MJ (eds) Behavioral neurology and neuropsychology. Mc-Graw-Hill, New York
37. Rorden C, Karnath HO (2004) Using human brain lesions to infer function: a relic from a past era in the fMRI age? Nat Rev Neurosci 5:813–819
38. Shahid H, Sebastian R, Schmur TT, Nanayik T, Hillis AE (2017) Important considerations in lesion-symptom mapping: illustrations from studies of word comprehension: lesion symptom mapping. Hum Brain Mapp 38(6):2990–3000
39. Rorden C, Fridrikson J, Karnath H-O (2009) An evaluation of traditional and novel tools for lesion behavior mapping. NeuroImage 44(4):1355–1362

Part I
Cognitive Functions and Their Interrelationships

Chapter 2
Sensation and Perception

2.1 Introduction

Sensation is a primordial act of taking cognizance of something that touches the body, is hot or cold, emits sound or light, and whose action in the sense organs is a stimulus that causes excitation of receptor cells. At the level of sensation, the living creature is already able to differentiate and generalize stimuli, notice their simple or complex character, and detect its meaning as a signal about isolated individual properties of objects and phenomena. The detection of the external thing as a whole and its meaning is a more complex cognitive process (perception), consisting in simultaneous synthesis of multiple sensory information, occurring mainly in the cerebral cortex.

2.2 Sensation

Sensation is the first step of cognition, the primary source of our knowledge about the world and its properties, movements, and changes. It is the subjective image of the objective world, the effect detected, consciously or not, by the central nervous system after the psychic integration of inputs originated in the peripheral receptors and used by the organism for its orientation and activity in the external world. The psychic integration of these sensory inputs allows us to detect sounds in the air pressure waves that reach our ears, light and colors in the electromagnetic waves that stimulate the retina of our eyes, and odors in the chemical substances that excite the smell receptors of our noses. Sounds, colors, and odors are mental constructions created by sensory processing in higher divisions (cerebral cortex) of the central nervous system (CNS). Obviously, these physical and chemical excitations also arrive at lower divisions of the CNS (spinal cord, brain stem), which integrate them and generate appropriate reactions, such as pupil constriction, eye blinking, or

B. Damasceno, *Research on Cognition Disorders*,
https://doi.org/10.1007/978-3-030-57267-9_2

salivation, but we cannot be certain that we have subjective experiences of touch, light, color, smell, or sound at these lower levels of the sensory pathways. The subjective experience (qualia) of sounds, odors, or colors (e.g., the redness of red roses) does not exist without the perceiving activity of a living being [1]. However, this does not mean that these subjective experiences do not authentically reflect the objective reality of the outside world, as sensed and acted upon by human beings [2].

2.2.1 The Question of the Authenticity of Our Sensations and Perceptions

This has been a subject of debate and controversies between materialist and idealist philosophy. The materialist point of view is that the external world exists objectively, independent of our consciousness, with its properties exciting our receptor organs and being reflected in our mind through our sensations and perceptions. The mere existence of different types of sensations with their respective peripheral receptor organs is an ample proof that the material world exists independently from ourselves and from our consciousness. Otherwise, why and for what purpose would life and the living organisms themselves develop sensory organs, such as eyes and ears, suited for detecting even distant objects and phenomena? The more convincing explanation is that there must be things of vital importance outside, with which the organism has to interact, exchanging substances and information for survival. This fact contradicts the thesis of the subjective idealism and solipsism, which considers that only I (my consciousness) exist, and that external objects are no more than sets of our sensations and ideas, only creations of our mind, without objective existence. Obviously, all things belonging to the world of culture, from artifacts and instruments to works of art, are creations of our mind, constituting a kind of objectified mind. We know the world through information from our receptor organs by processing this information in the whole aggregate of sensory analyzers mainly in the cerebral cortex and by verifying its authenticity by means of our actions and life experience, particularly by our joint *social practice* with other human beings [2]. As asserted by Marx [3], this social practice is the criterion of truth: "The question whether objective (*gegenständliche*) truth can be attained by human thinking is not a question of theory but is a practical question. It is in practice that man must prove the truth, i.e., the reality and power, the this-worldliness (*Diesseitigkeit*) of his thinking. The dispute over the reality or non-reality of thinking which is isolated from practice is a purely scholastic question."

2.2.2 Sensations Basic Properties

These are (1) *modality* (vision, hearing, touch, taste, smell, and others), each with its various subtypes (e.g., sweet, salty, sour, and bitter taste); (2) *intensity*, dependent on the strength of the stimulus, whose minimal detectable intensity may vary under the influence of experience, fatigue, or context in which the stimulus is presented; (3) *duration*, dependent on the duration and intensity of the stimulus, which may change due to adaptation to a repetitive or continuous stimulus; and (4) spatial *localization*.

Each sensory *modality* is processed in its respective *sensory-perceptive analyzer*. The concept of analyzer was introduced and defined by Pavlov as "an apparatus whose purpose is to decompose the complexity of the external world into separate elements," and "in addition to the analyzers related to external world, there must be internal analyzers, whose function is to decompose the enormous complexity of the internal phenomena arising within the organism itself, the most important of which is the motor analyzer, the analyzer of movement…which decomposes the motor act with its enormous complexity into a large number of the most delicate elements; this ensures the enormous variety and the precision of our skeletal movements." [4]

All analyzers have a similar functional structure constituted by (1) peripheral receptors (primary sensory neurons), (2) peripheral nerves and centripetal pathways in the spinal cord and brain stem conducting the peripheral excitation to the CNS, and (3) primary cortical areas for synthesis of different modalities or complex stimuli as well as efferent (centrifugal) pathways projecting from the cerebral cortex to the peripheral receptor organs. The concept of analyzer takes into account its active character in separating different characteristics of a complex stimulus or subtypes of a sensory modality and in acting upon the peripheral receptor organ, regulating its receptive function [5]. The visual analyzer, for instance, has afferent parallel pathways originating from retinal ganglion cells and projecting to the CNS with information on form and color (in the parvocellular pathways, arisen from the small retinal ganglion cells) and on spatial relationships, depth perception (stereopsis), and motion (in the magnocellular pathways), and it has, additionally, efferent pathways projecting from the primary visual cortex to the lateral geniculate nucleus in similar way that the auditory analyzer has efferent projections from the brain stem (superior olivary complex) to the cochlea (hair cells) receptors. This conception of the visual system as a analyzer permits us to understand why only 10–20% of presynaptic connections of the lateral geniculate nucleus come from the retina, and the majority of its connections originate from other brain regions (feedback connections), mainly from the cerebral cortex and brain stem reticular formation [6]. The visual analyzer also includes the muscles of the eyes (the extrinsic muscles for moving the eyes in all directions and to all positions, and the intrinsic for constricting or dilating the pupils, or changing the form of the crystalline lens) as well as the proprioceptive and motor pathways for adjusting the movements and position of the eyes in such a way that the images of external objects are optimally projected onto the surface of the retina. So, the visual analyzer adjust itself to characteristics of the stimulus facilitating its reception, similarly to what occurs with the palpation movements of the hand fingers for tactile perception of an object without the help of vision. For achieving this, the sensory-perceptive analyzer requires the participation of cortical regions involved in processes of fine-tuning of the receptor organs and complex simultaneous synthesis for a more detailed and complete perception of the external object, which comprises both the object itself (its details of form and color, processed in the ventral, occipito-temporal pathways) and the context in which it is presented (spatial position and movement, in the dorsal, occipito-parietal pathways).

Sensory modality is genetically encoded in each specific receptor and its correspondent neural pathway (called *labeled line code*) in such a way that the subject always feels that sensory modality every time its receptor is stimulated, even when the stimulus is of another modality, for example, a blow to the skull or to the eye is felt as light [1].

Stimulus *intensity* and *duration* are codified by the receptor cell after its *transduction*, which consists in the conversion of the external stimulus energy (mechanical, electromagnetic) into electrochemical neural signals representing features of that stimulus. The energy of the stimulus leads to opening of ion channels (for sodium, potassium, and calcium) producing electric depolarization in a limited region of the cell membrane, with formation of a local *receptor potential* (RP). This RP is a graded response, and with increased strength of the stimulus, its amplitude becomes above the cell's threshold for firing, and so it reaches the sensory cell's trigger zone, where *action potentials* (APs) are generated and transmitted through the cell's axon to other neurons in the CNS.

Stimulus *intensity* is encoded by the frequency of discharges of APs by the sensory neuron (i.e., number of APs per unit of time, called *frequency code*). However, since the frequency of APs discharges by an isolated sensory neuron has a limit (called *saturation point*, given by the cell's limited transduction capacity and refractory period), a stronger stimulus activates greater number of neighboring receptor cells and is then represented by a *population code*, which makes possible for the individual to sense the maximal intensity of the stimulus.

Stimulus *duration* is encoded by the patterns of discharges of APs by two types of receptor cells: the rapidly adapting (which discharge transiently, only at the beginning and ending of the stimulation) and the slowly adapting receptors (fire continuously during the whole stimulation) .

The *minimal perceptible difference* (ΔS) between two stimuli of different intensities but of same modality is determined by Weber's law: $\Delta S = K \times S$, where ΔS is the minimal difference that can be noticed between a reference stimulus S and another stimulus, and K is a constant. As the intensity of a reference stimulus S increases, the greater the difference between it and a second stimulus must be for this difference to be noticeable, for example, we may easily detect the difference in weight between 1 kg and 2 kg but hardly between 30 and 31 kg, even though the difference remains the same (1 kg). For the intensity of a second stimulus to be detected as different, the constant K should be 1/30 of the reference stimulus S for weights, 1/10 for sounds, and 1/100 for lights [7]. The minimal detectable intensity and ΔS may vary under the influence of experience, fatigue, drowsiness, and conditions in which the stimulating object is presented [1]. Sensory-perceptive discriminative abilities are improved by social practice, particularly that of labor activities, for example, the Inuits (Eskimos) visual differentiation of many types of snow and the experienced taster's expertise in distinguishing different qualities of wine or tea.

Localization of a stimulus (e.g., in the skin), by discriminating it from other neighboring stimuli, depends on the size of the receptors *receptive field* and on *lateral inhibition* occurring in its neural pathway. Each sensory cell has a receptive field, defined as the area of the receptor organ (e.g., the skin or retina) in which the stimulation can excite the cell, leading it to produce action potentials. The size of the receptive field determines the receptor's capacity to detect the spacing between different stimuli reaching the same receptive surface. The smaller the size of the receptive field, the greater the cell's spatial resolution, making possible the detection of more details of the external object. For example, when reading the Braille alphabet by rubbing the index finger over the array of dots, the smaller receptive fields of Merkel skin receptors provide the most accurate distinction between the dots and the empty spaces between them. The dots cause the cell to fire action potentials, and the empty spaces silence the cell. The set of inputs from active and inactive skin receptors coming to postcentral gyrus area 3b constitutes a population code that represent a Braille letter or number.

Lateral inhibition is another neural mechanism that facilitates the precise localization of the stimulus, thus increasing the spatial resolution (Fig. 2.1).

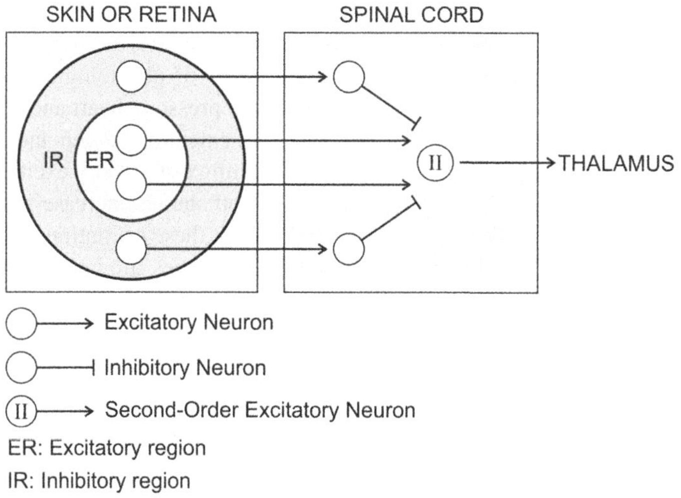

Fig. 2.1 In the neural pathway conducting the stimulus excitation, the axons of various peripheral sensory cells converge onto a single second-order sensory neuron in the CNS (spinal cord or brain stem), whose receptive field is constituted by the receptive fields of all the peripheral presynaptic cells, and it has a central excitatory region (ER) surrounded by a peripheral inhibitory zone (IR), which facilitate the delimitation and localization of the point with maximal stimulation

As regards localization of sounds in the surrounding space, this is done through a neuronal population code based on the responses of ensembles of neurons which are tuned to interaural time difference of incoming signals (i.e., the interval between the arrival of the same sound at the right and left ear), becoming more accurate as the signals ascend through the auditory system, from the superior olivary complex to the inferior colliculus, auditory thalamus, and auditory cortex [8].

2.2.3 Sensory Information Contributes to Vital Bodily Functions

The workings of our body, particularly of our nervous system and mind, are based on exchange of information. The term *information* is difficult to be readily defined. According to *The International Webster's Comprehensive Dictionary of The English Language* [9], information is "any distinct signal element forming part of a message or communication, especially one assembled and made available for use by automatic machines...". Tulving (2000) conceived it as "simply the intangible, ineffable, unknown "stuff that is somehow created, transferred, transformed, preserved ("processed") in the mind/brain, which, when appropriately "converted," determines behavior and conscious thought" [10]. In other words, it would be any signal, sign, or meaning carrying element that is interpreted by something (machine, brain) or someone else as giving instruction for decision-making or behavioral change.

Sensory information contributes to relevant bodily functions, such as homeostasis, reflex reactions, motor control, arousal, and perception. Sensations from within the body (viscera, blood vessels, skeletal muscles, and joints) are used by the CNS for automatically maintaining the relative constancy of physiological processes, called *homeostasis*, such as body temperature, blood pressure, heart and respiratory rates, and blood concentration of water, sugar, salt, calcium, oxygen and hydrogen ions, etc. These metabolic processes as well as the influx of sensory excitations into the ascending reticular activating system and hypothalamus increase our state of vigilance and readiness to respond (*arousal*). Without these excitations (as in cases of long-lasting sensory isolation), the individual becomes drowsy and then with altered state of consciousness, hallucinations, and delusions.

A new and unexpected sensory stimulus that appears suddenly in the environment, particularly if strong or biologically significant (potentially advantageous or threatening), causes orienting reactions of the organism, with turning of eyes, ears, and head in the direction of the source of the stimulus, so it can be appropriately perceived and attended to. This is the *orienting reflex*, a concept introduced by Pavlov [4].

Besides orienting reactions to stimulus first presentation, sequential stimuli or events occurring repeatedly in the environment can cause *conditioned reflexes*, which may be of two main types: the *classic* (Pavlovian), in which the animal learns to associate two or more external stimuli with each other, that is, the contingent or conditioned, and the unconditioned, innate stimulus, and the *operating* (Skinnerian), in which the animal learns, by trial and errors, to associate its own correct actions with the appearance of the innate stimulus (for instance, deployment of food when the level is pressed). The correct actions are gradually reinforced and the wrong ones, weakened (Thorndike's "law of effect").

Sensory information, particularly visual, vestibular, proprioceptive, and tactile, is crucial for *motor control* of voluntary goal-directed movements (e.g., reaching a cup of tea with the hand) as well as gait and posture. Even the automatic movements of walking need these sensory inputs to regulate stepping.

Sensation and perception are interconnected processes, inseparable from the organism's activity, with which they constitute a functional unit. In inferior animals, sensation is enough for adaptive sensory-motor reactions to isolated properties of vitally important objects, but in superior animals living in complex and highly changeable environments, perception is necessary for representing not only the object as a whole but also the conditions in which it is located (surrounding things, obstacles, etc.).

Rubinstein [5] pointed out that sensation, similarly to perception, is not only an image or sensitive representation but also a component of a living being's activity, which brings about stimuli and regulate them. Thus, the phylogenetic development of animal sensation and perception depends crucially on those biologically significant stimuli that arise in the process of the animal's vital activity, associated with its way to act and adapt to its environment. Dogs, for instance, are excellent in detecting the odor of organic acids (arising from living bodies and trails), but they hardly perceive aromatic odors of herbs and flowers; otherwise these aromas could impede them to perceive the odor of the prey or trail. As stated before, the sensitive-perceptive ability of humans is additionally influenced by the social character of their practical productive activity, mediated by language. Eskimos, for instance, are able to perceive 30 different types of snow to which are given 30 different names, since this differentiation is relevant for orienting their activity (hunting, gathering) in the Arctic environment. An individual's threshold of sensitivity as well as his/her discriminative ability vary depending on various factors such as type of professional activity, level of attention, degree of adaptation to repetitive or continuous stimuli, and influence of preceding stimulus (e.g., we feel an increase of the acid flavor after tasting sweets) [5].

2.3 Perception

As we saw, sensation detects only isolated properties of objects. Perception, on the other hand, discovers sets of relevant properties of these objects and phenomena which stimulate the sensory organs. In perception, the object is represented as a whole and understood not as a simple sum of sensations caused by it, but as a set of specific and constant relationships between each of its parts and properties, here included the relations between the subject that perceives and the thing that is perceived (as conceived by Max Wertheimer, Wolfgang Köhler, Kurt Koffka, and Kurt Lewin, founders of Gestalt Psychology). An object may vary its form when seen from different angles (from the front, back, above, bottom, and sides) or when presented in different colors or sizes. A melody can be sung, performed by a musical instrument, played in different tonalities, whistled or whispered, and speeded or slowed, but the relationships between its parts will stay constant (same pleasing succession of musical sounds, same rhythm), allowing the listener to recognize its meaning and, therefore, its affective value for him.

Perception is not passive or contemplative but active, creative, and dependent on the subject's perceptive activity. Alva Noë [11] has also emphasized this enactive view of perception: "What we perceive is determined by what we do; it is determined by what we are ready to do...We enact our perceptual experience; we act it out...Perception is not just a process in the brain...whereby the perceptual system constructs an internal representation of the world...but a kind of skillful activity on the part of the animal as a whole...Perceptual experience acquires content (meaning) thanks to the perceiver's skillful activity."

Soviet psychologists have emphasized the relevance of practical activity for the human perception, especially the social and productive practice mediated by language: (1) first, what human subjects perceive and how they perceive it depend on what they are doing and how they are doing it, as well as on the objective, content, and character of their practical activity, besides being influenced by their personal characteristics such as age, educational and cultural level, profession, and interests; (2) by establishing relationships with other persons by means of language, the subject assimilates and improves the experience accumulated by society and by his/her own past experience, and this allows him/her to perceive the stimuli acting on him/her as being determined objects of reality, which belong to certain categories, such as "trees," "houses," "tools," "persons," and their respective "functions," and not as undifferentiated and indeterminate things; (3) the authenticity of sensations and perceptions is proved by the socially shared practice of the subject with other subjects, and this practice is the criterion of the truth and of the objective character not only of perception but also of all knowledge [7].

Perception is not an isolated mental faculty or mere output of a computational process in a limited brain center but a complex functional system comprising various interconnected mental operations and brain regions [12]. In the visual perception of an object (e.g., a dog), we have: (1) *analysis* of fragmentary information (on color, angles of edges, movement, etc.) carried by parallel pathways from the retina through the primary visual area in the occipital lobe and its subsequent *synthesis* in the neighboring occipito-temporal and occipito-parietal secondary visual areas, where a temporary neuronal model (neuronal assembly) is created, which constitutes the neurophysiological basis of the object's image (percept) in construction; (2) comparison of this percept with templates of similar percepts previously existing in the long-term memory as product of the subject's experience, without which there is no recognition or categorization of the object; (3) active and selective search for new, task relevant information, with the purpose of testing hypothesis about the nature and meaning of the object (requiring frontal-occipital interactions); (4)

selection and verification of the most probable hypothesis about the meaning of the percept, by comparing it with the most congruent templates (neuronal models) existing in long-term memory; and (5) encoding of the perceived object in the phonological (dɔg) and semantic system of language. This requires a simultaneous synthesis of all essential characteristics of the object dog, both the functional (it barks, protects the owner's house, chases cats, etc.) and the categorical ones (living being, animal), all these characteristics being processed in several co-activated interconnected brain regions.

2.4 Conclusion

Sensation is cognition first step, by which the living organism detects isolated properties of an external object, not the object as a whole, even though it can differentiate and generalize stimuli, and notice their simple or complex character. Sensations authentically reflect the world, whose objective existence (i.e., independent of our consciousness) is given by the mere fact that the organism possesses peripheral receptor organs. Sensations main properties are *modality*, *intensity*, *duration*, and spatial *localization* of a stimulus. The smaller the size of the receptive field, the greater the cell's spatial resolution, allowing the detection of more details of the external object. The minimal perceptible difference (ΔS) between the different intensities of two stimuli of same modality is determined by Weber's law: $\Delta S = K \times S$, where S is a reference stimulus, and K is a constant, which is 1/30 for weights, 1/10 for sounds, and 1/100 for lights. Each sensory modality has a similar functional structure which constitutes its sensory-perceptive analyzer comprising (1) peripheral receptors, (2) afferent centripetal pathways to the spinal cord or brain stem, and (3) primary cortical areas as well as efferent centrifugal projections from the cortex to the peripheral receptor organs. Sensory information contributes to relevant bodily functions, such as homeostasis, reflex reactions, motor control of voluntary goal-directed movements, arousal (vigilance and readiness to respond), and perception. Perception is the abstract representation of the object as a whole, as a set of specific and constant relationships between its parts and properties as well as between the perceiving subject and the object. The meaning of the object is grasped by means of a complex mental-cerebral functional system comprising (1) analysis of sensory information and their synthesis in an abstract percept, (2) comparison of this percept with similar percepts memorized from the previous experience, (3) selection of the most probable hypothesis about the meaning (category) of the object, and (4) its phonological and semantic encoding. Perception is not a passive reflection (as in a mirror) but a creative process, dependent on the subject's perceptive actions, ontogenetically constructed in the joint social-cultural practice mediated by language, which allows the object to be perceived as belonging to a certain category ("tree," "house," "dog").

References

1. Kandel ER, Schwartz JH, Jessel TM (eds) (1995) Essentials of neural science and behavior. Prentice Hall International, Inc., London
2. Babsky E, Khodorov B (1970) Chapter 17: Higher nervous activity. In: Babsky E, Khodorov B, Kositsky G, Zubkov A (eds) Human physiology. MIR Publishers, Moscow, pp 329–379
3. Marx K (1976) Theses on Feuerbach. In: Marx K, Engels F (eds) The German ideology (1845–1846). Progress Publishers, Moscow
4. Pavlov IP (1949) Complete works. Academy of Sciences of the USSR, Moscow/Leningrad
5. Rubinstein SL (1972) Princípios de Psicologia Geral, 2nd edn. Estampa Editorial, Lisbon (translated from the original title in Russian: Osnovy Obschei Psijologuii)
6. Kandel ER, Schwartz JH, Jessel TM, Siegelbaum SA, Hudspeth AJ (eds) (2013) Principles of neural science, 5th edn. The McGraw-Hill Global Education Holdings, New York
7. Sokolov EN (1969) Las sensaciones. In: Smirnov AA, Leontiev AN, Rubinshtein SL, Tieplov BM (eds) Psicologia. Editorial Grijalbo S.A, Mexico (translated from Russian)
8. Fitzpatrick DC, Batra R, Stanford TS, Kuwada S (1997) A neuronal population code for sound localization. Nature 388:871–874
9. The International Webster's Comprehensive Dictionary of The English Language (1996) Encyclopedic edition. Trident Press International, Naples
10. Tulving E (2000) Memory: introduction. In: Gazzaniga MS (ed) The new cognitive neurosciences, 2nd edn. The MIT Press, Cambridge, MA, pp 727–732
11. Noë A (2004) Action in perception. Massachusetts Institute of Technology Press, Cambridge
12. Luria AR (1973) The working brain: an introduction to neuropsychology. Basic Books, New York

Chapter 3
Attention

3.1 Introduction

Animals, particularly humans, live in a complex natural environment, rich in stimuli of different modalities, intensities, and values (both biological and social values), in which they have to orientate to perform their activities and survive. Many of these stimuli are not detected or they are perceived in an imprecise, vague way. In reality, from the point of view of the animal, the environment should be better understood as *Umwelt* ("environment," in German), a concept introduced by von Uexküll (1940) [1]. This concept means, not the whole set of all stimuli or external objects surrounding the individual, but only those that indicate food, sexual partner, protection, friend, enemy, or anything vitally important for that animal living in those conditions.

Attention is the orientation, directionality and selectivity of cognitive acts (from perception to thinking), volition, and emotion toward the object (or idea) perceived, thought, imagined, or wished. Attention has no own object, since it is simply the directional and selective character of the other mental-cognitive functions, allowing the subject to focus these other mental functions on any of their respective objects (ideas). In this regard, as emphasized by Rubinstein [2], that who attends to and focuses is the subject and not the mental process itself, in the same way that "it is not the perception itself that which perceives neither the thought that which thinks; but it is the human being that does it, it is the person (personality) that who perceives and thinks." This author considers attention as being a bidirectional correlation between subject and object: "On the one hand, attention directs itself to the object; on the other hand, it is the object that attracts the attention upon itself. The motive why attention orientates itself to a particular object and no to others does not reside only in the subject but also in the object and precisely in this object, in its characteristics, in its qualities...resides in the object that presents itself in its relation with the subject, as well as in the subject, in its relation with the object." In other words, the motive of the attention directed to the object is, at the same time, an internal desire

B. Damasceno, *Research on Cognition Disorders*,
https://doi.org/10.1007/978-3-030-57267-9_3

or emotion of the subject and a need that is objectified in the form of something that attracts the attention of the subject and can satisfy his need.

3.2 Types of Attention

There is an elementary, undifferentiated type of attention, manifested as the awake and alert state that accompanies the sleep-wake cycle regulated by the brain activating reticular system. Attention proper is selective, and it can be (1) involuntary, reflex, stimulus-driven, or exogenous (bottom-up) or (2) voluntary, goal-directed, or endogenous (top-down).

The most primitive type of selective attention is the *orienting reflex* (OR) consisting in a sudden redirection (reorienting) of attention to the source of a new external or internal stimulus (a sound, something luminous, sudden pain in some part of the body). The OR is a reaction to "novelty," occurring when a stimulus is first presented or when the parameters of an already habitual stimulus are changed (its quality, appearance at an unusual moment, or absence in the usual place), but "factors other than novelty can influence the OR, specifically the significance of the stimulus, and the probability of emergence of a signaling or unknown stimulus within a given space of time" [3, 4].The OR also leads to stop irrelevant forms of ongoing activity and is accompanied by emotional and autonomic (cardiovascular, respiratory) reactions, increased sensitivity of the correspondent sensory analyzer and of its respective cortical evoked potentials, besides inhibition of alpha rhythm of the electroencephalogram (desynchronization) [5, 6]. The OR makes the individual ready to choose and execute the appropriate action in the given situation (e.g., to fight or flight) and is highly relevant for survival of animals living in environments that change rapidly and require increased vigilance. The involuntary or reflex attention may vary depending on characteristics of the stimulus (intensity, novelty, biological value) as well as of states or conditions of the subject (humor state, tiredness, interests, needs).

Contrary to the involuntary attention, which is provoked by the object that attracts it (primacy of the object), *voluntary attention* is an act of the subject (primacy of the subject) who directs it to a certain object, phenomenon, or property, which is consciously chosen because it is highly relevant for fulfillment of determined task or objective. One of its main characteristics is selectivity, as brilliantly first defined by William James [7]: "Millions of items...are presented to my senses which never properly enter my experience. Why? Because they have no interest to me. My experience is what I agree to attend to... Everyone knows what attention is. It is the taking possession by the mind, in clear and vivid form, of one out of what seem several simultaneously possible objects or trains of thought. Focalization, concentration, of consciousness are of its essence. It implies withdrawal from some things in order to deal effectively with others...". This kind of attention is what we call *concentration*. The concentrated focusing on determined object or task requires the subject to be able to inhibit and ignore all types of interferences, be them internal or external stimuli, reminiscences, and ideas that are considered as irrelevant from the point of view of the current activity and final objective to be achieved.

Also differently from involuntary attention, which is biologically inherited and shared with other animals, voluntary attention is product of the individual's social-cultural experience, typical of humans. As pointed out by Vygotsky [8] and Luria [9], in the initial stages of the child development, this complex psychological function is shared by two persons: the adult and the child. The adult starts the psychological process of attention when he/she names and points to an object, and the child attends to his/her pointing gesture by looking at the object or grasping it with the hand. When the mother shows the child a pet bear surrounded by other objects and says "this is a bear," the indicative function of the word "bear" (denoting the object bear) leads to a reorganization of the child's perceptive field and allows the child to dedicate more attention to the named object, even when it is visually less attractive, for example, a gray small bear put among other brightly colored bears and things. Posteriorly, when the child has learned to speak and then names an object it wants, the word used is directed both to itself and to the adult (mother), as a kind of social interactional instrument. Thus, by means of language (first external and then internal), the child learns to direct both its and the adult's attention to that object (Tomasello's "joint attention") [10], now consciously, voluntarily. The acquisition of language (linguistic signs, words, called by Pavlov "second system of signals") and internal speech self-regulating function makes possible for the child to overcome and analyze natural stimuli or signals ("first system of signals") present in its visual-spatial field and to give more value and dedicate more attention to stimuli and objects that are socially considered to be more important, that is, more valued from the point of view of other persons.

Voluntary attention has mediated nature, while the involuntary is immediate, reflex. When learning language, the child appropriates the words and verbal instructions used by the adults for controlling its attention, actions, and behaviors, and now the child itself uses them to regulate its own attention and actions, as if the child was "another-itself." This is the origin of the voluntary, conscious act. Other animals, as the predators, are able to maintain their visual attention focused on the prey while chasing it, but here everything indicates we are dealing with an instinctive behavior.

Voluntary attention can be manifested as:

(1) *Concentrated attention*, selectively focused on a single item (object, phenomenon, property, action, idea), whose external manifestation may be *explicit*, with eyes and head directed to the object, or *undefined*, with wandering look at the environment, as when a student is concentrated in solving a problem, or *covert*, paying attention to something without directing the eyes to it, which may present in *disguised* form, for example, pretending to be looking with great interest to something but in fact paying attention to something else [11].
(2) *Divided attention*, distributed to different items, comprising various simultaneous stimuli and actions, for instance, the divided attention of a car driver in a very busy street, having to take various simultaneous driving actions (to watch the traffic lights, look at the rearview mirror and speedometer, step on the

accelerator, brake and clutch, etc. while talking about a problem with its traveling companion).

(3) *Vigilance*, a kind of concentrated attention maintained during long period of time, trying to detect relevant stimuli that may appear anywhere and anytime (e.g., the vigilance of a sentry guard in a military camp).

3.3 Attention Is Carried Out by a Complex Functional System

Involuntary attention (OR) is elicited by a stimulus that is new or that has changed some of its characteristics. Every new stimulus pass through a process of filtering or selection in which participate hippocampal neurons (novelty detectors) comparing the new stimuli with the old ones, inhibiting irrelevant stimuli and habituating to continuous or repetitive stimuli. Change in any parameter of an old stimulus provokes an OR, since the stimulus now does not coincide with its neuronal model previously created. The concept of *neuronal model of the stimulus*, introduced by Sokolov [5], means "a certain cell system (neuronal assembly) whereby the information is stored concerning the properties of a stimulus which has been applied many times," thus producing "an exact model of the properties of external objects acting on the sense organs." The OR depends on limbic regions and upper brain stem, mainly the superior colliculi, hippocampus, amygdala, and caudate nucleus, besides other structures such as lateral pulvinar, posterior parietal, and frontal dorsolateral (frontal eye fields, FEFs), particularly involved in the visual orientation reaction [12]. Hippocampal-limbic damage causes loss of selectivity of stimuli, increased distractibility, impairment of episodic memory, emergence of irrelevant associations, and even mental confusion. On the other hand, unilateral lesion of posterior parietal region or pulvinar, particularly in the nondominant hemisphere, usually results in neglect syndrome (inattention for stimuli in the contralateral hemi-space).

Voluntary attention is highly dependent on the frontal lobes, both dorsolateral and medial regions (including the anterior cingulate), given the importance of these regions for (1) inhibition of reactions to irrelevant stimuli, intrusive reminiscences, impulsive actions and behaviors, and all kinds of interferences able to affect a programmed, goal-directed activity; (2) maintenance of the awake state and optimal tone of cortical activation according to what is required by the individual's immediate tasks; and (3) for the directive and regulatory role of inner speech in human voluntary actions and behaviors [6]. Bilateral frontal lesions impair voluntary attention but leave intact ORs even to irrelevant stimuli, in this way resulting in increased distractibility. Neuroimaging, neurophysiological, and neuropsychological studies have shown that the control of selective attention (both involuntary, stimulus-driven, bottom-up, and voluntary, goal-directed, top-down) engages a right hemisphere dominant frontoparietal network (Fig. 3.1) comprising the dorsal attention network

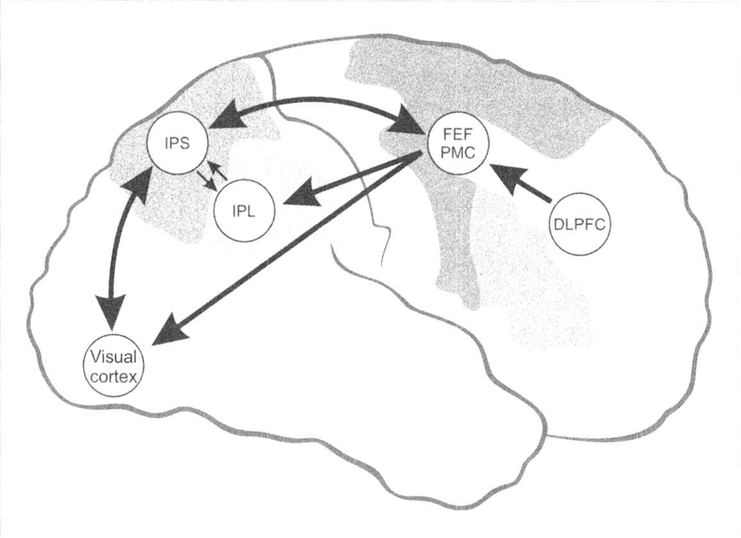

Fig. 3.1 Neuroanatomical implementation of Ptak's model of attentional selection based on a complex functional interaction between frontal and parietal regions. In this model, feature maps computed in the sensory cortex (e.g., visual) as well as current behavioral goals and abstract representations of associated actions generated in the dorsolateral prefrontal (DLPFC) and premotor cortex (PMC, including frontal eye fields FEF), feed into the parietal priority map (*IPS* intraparietal sulcus, *IPL* inferior parietal lobe). (From Ptak 2012, with permission)

(dorsolateral frontal cortex, frontal eye fields, and intraparietal sulcus) and the ventral attention network, located around the temporoparietal junction (TPJ) on the right caudal supramarginal gyrus and posterior superior temporal gyrus [13–15].

According to Patel et al. [15], "during top-down or goal-directed control of attention, the dorsal attention network is activated, enhancing the selected stimulus in visual cortex, and the temporoparietal junction (TPJ) is deactivated, suppressing the orienting of attention to potentially distracting stimuli; but when a behaviorally relevant stimulus is presented, the TPJ is activated, causing attention to be focused on this stimulus," which is "a characteristic that might be useful in social situations for picking out subtle changes in visual features, like eye-gaze direction."

3.4 Conclusion

Attention is the directionality and selectivity of mental acts (from perception to thinking) toward the object (or idea) perceived, thought, imagined, or wished. It is classified in involuntary, manifested as a stimulus-driven orienting reflex (bottom-up), and voluntary, as a goal-directed act of the subject (top-down). Involuntary attention is biologically inherited and shared with other animals, while the voluntary one is learned in the social-cultural practice with other humans, mediated by language. In this practice, the child first appropriates the words and verbal instructions used by adults for controlling its attention and behaviors, and then the child itself uses them (as internal language) to regulate its own attention and actions. Voluntary attention can be manifested as (1) concentrated attention, by maintaining the focus selectively on a single item (object, phenomenon, idea), and whose external manifestation may be explicit, undefined, covert, or disguised; (2) divided attention, distributed to different items; or as (3) vigilance, a kind of watchful concentration on any relevant stimuli that may appear anywhere and anytime.

The functional system involved in involuntary attention (orienting reaction) comprises hippocampal neurons (novelty detectors) in connection with other limbic regions and upper brain stem (superior colliculi), posterior parietal, and frontal dorsolateral (frontal eye fields). Voluntary attention depends mainly on dorsolateral and medial frontal regions for inhibition of irrelevant stimuli, intrusive reminiscences and all kinds of interferences that could affect a programmed goal-directed activity. Control of selective attention (involuntary or voluntary) engages a right hemisphere dominant network comprising two main components: a dorsal (dorsolateral frontal cortex, frontal eye fields, intraparietal sulcus) and a ventral (inferior parietal lobe, caudal supramarginal gyrus, posterior superior temporal gyrus).

References

1. von Uexküll J (1982) The theory of meaning. Semiotica 42(1):25–82
2. Rubinstein SL (1972). Princípios de Psicologia Geral, 2nd edn. Estampa Editorial, Lisbon (translated from the original title in Russian: Osnovy Obschei Psijologuii)
3. Voronin LG, Bonfitto M, Vasilieva VM (1975) The interrelation of the orienting reaction and conditioned reflex to time in man. In Sokolov EN, Vinogradova OS (eds) Weinberger NM (editor for the English edn) Neuronal mechanisms of the orientig reflex. Lawrence Erlbaum Associates, Publishers, Hillsdale
4. Sokolov EN (1975) The neuronal mechanisms of the orienting reflex. In Sokolov EN, Vinogradova OS (eds), Weinberger NM (editor for the English edn) Neuronal mechanisms of the orienting reflex. Lawrence Erlbaum Associates, Publishers, Hillsdale
5. Sokolov EN (1963) Perception and the conditioned reflex. Pergamon Press, Oxford
6. Luria AR (1973) The working brain: an introduction to neuropsychology. Basic Books, New York
7. James W (1890) The principles of psychology. Henry Holt and Company, New York
8. Vygotsky LS (1978) In: Cole M, John-Steiner V, Scribner S, Souberman E (eds) Mind in society: the development of higher psychological processes. Harvard University Press, Cambridge
9. Luria AR, Fla Yudovich (1959) In: Simon J (ed) Speech and development of mental processes in the child. Staples Press, London
10. Tomasello M (1999) The cultural origins of human cognition. Harvard University Press, Cambridge
11. Smirnov AA (1969) La atencion. In: Smirnov AA, Leontiev AN, Rubinstein SL, Tieplov BM (eds) Psicologia. Editorial Grijalbo S.A, Mexico (translated from Russian)
12. Chelazzi L, Corbetta M (2000) Cortical mechanisms of visuospatial attention in the human brain. In: Gazzaniga MS (ed) The new cognitive neurosciences. MIT Press, Cambridge, pp 667–686

13. Corbetta M, Patel G, Shulman GL (2008) The reorienting system of the human brain: from environment to theory of mind. Neuron 58(3):306–324
14. Ptak R (2012) The frontoparietal attention network of the human brain: action, saliency, and a priority map of the environment. Neuroscientist 18(5):502–515
15. Patel GH, Yang D, Jamerson EC, Snyder LH, Corbetta M, Ferrera VP (2015) Functional evolution of new and expanded attention networks in humans. PNAS 112(30):9454–9459

Chapter 4
Memory

4.1 Introduction

The temporal and spatial organization of the world, with its sequential, recurrent, and rhythmic events, made possible the emergence of life and, with life, the development of memory, both that of the species (genetic, innate) and that of the individual (learned). In a chaotic world, constituted by phenomena that never happen again, without regularities or natural laws, it would not be possible and even not necessary a memory.

Memory is not an isolated mental faculty nor a passive deposit of information and images, but a complex functional system made up of processes and procedures that unfold in successive temporal stages, diverse levels of mental organization, and various interconnected brain regions, allowing us to recall information, actions, and past experiences for using them in our daily life. *Learning* refers to the method or way by which new knowledge or skill is acquired, usually through training or repeated experience.

The study of memory started with the researches of Ebbinghaus (1885) on the formation of associations [1]. Posterior studies by Bartlett, Milner, Talland, Norman, Wickelgren, Miller, Tulving, Luria [2–9], and several others advanced our understanding of the human memory, particularly the memorization and learning of new information that constitute the episodic and semantic memory.

4.2 Memory Processes

The initial phase of the memory process is called *ultrashort*, relatively short and transitory (fractions of second), comprising the register of elementary traces of the information (mostly sensory) which will constitute the percept, in this way representing an extension of the process of perception. In reality, this initial memory

B. Damasceno, *Research on Cognition Disorders*,
https://doi.org/10.1007/978-3-030-57267-9_4

phase involves processes of perception, attention, and memory constituting a functional unity, as a kind of attentive perception, perceptive attention, and perceptive memory.

The next phase, *short-term* or *working memory* (seconds), makes possible the construction and stabilization of the percept and its subsequent encoding in a system of conceptual connections, through which occurs its categorization and consolidation in the *long-term memory*. Although these phases entail a serial processing, the use of memory in real-life activities requires a reciprocal interaction and coordination between its different phases and subtypes.

Consolidation is not the maintenance of invariable and indelible traces in the mind. On the contrary, it implies a transformation of the new information, which occurs even when this is not being recalled. When remembered afterward, the information becomes more vulnerable to modifications and is reconstructed and rebuilt, as first demonstrated by Bartlett [2] in his experiments of cognitive psychology and more recently by studies of episodic memory reconsolidation [10]. Several factors (both social and personal, affective, motivational) can influence the way our memories are transformed and reconstructed with the passage of time.

Recall is not simply the spontaneous emergence of images, but a complex mental activity comprising (1) an active search and selection of the necessary connections (sensory, conceptual) consisting in a commutative process of excitation of those that are relevant as well as inhibition of those that are irrelevant and inadequate for the task at hand; (2) comparison of the search results with the material originally memorized; and (3) verification and decision about the result found, whether it is correct, congruent, or not [9, 11].

Recognition consists in the subject judging whether or not determined item or information matches with or is the same as the one that has been perceived or remembered before. To be recognized, the item has to be encoded again in the same way it was in the initial presentation, so it can excite the same percept or prior memory traces (*encoding specificity principle*) [12]. Visual recognition of any object takes into account the spatial relations among its parts and the extent to which these spatial relations deviate from the prototype object, as has been evidenced in studies of face recognition and prosopagnosia (*configural model*) [13, 14]. Recognition is similar but generally easier than recall by having cues and requiring less searches; nevertheless, it involves more active comparison and decision-making regarding the congruence or discordance of the item with the one previously memorized, particularly in multiple-choice tasks with items that are like but not exactly the same.

Memory presupposes *forgetting*, which is necessary for us to focus our mind in what is more relevant in our daily living, as evidenced in studies by Storm, Bjork, and Bjork [15] and beautifully exalted by Bertolt Brecht in his poem "Praise of Oblivion":

> Good is forgetfulness,
> otherwise how would the
> motherfucker
> who breastfed him stay away?

That gave you the strength of the
limbs
and prevents you from experiencing
it.

Or how would the student leave the
teacher who gave him the knowledge?
When knowledge is given,
the student has to start on his way. The new residents move into
the old house.

If those who built it still lived there,
the house would be too small.

The oven heats up. It is no longer known
who the potter was. The planter
does not recognize the bread.

How would the man get up in the morning
without remembering the night that undoes the trail?
How would the
one who felled six times stand up for the seventh time
to plow the stony ground, fly
the dangerous sky?

The weakness of memory
gives man strength.

The mechanism of forgetting has been a debated issue. The first and dominant view, since the studies of Ebbinghaus [1], was that the memory traces would gradually fade away and extinguish (the theory of *trace decay*). However, already in 1900, Müller and Pilzecker [16] proposed another explanation, nowadays more adopted – the theory of *interference* of the items in each other through proactive and retroactive inhibition. Forgetting would result from the inhibitory influence of the preceding items on the subsequent ones and vice versa. This is clearly observed in tests of word list learning. The words in the middle of the list are more forgotten due to the proactive inhibition of the preceding ones and retroactive inhibition of the subsequent ones. In fact, this effect of interference has also been observed in other tests for memorizing series of verbal or visual items, sentences, and even narratives.

Episodic, retrospective memory is usually evaluated by means of tests using word lists (verbal memory) or series of figures (visual memory). One of the most used is the Rey Auditory Verbal Learning Test (RAVLT), which consists of 15 unrelated words read aloud by the examiner for five consecutive trials (list A), followed by a free-recall test. After the fifth trial, a new interference list of 15 words is presented (list B) followed by a free-recall of that list. Soon afterward, a free-recall of the first list is tested without new presentation. After a 20-min delay period, subjects are again required to recall words from list A. Finally, the patient must identify (recognize) list A words from a list of 50 words which includes lists A and B and 20 other words phonemically or semantically related to lists A and B.

4.3 Memory Systems

Memories have been classified in two main types, *explicit* (also known as *declarative*) and *implicit* (*nondeclarative*), the main difference between them being whether or not it requires conscious or intentional recollection of previous experiences [8, 17]. Implicit memories are predominantly reflex and automatic, being registered and recalled independently of awareness or complex cognitive processes. Here are included the conditioned reflexes, priming, and procedural memory.

Procedural memory is the learning of behavioral and cognitive abilities, whose mastering is later performed at an automatic and unconscious level. It refers to various skills learned by repetition and practice, such as perceptual (mirror reading), motor (dancing, bike riding), and cognitive skills (syntactic rules, reading). Although most skills are classified as nondeclarative or implicit memory, their acquisition may be mediated by verbal instructions, for example, when learning to drive a car. The neurofunctional system of procedural memory is distinct from that of episodic and semantic memories. Procedural memory may be spared in cases of severe amnesia associated with bilateral hippocampal lesion as in the case H.M. submitted to bilateral medial temporal lobectomy [18] and in patients with mild to moderate Alzheimer's dementia. On the other hand, it can be impaired in cases of basal ganglia lesions which leave intact the hippocampal system, preserving episodic memory, such as Parkinson's and Huntington's diseases. Learning of new motor skills is also impaired in such diseases. In neuroimaging studies, the brain regions most involved in procedural memory have been the basal ganglia, cerebellum, and supplementary motor area [19, 20].

Priming is a kind of subliminal activation that spreads among interrelated stimuli or items of a whole system of associations, so that the presentation of one of the items facilitates the recall of the others, often without the individual being aware of the previous exposure to the items, as observed in the patient H.M. with severe amnesia due to bilateral hippocampal damage. This patient could remember a list of words when only their first syllables were shown to him for completing the name (cued recall; e.g., *ele* _____ for *elephant*), though he was unable to recall them spontaneously, without cues (by free-recall). For verbal memory, priming may be based on meaning (semantic priming, e.g., the prime *school* for the target *teacher*) or based on sound (phonological) or on the first letters, as cues.

Explicit or declarative memories involve deliberate and conscious encoding and recall of information, which can be expressed verbally as when we memorize everyday events and personal experience (*episodic memory*) or when we learn new concepts (*semantic memory*). Depending on the temporal processing, explicit memory can be long-term (episodic or retrospective, prospective, and semantic) or short-term (working memory).

Episodic memory, also called *retrospective* or *autobiographic*, consists in the conscious recollection of episodes or events in the personal biographic history, with the self mentally traveling back in time and re-experiencing one's past [21]. The detailed remembering of everything involved in the past episode requires inhibition not only of irrelevant associations but also of the attentive perception of things present in the here and now of the person who is remembering, as a kind of detachment from his/her current surrounding world. The self is not here now but there in the past episode, re-experiencing it with a sense of presence and feelings for all events and actions. Imagine, for example, someone remembering the total eclipse of the sun he experienced: "It was a nice sunny afternoon, January 26, 1990. I was taking a walk together with my two boys in the banks of Paranã river (Goiás State, Brazil), enjoying the beautiful nature, when unexpectedly, around 5 PM, darkness started coming slowly, as if it was going to be nightfall. My first reaction was of strangeness and fear, I did not know what that could be, but soon afterward I realized it was an eclipse of the sun and observed it with pleasure."

Episodic memory is highly dependent on the medial temporal lobe, especially the hippocampal system (hippocampus, entorhinal and perirhinal cortices), which facilitates the long-term register of new information (consolidation) in the associative neocortex. Lesions of the hippocampal system cause *amnesia* or *amnesic syndrome*, characterized by (1) the patient not remembering events that happened immediately previous to the lesion (*retrograde amnesia*) nor does he retain new information after the lesion (*anterograde amnesia*); (2) it is multimodal, affecting information of any sensory modality; (3) it is worsened by interferences and distractions; and (4) it leaves intact the short-term working memory, priming, and procedural memory. Events that occurred just before the lesion are most vulnerable to forgetting, while remote events are more resistant (Ribot's law). Amnesia associated with bilateral hippocampal damage impairs not only the recollection of the past but also the ability to imagine and experience specific events in the future, since the hippocampus is critical for provisioning the spatial context and binding together disparate elements of the imagined scene, in similar ways as it does in re-experiencing past events [22]. Dysfunction of episodic memory may be caused by lesion of other structures of the "Papez circuit," which includes the presubiculum, fornix, mammillary bodies, mammillothalamic tract, anterior nucleus of the thalamus, medial septum, diagonal band of Broca, and retrosplenial cortex.

Thus, explicit long-term episodic learning is highly dependent on the hippocampus, particularly when a spatial component is present in the task situation. The hippocampus stores a cognitive map of the spatial layout of the environment [23], and the right hippocampus and parahippocampal cortex are crucial for learning the spatial location of objects, especially when the position of each object is registered automatically and unintentionally [24]. On the other hand, the neighboring amygdala is involved in implicit emotional memory as well as in fear conditioning, so that a selective and bilateral lesion of the amygdala prevents fear conditioning in humans, but does not impair the explicit memory for the events that occurred during the experimental testing [25].

Semantic memory constitutes our knowledge of objects, facts, concepts, words, and their meaning, for example, to know what the eclipse of the sun is. Tasks dependent on semantic memory include object naming, definition of spoken words, word-picture and picture-picture matching, and generation of exemplars on category fluency tests [26].

Semantic memory differs from episodic memory by not being personal or temporally specific, but culturally shared, since it is acquired through language-mediated social practice with other persons. Semantic memory is necessary but not sufficient for the discursive use of language, which requires a high degree of social cognition for implementing procedures and strategies in the process of enunciation during the interlocution (discursive memory). Semantic memory is relatively spared in patients with severe amnesia due to bilateral lesion of the hippocampus or Papez circuit [18], but it may be impaired in cases of semantic dementia associated with anterior-lateral temporal lobe degeneration, which spares the hippocampal system and episodic memory [27].

On the other hand, semantic and episodic memories share interdependences and interrelationships. Acquisition or encoding of new episodic memories depends on information in semantic memory, particularly on the binding of semantic concepts to the specific context in which they appear [8, 28, 29]. For instance, if someone sees a street demonstration with people walking together in the same direction, carrying placards and crying out watchwords demanding higher pay, it will be easier to remember this episode afterward if it is understood as a strike of city hall workers. On the other hand, semantic memory depends on the episodic one. According to Greenberg and Verfaellie [29], episodic memory facilitates the acquisition of new semantic memory as well as the transfer and consolidation of information into neocortical regions. For example, a child learns the concept of restaurant by eating meals with its family in different restaurants (Italian, Japanese, Brazilian, Arab), each one with its specificities and own characteristics (kind of dishes, music, clothes of the waiters, etc.), but each time constituting a unique episode. In all these restaurants, the child learns that there is a common ritual (restaurant script) which constitutes the concept of restaurant (to sit at the table, to call the waiter, to choose the dish in the menu, etc., and at the end, to pay and leave). Episodic and semantic memories interact with each other not only at encoding but also at retrieval. As shown in studies of semantic verbal fluency, when the names to be retrieved are linked to a memory of specific events (episodic memory) and thus autobiographically significant, episodic memory facilitates semantic retrieval by providing an organizational strategy or an efficient route of access [29–31].

Prospective memory (PM) is the memory of the future, which makes possible for us to remember to carry out intended actions at a determined time in the future, for example, to keep appointments, pay bills, and take medicine, being crucial for our functioning in everyday living. PM tasks can be either time-based (to make an intended action at a particular time of day or after a certain period of time has elapsed), event-based (to execute the intended action upon the occurrence of a particular environmental event), or activity-based (to do something when a particular activity has been completed). As proposed by McDaniel and Einstein (2007), a typical and informative PM task should (1) not to be executed immediately after the intention; (2) to be embedded in another ongoing activity; (3) to have constrained time window of opportunities for initiating the intended action; (4) to have limited time frame for accomplishing the action; (5) to be based on an consciously formed intention or plan; and (6) the formed intention should not be maintained in the focus of consciousness (working memory) but has to be temporarily forgotten by performing other activities; otherwise, it would constitute a vigilance task, not a PM task [32].

PM tasks require one to remember there was an intention (the prospective component) and also to remember the contents of the intention, "what to do" (the retrospective component). The prospective component or memory of intention is essential for goal-directed behaviors and depends mainly on the prefrontal regions. Positron emission tomography (PET) studies of young adults performing PM tasks have found brain activations particularly in the right dorsolateral and ventrolateral prefrontal cortices, anterior cingulate gyrus, left parahippocampal gyrus, and midline medial frontal lobe [33]. The retrospective component, on the other hand, is highly dependent on the medial temporal lobe structures, and it is what makes PM (to memorize a list of things to do in the future) to be similar to retrospective memory (to remember a list of events or items from the past) and constitutes one of the reasons why prospective and retrospective memories are usually impaired in the early stages of Alzheimer's disease [34–36].

The memory of intention is a complex mental process which, according to Karantzoulis et al. (2009), involves at least four stages: (a) intention formation, to plan the future activity, i.e., what to do and when to do it; (2) intention retention, to hold the intention in memory while other activities are occurring, i.e., during the ongoing task; (3) intention initiation, the point at which the appropriate cue (e.g., an event) triggers an effortful and controlled search of memory for the intention; and (4) intention execution, when the retrieval context actually occurs and the action of the intended action is executed [37].

Working memory is a kind of attentional and executive short-term memory that holds temporarily in the focus of consciousness (for 5–20 s) several types of information (sensory, perceptual, spatial, verbal-phonological), both the new ones (just received from the external world) and the old ones (recalled from long-term, episodic, and semantic memory), enabling us to operate on them simultaneously (online) when solving a problem, making a decision, and interpreting or producing a discourse. An example of WM test is the Paced Auditory Serial Addition Test (PASAT), in which the subject listens to 61 digits presented every 3 s, adds each new digit to the one immediately prior to it, and gives orally each sum as quickly as possible [38].

In the last four decades, various studies have investigated the complex psychological structure of WM. The Baddeley-Hitch model of WM (reviewed in Baddeley 2007, 2012) has been the dominant theory in this regard, supported by evidence from behavioral, neuropsychological, developmental, and neuroimaging studies [39, 40]. According to this model, WM is not a simple passive store of information, but a dynamic multiple-component framework comprising limited-capacity short-term subfunctions: (1) the *phonological loop* that deals with sounds and phonological information and consists in two subcomponents: a store of auditory memory traces and phonological codes, which is coupled with a subvocal ("inner speech") articulatory rehearsal component for maintaining these memory traces and codes; otherwise, the activation of these traces would decay spontaneously with the passage of time; (2) the *visual-spatial sketchpad* that holds visual and spatial information whose mental image is inspected, navigated, and cognitively manipulated; (3) the *episodic buffer* is a short-term store that integrates short-term and long-term memories and binds together and manipulates multimodal complex information, sequencing episodes spatially and temporally (e.g., when memorizing a story) [41, 42]; and (4) the *central executive* is a supervisory system comprising diverse cognitive functions such as selectively focusing and maintaining attention, coordinating and binding information from the other short-term buffers, inhibiting irrelevant information, and flexibly shifting between tasks or retrieval strategies [39].

Neuropsychological and neuroimaging studies have yielded enough evidence that WM, as a multiple-component framework, engages complex cortico-subcortical brain networks which may vary depending on the particular task, but almost all tasks require the participation of the prefrontal cortex (PFC) for the attentional, goal-focused executive components, mainly the dorsolateral prefrontal, anterior cingulate, and orbital cortical regions [43, 44]. Other crucial regions of WM fronto-parietal and fronto-subcortical networks are the posterior visual association areas, particularly posterior right parietal in connection with right PFC for the visual-spatial short-term memory; the left angular and supramarginal gyri as well as Broca's area for the verbal component [45–47]; subcortical structures subserving motivation, such as the basal ganglia (bilateral caudate, nucleus accumbens) and thalamus (bilateral mediodorsal nucleus) reciprocally connected to the PFC [48–50]; the subthalamic nucleus role in decision-making [51]; and in cases of affectively charged stimuli, also the amygdala with its projections to the anterior cingulate and orbital cortex [52]. Usually, more complex and difficult WM tasks require bilateral and more widespread brain activation [53]. In such cases, PFC activation increases as a function of the memory load and the level of representational abstraction of the information being processed [54].

The Baddeley-Hitch multiple-component WM model has been the most influential and the one that has most contributed to our understanding of human working memory. Notwithstanding, there remain some unresolved issues. The first problem is the lack of a conscious self or subject of the mental actions involved, which is common in most Cartesian-Kantian, computational, or purely biological approaches of the human mind. There is no memory or thought as isolated mental faculties, but a real human being with its needs and motives, having to memorize and think for solving new or difficult situations. Baddeley [40] tackles this issue by introducing the central executive in the model, assumed to be "the most complex component,... capable of attentional focus, storage, and decision making, virtually a homunculus, a little man in the head, capable of doing all the clever things that were outside the competence of the two subsystems (phonological loop and visual-spatial sketchpad)". In the two sentences that follows this one, he seems to recognize the need of such a conscious self or subject: "Although our model tended to be criticized for taking this approach, like Attneave (1960) I regard homunculi as potentially useful if used appropriately. It is important that they are not seen as providing an explanation, but rather as a marker of issues requiring explanation" [40, 55]. What we need in the model is not a homunculus or series of homunculi acting in Cartesian theaters, but a conscious self or self-aware subject with its first-person givenness or "myness" dimension of experience [56], that is, an "I" as the invariant and persisting subject pole of experience and action, with its feelings of agency, coherence, unity, temporal identity, and demarcation [57]. This conscious self is an emergent property of the self-organizing system of the mind, which is not a priori established but socially mediated and constructed in the interactions of the individual with persons, tools, and objects (see more on this topic in the chapter on the ontogenetic development of the mind). As emphasized by Gärdenfors (2005), this kind of self-awareness is developed with the previous establishment of a representation of the inner world of other individuals, so that an "I" experience is preceded by a "you" experience [58].

As second problem, the model establishes the primacy of WM over the executive function, which is understood as just one of the components of WM. On the contrary, as proposed by other authors [59], WM is one of the core components of our executive functions (EF), besides *inhibition* for controlling one's attention, behavior, thoughts, and emotions, and *cognitive flexibility*, for shifting sets, switching from one task to the other, and changing perspectives and ways to think, which are needed for higher-order intellectual and executive functioning as in problem-solving, logical and discursive reasoning, decision-making, and creativity. As a component of EF, WM is the holding of information in mind for working with it, for relating what happened earlier with what comes later [59]. Without being kept simultaneously in mind by WM, information from multiple domains cannot be appropriately related with each other in the goal-directed course of the executive activity. Even though WM is necessary, it is not sufficient for the executive task as a whole to be successful. WM is just one among other mental operations belonging to the thinking or intellectual process, which are required for a successful task. Real-life tasks require reciprocal interactions between the subtypes of memory, which are coordinated by our executive functions (Baddeley's "central executive"; Fig. 4.1).

Pioneering studies of the intellectual-executive function by Köhler (1917), Vygotsky (1934), Piaget (1936), Bruner et al. (1956), Leontiev (1959), Galperin (1966), Miller (1960), Luria [9, 60–66], and other psychologists have shown that it is a highly complex mental process required when the subject confronts a new or problematic situation for which he doesn't have an innate, habitual, or automatic

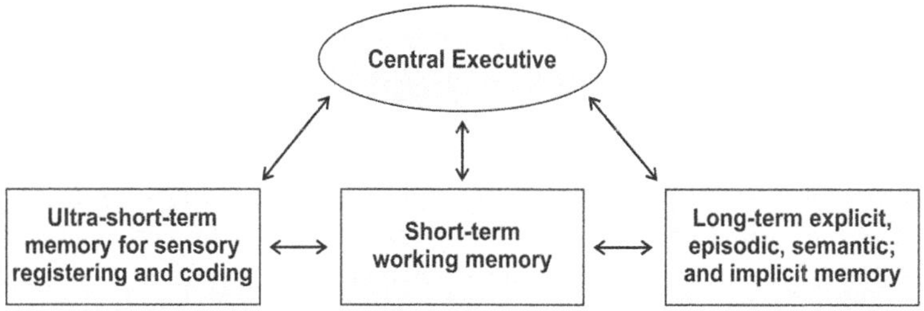

Fig. 4.1 Relationships between ultrashort, short, and long-term memories, coordinated by the executive functions

solution. Luria's [9] detailed neuropsychological investigation has disclosed the complex and dynamic internal structure of the thinking process both in concrete-active (e.g., chess game) and in verbal, logical, or discursive thinking (e.g., arithmetical problem-solving). Luria has shown the main components and the corresponding brain mechanisms of the intellectual function, as well as its dependency on the meaning of words, which constitute its logical and discursive matrix. The first step and component is to establish a goal whose attainment would satisfy a need or motive of the subject in the given conditions. The second step is to inhibit premature impulsive responses and to analyze the conditions in which the goal is given and to recognize the most relevant and essential components of the problematic situation and their reciprocal correlations. The third step is the establishment of hypotheses, selecting the one that most probably would solve the problem, and forming the corresponding scheme of action or strategy. The fourth step is to choose the methods and operations that would be most appropriate to implement the general scheme of action, based on previous learning experience with linguistic, logical, and numerical algorithm used to solve similar problems. The fifth step is the solution of the problem, which is followed by the final phase, namely, comparison of the results so far obtained with the original conditions of the task, and correction of any wrong solution or response. As shown in neuropsychological studies, the frontal lobes are the most crucial brain region for programming, executing, and verifying the intellectual activity as a whole, while the posterior (temporal-parietal-occipital) regions are responsible for the necessary operations and methods, particularly when the operations require simultaneous syntheses.

4.4 Conclusion

Memory and learning are complex processes that unfold in successive temporal stages, various levels of mental organization, and interconnected brain regions. After the initial ultrashort register of elementary traces of the information (fractions of seconds), the short-term (seconds) or working memory allows the construction and stabilization of the percept and its consolidation in long-term memory, on the basis of interaction and coordination between these different phases. Afterward, processes of recall and recognition allow relevant information to be recovered and used in real-life activities. Memory presupposes forgetting for the mind to focus on the information that is more relevant for the task at hand. Memory may be explicit, conscious, and declarative, such as the episodic, semantic, prospective, and working memories, and implicit, predominantly reflex and automatic, for example, the procedural memory, conditioned reflexes, and priming. Procedural learning (e.g., car driving) has an initial explicit conscious phase, mediated by verbal instructions, which engages various cortical areas, but then becomes implicit and automatized to the extent that the supplementary motor area, basal ganglia, and cerebellum take over it. Episodic memory (EM) is the conscious recollection of one's past life episodes or events, requiring the self to travel back in time and re-experience them even affectively. EM is highly dependent on the medial temporal lobe (hippocampal system), whose lesion causes amnesia. Semantic memory (SM) constitutes our culturally shared conceptual knowledge about objects, facts, words, and their meaning. SM is preserved in amnesia (hippocampal lesions), but usually impaired in cases of widespread neocortical lesions, particularly in left-sided anterior inferolateral temporal lesions. Prospective memory (PM) is the act of remembering to carry out intended actions in the future, and it can be time-based, event-based, or activity-based. PM has two main components: the prospective (memory of the "intention to do" something in the future), crucially dependent on prefrontal regions, and the retrospective ("what to do"), reliant on the medial temporal lobe structures. Working memory (WM) is a kind of short-term memory that holds temporarily (5–20 s) in the focus of consciousness both new and old information that needs to be simultaneously worked out for solving problems or making decisions. WM attentional and central executive components depend mainly on the dorsolateral prefrontal, anterior cingulate, and orbital cortices in connection with posterior cortical regions involved with language and visual-spatial components.

References

1. Ebbinghaus H (1885) Über das Gedächtniss: Untersuchungen zur experimentellen Psychologie. Dunker u. Humboldt, Leipzig
2. Bartlett FC (1932) Remembering: a study in experimental and social psychology. Cambridge University Press, Cambridge
3. Milner B (1958) Psychological defects produced by temporal lobe excision. Res Publ Assoc Res Nerv Ment Dis 36:244–257
4. Talland GA (1965) Deranged memory. Academic Press, New York
5. Norman DA (1969) Memory and attention. John Wiley, New York
6. Wickelgren WA (1977) Learning and memory. Prentice-Hall, Englewood Cliffs
7. Miller GA (1956) The magical number seven plus or minus two: some limits on our capacity for processing information. Psychol Rev 63:81–97
8. Tulving E (1972) Episodic and semantic memory. In: Tulving E, Donaldson W (eds) Organization of memory. Academic Press, New York
9. Luria AR (1966/1980) Higher cortical functions in man. New York: Basic Books
10. Nader K (2015) Reconsolidation and the dynamic nature of memory. Cold Spring Harb Perspect Biol 7:a021782. https://doi.org/10.1101/cshperspect.a021782
11. Kintsch W (1970) Models for free recall and recognition. In: Norman DA (ed) Models of human memory. Academic, New York
12. Tulving E, Thompson DM (1973) Encoding specificity and retrieval processes in episodic memory. Psychol Rev 80:352–373
13. Rhodes G, Brennan S, Carey S (1987) Identification and ratings of caricatures: implications for mental representations of faces. Cogn Psychol 19:473–497
14. Smith EE, Kosslyn SM (2007) Cognitive psychology – mind and brain, 1st edn. Pearson Prentice Hall, Upper Saddle River
15. Storm BC, Bjork EL, Bjork RA (2008) Accelerated relearning after retrieval-induced forgetting: the benefit of being forgotten. J Exp Psychol Learn Mem Cogn 34(1):230–236
16. Müller GE, Pilzecker A (1900) Experimentelle Beiträge zur Lehre vom Gedächtnis. Z Psychol Ergänzungsband 1:1–300

17. Schacter DL (1987) Implicit memory: history and current status. J Exp Psychol Learn Mem Cogn 13:501–518
18. Corkin S (1984) Lasting consequences of bilateral medial temporal lobectomy: clinical course and experimental findings in H.M. Semin Neurol 4:249–259
19. Daselaar SM, Rombouts SA, Veltman DJ, Raaijmakers JG, Jonker C (2003) Similar network activated by young and old adults during the acquisition of a motor sequence. Neurobiol Aging 24(7):1013–1019
20. Censor N, Dayan E, Cohen LG (2014) Cortico-subcortical neuronal circuitry associated with reconsolidation of human procedural memories. Cortex 58:281–288
21. Tulving E (2002) Episodic memory: from mind to brain. Annu Rev Psychol 53:1–25
22. Hassabis D, Kumaran D, Maguire EA (2007) Using imagination to understand the neural basis of episodic memory. J Neurosci 27(52):14365–14374
23. O'Keefe J, Nadel L (1978) The hippocampus as a cognitive map. Oxford University Press, Oxford
24. Smith ML, Milner B (1981) The role of the right hippocampus in the recall of spatial location. Neuropsychologia 19:781–793
25. Bechara A, Tranel D, Damasio H, Adolphs R, Rockland C, Damasio AR (1995) Double dissociation of conditioning and declarative knowledge relative to the amygdala and hippocampus in humans. Science 269(5227):1115–1118
26. Hodges JR, Patterson K (1995) Is semantic memory consistently impaired early in the course of Alzheimer's disease? Neuroanatomical and diagnostic implications. Neuropsychologia 33(4):441–459
27. Hodges JR (2001) Frontotemporal dementia (Pick's disease): clinical features and assessment. Neurology 56:S6–S10
28. Reder LM, Park H, Kieffaber PD (2009) Memory systems do not divide on consciousness: reinterpreting memory in terms of activation and binding. Psychol Bull 135:23–49
29. Greenberg DL, Verfaellie M (2010) Interdependence of episodic and semantic memory: evidence from neuropsychology. J Int Neuropsychol Soc 16(5):748–753
30. Greenberg DL, Keane MM, Ryan LR, Verfaellie M (2009) Impaired category fluency in medial temporal lobe amnesia: the role of episodic memory. J Neurosci 29:10900–10908
31. Westmacott R, Black SE, Freedman M, Moscovitch M (2004) The contribution of autobiographical significance to semantic memory: evidence from Alzheimer's disease, semantic dementia, and amnesia. Neuropsychologia 42:25–48
32. McDaniel MA, Einstein GO (2007) Prospective memory: an overview and synthesis of an emerging field. Sage, Thousand Oaks
33. Burgess N, Maguire EA, Spiers HJ, O'Keefe J (2001) A temporoparietal and prefrontal network for retrieving the spatial context of lifelike events. NeuroImage 14(2):439–453
34. Jones S, Livner Å, Bäckman L (2006) Patterns of prospective and retrospective memory impairment in preclinical Alzheimer's disease. Neuropsychology 20(2):144–152
35. Martins SP, Damasceno BP (2008) Prospective and retrospective memory in mild Alzheimer's disease. Arq Neuropsiquiatr 66(2B):318–322
36. Damasceno BP (2012) Prospective and retrospective learning in mild Alzheimer's disease. In: Seel NM (ed) Encyclopedia of the sciences of learning. Springer, Boston
37. Karantzoulis S, Troyer AK, Rich JB (2009) Prospective memory in amnestic mild cognitive impairment. J Int Neuropsychol Soc 15(3):407–415
38. Gronwall DM (1977) Paced auditory serial-addition task: a measure of recovery from concussion. Percept Mot Skills 44(2):367–373
39. Baddeley AD (2007) Working memory, thought and action. Oxford University Press, Oxford
40. Baddeley AD (2012) Working memory: theories, models, and controversies. Annu Rev Psychol 63:1–29
41. Baddeley A (2000) The episodic buffer: a new component of working memory? Trends Cogn Sci 4(11):417–423
42. Logie RH (1995) Visuo-spatial working memory. Erlbaum, Hove

43. Goldman-Rakic PS (1992) Working memory and the mind. Sci Am 267(3):110–117
44. Fletcher PC, Henson RNA (2001) Frontal lobes and human memory: insights from functional neuroimaging. Brain 124:849–881
45. Rogalsky C, Matchin W, Hickok G (2008) Broca's area, sentence comprehension, and working memory: an fMRI study. Front Hum Neurosci 2(14). https://doi.org/10.3389/neuro.09.014.2008
46. Logie RH (2011) The functional organization and capacity limits of working memory. Curr Dir Psychol Sci 20(4):240–245
47. Elmer S Broca pars triangularis constitutes a "hub" of the language-control network during simultaneous language translation. Front Hum Neurosci. 29 September 2016. https://doi.org/10.3389/fnhum.201600491
48. Dagenbach D, Absher JR, Kubat-Silman AK (2001) Human working memory impairments associated with thalamic damage. Int J Neurosci 111:67–87
49. Watanabe Y, Funahashi S (2012) Thalamic mediodorsal nucleus and working memory. Neurosci Biobehav Rev 36:134–142. https://doi.org/10.1016/j.neubiorev.2011.05.003
50. Moore AB, Li Z, Tyner CE, Hu X, Crosson B (2013) Bilateral basal ganglia activity in verbal working memory. Brain Lang 125(3):316–323. https://doi.org/10.1016/j.bandl.2012.05.003
51. Whitmer D, White CN (2012) Evidence of human subthalamic nucleus involvement in decision making. J Neurosci 32:8753–8755
52. Armony JL, LeDoux JE (2000) How danger is encoded: toward a systems, cellular, and computational understanding of cognitive-emotional interactions in fear. In: Gazzaniga MS (ed) The new cognitive neurosciences, 2nd edn. The MIT Press, Cambridge, MA, pp 1067–1079
53. Newman SD, Carpenter PA, Varma S, Just MA (2003) Frontal and parietal participation in problem solving in the tower of London: fMRI and computational modeling of planning and high-level perception. Neuropsychologia 41:1668–1682
54. Nee DE, D'Esposito M (2018) The representational basis of working memory. Curr Top Behav Neurosci 37:213–230
55. Attneave F (1960) In defense of homunculi. In: Rosenblith W (ed) Sensory communication. MIT Press, Cambridge, MA, pp 777–782
56. Parnas J, Zahavi D (2002) The role of phenomenology in psychiatric classification and diagnosis. In: Maj M, Gaebel W, Lopez-Ibor JJ, Sartorius N (eds) Psychiatric diagnosis and classification. John Wiley, New York, pp 137–162
57. Parnas J (2003) Self and schizophrenia: a phenomenological perspective. In: Kircher T, David A (eds) The self in neuroscience and psychiatry. Cambridge University Press, Cambridge, pp 217–241
58. Gärdenfors P (2005) The detachment of thought. In: Erneling CE, Johnson DM (eds) The mind as a scientific object – between brain and culture. Oxford University Press, Oxford, pp 323–341
59. Diamond A (2013) Executive functions. Annu Rev Psychol 64:135–168
60. Köhler W (1917) Intelligenzprüfungen an Anthropoiden. Königlich Akademie der Wissenschaften, Berlin
61. Vygotsky LS (1934/1962) Thought and language. The MIT Press, Cambridge, MA
62. Piaget J (1936) Origins of intelligence in the child. Routledge & Kegan Paul, London
63. Bruner JS, Goodnow JJ, Austin GA (1956) A study of thinking. Wiley, New York
64. Leontiev AN (1959/1981). Problems of the development of the mind. Progress Publishers, Moscow
65. Galperin PY (1966). The psychology of thinking and the study of the stage formation of mental actions. In: The investigation of thinking in Soviet psychology 196. Nauka, Moscow (in Russian)
66. Miller GA, Galanter E, Pribram KH (1960) Plans and the structure of behavior. Henry Holt, New York

Chapter 5
Language

5.1 Introduction

Language is a cognitive function based on the conscious use of signs (words, symbols) for communication, social interaction, and representation of the world. It is functionally organized in diverse components (phonologic, morphologic, syntactic, semantic, and discursive-pragmatic), which will be succinctly defined. These components are interrelated in the everyday real-life use of language. The *phonologic* component is concerned with sounds understood not as physical phenomena detected and produced by the body (object of study of phonetics) but as abstract entities called *phonemes*, considered to be the minimal meaning bearing elements of spoken language, functioning to distinguish one morpheme from another, for example, *pat* from *bat* by exchanging the phoneme /p/ for /b/. As an abstract construct, a phoneme can be perceived as the same when spoken with different sound frequencies or intensities, or even when whispered, in similar way that a letter (e.g., *b*) can be recognized when written in different formats (B, b, ʙ, ь). The phonologic component includes *prosody*, which is the prominence (accent) given to a syllable in a word or to a word in a phrase, being manifest in its intonation, stress, and rhythm. Prosody indicates the emotional state of the speaker, the form of the utterance (whether it is a question, command, irony, or sarcasm). With prosody the speaker intentionally modifies the meaning of words by uttering them with different intonation and emotional load, in order to influence the interlocutor in the conversational, discursive interaction. The *morphologic* component is the formation of *morphemes* as the smallest lexical units of a language, for example, a word or its parts (roots, stems, prefixes, suffixes). The *syntactic* comprises a set of structural rules and principles that control the interrelationship of words, specifically grammar and word order, for the construction of phrases and sentences, for example, the sequence subject, verb, and object. The *semantic* deals with the meaning of signs, words, phrases, and symbols, with what they denote or represent. Words and phrases are not codes with rigidly fixed meaning but dynamic structures whose sense is jointly

B. Damasceno, *Research on Cognition Disorders*,
https://doi.org/10.1007/978-3-030-57267-9_5

constructed by the interlocutors on the basis of the immediate context of communication and the social-historical conditions of the interlocution. The word is polysemous; it can have several different meanings or senses depending on the contexts of its use, the intention of the speaker, and in what way it is interpreted by the listener. The semantic level can be subdivided into *lexical semantic*, referring to lexical units (words, affixes, compound words, phrases) and how their meanings correlate with the syntactic structure of language, and *discursive semantic* or *pragmatic*, mediating the social interaction between individuals by means of language, using metaphors, proverbs, jokes, ironies, and sarcasms, as occur in a common conversation. This level unfolds in two aspects: the *enunciation*, the utterance, the act of speaking, by which the subject appropriates the language, and the *statement* (the enunciated, Benveniste's *énoncé*), the result of the act of enunciation, the oral or written text [1].

5.2 Discourse and Pragmatics

Discourse and pragmatics have been tackled by several approaches, such as those of discourse analysis, pragmatics, theory of enunciation, theory of speech acts, analysis of conversation, textual linguistics, discursive psychology, and others, which have contributed to our better understanding of real-life language functioning.

The pragmatic and discourse level of language is the most complex and requires a high degree of social cognition, whose basis is constructed in the 3–4-year-old child as theory of mind, which is the ability to infer other people's mental states (perceptions, thoughts, feelings, intentions, and desires), to predict their behavior and interact with them accordingly. In the social interaction mediated by language, the speaker and listener take into account not only their knowledge of the lexicon, syntactic rules, and grammar but also what they know about the context, the reciprocal images (points of view) they have of each other, the inferred intention of the speaker, as well as the presuppositions and implicatures of the utterances. This knowledge reduces polysemy and ambiguity, and the interlocutors can infer with more confidence the real meaning of every utterance. Additionally, the interlocutors have to observe conversational rules, such as to respect the turn of each other, to attend to and follow the relevant topic, allowing temporary interruptions for explanations, illustrations, corrections, paraphrases, and digressions, which contribute to the coherence and better understanding of the statement. The interlocutors also have to take into account and to adjust themselves not only to the paralinguistic aspects (gestures, facial emotional expressions, and the like) but also to the linguistic markers of the conversation used by each other, such as those that mark agreement ("ok," "yes," "yeah"), confirmation ("I know," "yes"), disagreement ("no," "but"), checking understanding ("right?", "ok?"), sequencing of narrative ("then," "next"), and beginning or end of a digression (e.g., "by the way" and "to return to the subject," respectively).

Discourse (as in conversation, dialogue) is not a simple communication or transmission of messages, but a negotiation and "effect of senses" between speakers [2, 3].

The relation established between speakers as well as the context of the enunciation is constitutive of the meaning or sense of the utterance. The context may be understood as the immediate situation or circumstances of the enunciation, the here and now of the saying (e.g., a classroom with teacher and pupils), as well as the more detached social-historical and ideological conditions of production of the discourse, which also include the so-called interdiscourse and intertext, that is, the discursive memory of the speaker, his/her argumentative evidences based on what has already been said or written by others. When engaged in discursive social interaction (as in common conversation), the speaker and listener have to handle Pêcheux's "imaginary formations" [2], which are the images or conceptions they have of their own position and of the position of the other, that is, the image the speaker has of himself, the image he has of his listener, and the image he has of the object of discourse and, at the same time, the image the listener has of himself, the image he has of the speaker, and the image he has of the object of discourse (more on this topic in the chapter on "Ontogenetic Perspective").

The subject of the discourse is heterogeneous, divided as a kind of himself-another. According to Benveniste [1], in the discursive use of language (enunciation), the basis of subjectivity, person, and self-consciousness is constructed: "Consciousness of self is only possible if it is experienced by contrast. I use *I* only when I am speaking to someone who will be a *you* in my address. It is this condition of dialogue that is constitutive of *person*, for it implies that reciprocally *I* becomes *you* in the address of the one who in his turn designates himself as *I*." Additionally, in enunciation the subject (represented by the pronoun *I*) becomes temporally divided in himself as the subject (the *I*) who is speaking and whose speaking act is continuously fading away and the subject (the *I*) of the statement (the text) who lives on beyond the *I* who speaks.

5.3 Brain Lesion and the Classical Aphasia Syndromes

Most neuropsychological studies of language have been limited to the phonologic, syntactic, and lexical semantic levels, starting in the nineteenth century with the pioneering contributions of Dax, Broca, and Wernicke [4–6]. Impairment of enunciation and discourse has been less studied, although long ago recognized by Hughlings Jackson [7] and later on partially analyzed and described by Luria [8, 9].

Neurological investigations on the classical aphasia syndromes and their associated lesions have contributed to our knowledge of the cerebral organization of language, especially regarding the left hemisphere dominance, with damage to its anterior regions (particularly left posterior inferior frontal cortex) impairing language fluency and articulation and to its posterior regions (left temporal lobe) causing meaningless speech with poor comprehension, but well articulated.

Aphasia is a linguistic-cognitive syndrome due to a primary language disturbance associated with lesion in the left hemisphere peri-Sylvian sensu stricto "brain language area." It is characterized by difficulties to understand, interpret, and/or produce words, texts, or discourse; production of paraphasias, which can be phonemic (e.g., "papple" for apple or "ragon" for wagon) or semantic (e.g., "table" for chair, "lion" for tiger, or "fruit" for apple); syntactic and grammatical errors; difficulties with naming and finding words during conversation; and the occurrence of these symptoms also in motor-visual (sign) language, as well as in reading and writing. These disturbances characterize what Ardila [10] calls "primary or central" aphasias (typically Broca's and Wernicke's). Language may also be secondarily impaired due to a primary defect of another cognitive function, for instance, a failure of speech ignition or initiation ("speech arrest") by an epileptogenic focus in the supplementary motor area (SMA) or loss of the executive control of voluntary speech production by lesion in the left dorsolateral prefrontal region [11].

Aphasia classification by the Boston Group [12–15] and Luria [8, 9, 16] has been the most adopted (Table 5.1). Boston Group aphasias (Broca's, Wernicke's, global, conduction, anomic, and transcortical) have been more recently considered as vascular syndromes reflecting dysfunction of brain regions supplied by a particular artery [17]. Indeed, cerebrovascular disease is the most common etiology, but there are other causes, such as neoplasia, encephalitis, and neurodegeneration (e.g., primary progressive aphasia), which do not follow vascular territories and can give different aphasia syndromes. On the other hand, Luria's classification takes into account the specific level or basic mechanism that is impaired in language functioning. There are clinical similarities and correspondences between "efferent motor" and "Broca's," "sensory or acoustic-agnosic" and "Wernicke's," "afferent motor" and "conduction," "semantic amnesic" and "anomic," and "dynamic" and "transcortical motor" aphasias (Table 5.1).

Jakobson and Halle [18] and posteriorly Luria [16] proposed a classification of aphasias based on the impairment in one of the two language axes: (1) the paradigmatic axis (similarity or substitution disturbance), with difficulties to select phonemes (as in sensory or Wernicke's aphasia) and words (as in amnesic or anomic aphasia), being mostly difficult for finding specific or coordinate nouns (e.g., dog), which are usually substituted by superordinate nouns ("animal") or circumlocutory explanations ("it barks"), and (2) the syntagmatic axis (contiguity disorder), with inability to combine or sequence words (in efferent motor or Broca's aphasia) and sentences (in dynamic or transcortical motor aphasia).

Table 5.1 Most used classifications of aphasia syndromes

Luria (1966)	Boston Group (Benson 1979)
Motor efferent or kinetic	Broca's
Sensory or acoustic-agnosic	Wernicke's
Motor afferent or kinesthetic	Conduction
Semantic amnesic	Anomic
Dynamic	Transcortical motor
	Transcortical sensory
	Transcortical mixed
	Global

5.3.1 Boston Group Classification of Aphasias

In *Broca's aphasia*, usually caused by vascular lesion in the territory of the superior division of the left middle cerebral artery (MCA), spontaneous speech and repetition is nonfluent, with poor articulation, agrammatic sentence production, but relatively spared comprehension, except for sentences with complex grammatical or syntactic structure.

Wernicke's aphasia is characterized by meaningless spontaneous speech, with jargons and sometimes neologisms (nonwords), and poor repetition and comprehension of words, and the patient is not aware of the errors in the acute phase. The damage is usually an acute cortical-subcortical infarct in the territory of the inferior division of left MCA, in the left posterior superior temporal gyrus (Wernicke's area), which has been classically considered crucial for word and sentence comprehension. However, more recent studies with primary progressive aphasia (PPA) by Mesulam et al. [19] have shown that comprehension of word and sentence is controlled by different brain areas, with single-word comprehension being processed entirely outside of Wernicke's area, in the left anterior temporal lobe, differently from what has classically been found in stroke patients. Most of their patients with atrophy, cortical thinning, or neuronal loss in Wernicke's area had word comprehension completely spared [19]. On the other hand, sentence comprehension was more widespread in the language network, including even left prefrontal and Broca's areas. Mesulam's (2015) explanation is that "stroke destroys not only the cortex in Wernicke's area, but also the underlying fiber pathways that interconnect language centers that work with one another."

Global aphasia (lesion in the whole territory of left MCA), the most severe, is a kind of combination of Broca's and Wernicke's aphasia, sometimes with initial mutism or output limited to a single stereotype (word or nonword). In *conduction aphasia*, (damage to the left supramarginal gyrus and/or deep parietal white matter), spontaneous speech and comprehension are relatively preserved, but repetition is disproportionally impaired, besides presenting phonemic paraphasias. *Transcortical motor aphasia* (TMA) is similar to Broca's aphasia but with preserved repetition and is associated with lesion just anterior and superior to Broca's area due to occlusion of frontal dorsal-lateral division of anterior cerebral artery (ACA) or borderzones ("watershed areas") of ACA and MCA. *Transcortical sensorial aphasia* (TSA) is similar to Wernicke's aphasia, but with intact repetition and less phonemic paraphasias, usually associated with damage to the region posterior to and surrounding Wernicke's area, in the borderzones of the territories of left MCA and posterior cerebral artery (PCA) [17, 20]. *Mixed transcortical aphasia* is a combination of TMA and TSA, associated with a more widespread lesion in the borderzones of MCA and ACA, and MCA and PCA, preserving the language area sensu stricto.

5.3.2 Luria's Classification

In Luria's classification, *efferent (kinetic) motor aphasia* (caused by lesion in areas 44 and 45, or Broca's area, in the inferior part of the left premotor region) is characterized by a disturbance of the commutative processes of excitations and inhibitions of consecutive articulations (syllables or words), due to lack of inhibition of preceding articulations, which is necessary for a smooth transfer from one articulation to the next. The result is a pathological inertia (with perseveration) of one syllable or word, similar to stuttering. In *afferent (kinesthetic) motor aphasia* (by damage of inferior portions of postcentral cortical areas of the left hemisphere), the basic defect is the inability to determine the positions of the lips and tongue necessary for articulation of the required sounds (articulemes), thus affecting particularly sounds with similar articulation, for example, confounding the prepalatolinguals "*l*," "*n*," and "*d*" or the labials "*b*," "*m*," and "*p*". *Sensory aphasia* (by lesion of the secondary zones of the auditory cortex, especially of the posterior third of the left superior temporal gyrus) is a kind of acoustic agnosia specific for speech sounds (preserving the hearing and understanding of nature sounds), due to a failure of the analysis of the sound flow and synthesis of phonemes, being particularly difficult to discriminate similar sounds (phonemes), such as *d-t*, *b-p*, and *s-z*. Acoustic-amnesic aphasia is due to lesion in the middle parts of the left temporal cortex and deep white matter connecting it to the hippocampus (areas 21 and 37), with the basic defect affecting specifically the audioverbal memory, but leaving relatively intact phonemic hearing. The main difficulty is to memorize a short series of phonemes, syllables, or words orally presented, due to an increased mutual inhibition (proactive and retroactive) of audioverbal traces. A similar syndrome is the *amnesic aphasia* (by left inferior parietal-occipital-temporal lesion), characterized by naming difficulties (anomia) in which giving the patient the first syllable of the required name does help him, differently from the acoustic-amnesic and sensory aphasias. In *semantic aphasia* [by left inferior posterior parietal (area 39) or parietal-temporal-occipital lesion], the disturbance impairs not only naming and word finding but also simultaneous quasi-spatial reasoning and synthesis, with difficulties to understand complex logical-grammatical structures (e.g., "the father's brother," "the broder's father," "above," "between," "before") and sentences with embedded relative clauses ("The dog that was chased by the hyena is entering in its burrow now"), besides acalculia (mainly with subtractions, e.g., 41–14), constructive apraxia, and left-right disorientation. *Dynamic aphasia* is similar to TMA (lesion just anterior and superior to Broca's area), with difficulties in recalling verbs, but not in naming objects or repeating words or phrases [21]. The main disturbance is poor speech initiative manifesting as absence of spontaneous expressions by the patient (Kleist's "Spontanstummheit" or "Antriebsmangel der Sprache," "defect of speech initiative") [22], presenting long pauses both before the beginning of a narrative and between subsequent spoken expressions. The basic underlying defect affects the predicative function of inner speech, with disintegration of the linear scheme of the sentence, which is necessary for implementing the general abstract narrative plan [21, 23].

5.4 Brain Lesion and Disorders of Discourse

Discourse has deserved less attention of neuropsychological and neurolinguistic studies. Discursive disorders were analyzed by Luria (1976) and interpreted as disturbances of the sphere of thinking ("discursive intellect") or of nonverbal behavior, since at his time linguistics was restricted to the study of the relation between signs (syntax) or between signs and the world (semantics), leaving aside the relations between signs and their user, between language and its exteriority or conditions of its production (speaker, listener, communicative or interactive situation, and social-historical-ideological context).

In spite of these limitations, Luria contributed to outline some of the most relevant neuropsychological and cognitive processes involved in the discursive intellectual activity applied to problem-solving, which we could extend to the pragmatic-discursive activity in its varied forms, even to an everyday conversation: (1) motivation, intention, and goal(s) of the speaker/listener; (2) investigation of and orientation in the conditions of production and interpretation of discourse; (4) inhibition of impulsive responses, associations, or hypotheses; (5) elaboration of the discourse strategy as well the selection of one among various alternative hypotheses of production and interpretation of the act of enunciation and the statement, in an activity requiring highly dynamic, polysemous, and stochastic moves; (3) selection, comparison, and synthesis of the significant semantic and pragmatic components on the basis of their relevance, given by the goal(s) and the context; and (6) comparison and correction (by the speaker) of the statement, on the basis of the initial intention, goal(s), strategy, and conditions of production of the discourse. Such a complex mental activity would require additionally a stable working memory as well as a high-level executive function and visual-spatial-symbolic reasoning.

Other authors have also studied discourse in brain-damaged patients based on the theoretical constructs of pragmatics and textual linguistics, such as Ulatowska et al. [24] with production of narrative and procedural discourse in aphasics, and Bihrle et al. [25], Brownell et al. [26], Joanette et al. [27], and Gagnon et al. [28], showing the participation of the right hemisphere in the interpretation and production of metaphors, narrative and conversational discourse, as well as indirect requests (pragmatics) and humor (jokes).

In a study of 24 patients with frontal lesions (8 right, 6 left, and 10 bilateral), the majority traumatic, we found discursive-pragmatic disturbances without classic aphasic symptoms or impairment of fluency, naming, repetition, and understanding [29].Those patients with bilateral frontal lesions involving particularly medial-basal regions presented, after the coma, an initial stage with apathy, lack of communicative intention (or mutism), sometimes a dreamlike state, and confused nonsense statements with decontextualized associations, which were irrelevant for the interactional and pragmatic purposes and interfered with the recall and production of the needed semantic elements. Afterward, in the recovery phase, they presented a prolix enunciation characterized by perseveration of complex verbal stereotypes originated from their former experience with the social-occupational use of language. The discourse of some patients caused strangeness in the interlocutor, which could not see coherence in what he/she said, sometimes considering the patient as psychotic. These discursive disorders with lack of coherence were observed mainly when the patient confronted with new or problematic situations, but tended to disappear or not occur when he/she was dealing with habitual tasks that belonged to his/her occupational experience. Luria had already noted similar intellectual-discursive changes in such patients "...when the intellectual operations demanded the creation of a program of actions and the selection of one among various equally probable alternatives" [30].

In our study, these patients had severe discursive-pragmatic changes, with loss of social-interactional schemes, and violation of conversational rules, particularly with disrespect for the turn of the interlocutor and disregard for the relevant topic, besides presenting semantically incoherent statements. The strategy of interpretation and production of the discourse was unstable, and the self-regulation of behavior by means of speech (both own, internal speech, and the other's, external speech) was weakened. In this way, the disorder affected the subject's own social functioning. Our case VB is quite illustrative in this regard.

VB was a 47-year-old lawyer with bilateral frontal traumatic lesion and prolonged coma in October 1987, recovering without motor, sensory, or classic aphasic symptoms, but with social behavioral problems. Neuropsychological and neurolinguistic evaluation (September 1988) showed impulsivity, inattention, disinhibition, increased psychic fatigability, intellectual deficit manifested in problem-solving tests and visual-constructional tasks, and linguistic disturbances restricted to the discursive level. He had difficulties with interpretation of proverbs and the implicated senses, non-observation of topic relevance, deficient epilinguistic (self-corrective) function, and lack of insight for his errors. He was evasive and had difficulties to adapt his language to his interlocutor's reciprocal virtual images (Pêcheux's "imaginary formations"). In a test of logical memory, he was able to fully reproduce the story "The Lion and the Fox" (which says: "The lion had grown old and could no longer hunt game. And so he decided to live by cunning. He lay in his den and pretended to be ill. The wild animals came to see him, but the lion seized and ate every one that came into his den. One day a fox came up to the entrance to his den and asked: "How are you?" "Not so well. Why don't you come inside?" But the fox replied: "I can see footprints. Many animals have gone into your den but none has come out again."). However, when interpreting the moral sense of this story, he produced the text below, whose incoherence contrasted with what was found in statements and texts that were part of his professional repertoire.

"I think that this in reality...reflects a...a condition of life. When someone intends...to do the realization of something in life...he always has that more incoherent sense of everything, is it not so? I think that in this case...even the age brings more reflection...but it is a sense of...organization...in every sense...of elucidation... of what is necessary. Everyone who needs some information, he should not be shy... feigning a position, but always search for someone who can give him all senses...of recovery."

VB's inability to access the culturally crystallized sense of this story is due to the emergence of inappropriate uninhibited associations as well as perseverative reproduction of complex verbal stereotypes, such as "sense," "every sense," "life," "condition of life," and others that were also manifested in the interpretation of the story "The Ant and the Dove" and even during problem-solving and tasks of visual perception of complex thematic figures. The patient did neither recognize his failures nor attempted to correct them. The impairment at the linguistic discursive level of this and other frontal lesion patients (loss of epilinguistic function) is due to a basic defect, that is, the deficit of critical insight and self-correction, "the lack of final comparison of the methods used and results obtained, on the one hand, and the initial question and conditions of the problem, on the other" [31]. This component of the discursive thinking is presupposed but not made explicit in the models of interpretation and production of discourse of other authors as Beaugrande and Dressler [32], van Dijk and Kintsch [33], Bernardez [34], and Charolles [35]. According to van Dijk and Kintsch's model, the interpretation and production of discourse is a strategic process in which the language user takes effective and flexible interpretative steps at different language levels (syntactic, semantic, pragmatic, etc.) and make use of various types of information simultaneously (textual, contextual, scriptal, etc.), besides presupposing the occurrence of errors, misunderstandings, and reinterpretations. Their model lacks the self-correction component for readjusting the plan currently in action with the initial plan or intention as well as with the changing context.

5.5 Conclusion

Language is a cognitive function based on the conscious use of signs (words) for social interaction and representation of the world. It is organized in different interacting levels of abstraction: phonologic-morphologic, syntactic, semantic, and discursive-pragmatic. Discourse (e.g., in common conversation) unfolds as enunciation (the utterance) and statement (the enunciated, the text). Brain lesions, particularly in left peri-Sylvian language areas, may impair any language level, leading to various types of aphasia. Most used aphasia classifications are those of the Boston Group (Broca's, Wernicke's, conduction, anomic, transcortical motor, transcortical sensory, transcortical mixed, and global) and Luria's (motor efferent or kinetic, motor afferent or kinesthetic, sensory or acoustic-agnosic, semantic amnesic, and dynamic). Another classification is based on the impairment of one of the two axes of language: paradigmatic aphasia, a substitution disturbance with difficulties to select phonemes and words, especially for finding specific or coordinate nouns (e.g., "dog"), which are substituted by superordinate nouns ("animal") or circumlocutions ("it barks"), and syntagmatic aphasia, a contiguity disorder, with inability to combine or sequence words and sentences. Discourse functioning requires cognitive processes similar to those involved in problem-solving, such as (1) intention, motivation, and goal(s) of the speaker/listener; (2) orientation in the context of production of the enunciation; (3) inhibition of impulsive moves, associations, or hypotheses; (4) elaboration of a strategy within a highly dynamic, polysemous, and stochastic activity; (5) selection and comparison of the semantic elements on the basis of their relevance for the given goal and context; and (6) correction (by the speaker) of the statement taking into account intention, goal, strategy, and context. Discourse disorders may be manifested in the production of narratives and metaphors, presenting semantically incoherent statements as well as disrespect for conversational rules, particularly for the turn of the interlocutor and for Grice's rules of mode and topic relevance. Language disorders restricted to the level of discourse (discursive aphasia) may be observed in cases with frontal, right hemisphere, and diffuse or multifocal causing mental confusion or dementia.

References

1. Benveniste E (1966) Problèmes de linguistique générale. N. R. F., Bibliothèque des sciences humaines, Paris
2. Pêcheux M (1969) Analyse automatique du discours. Dunod, Paris
3. Orlandi E (1996) A linguagem e seu funcionamento: as formas do discurso. Campinas, SP, Pontes
4. Dax M (1863) Soumet au jugement de l'Académie un Mémoire intitulé: 'Observations tendant à prouver la coïncidence constante des dérangements de la parole avec une lésion de l'hémisphère gauche du cerveau'. Compt rend hebdom séan l'Acad Scien 56:536
5. Broca P (1861) Remarques sur le siège de la faculté du langage articulé, suivies dúne observation dáphemie. Bull Soc Anat Paris 2:330–357
6. Wernicke C (1874) Das Aphasiche Symptomkomplex. Breslau, Cohn and Weigart
7. Jackson JH (1958) Selected writings of John Hughlings Jackson. Basic Books, New York
8. Luria AR (1947/1970) Traumatic Aphasia. Mouton, The Hague
9. Luria AR (1976) Basic problems of neurolinguistics. Mouton, The Hague
10. Ardila A (2010) A proposed reinterpretation and reclassification of aphasic syndromes. Aphasiology 24(3):363–394
11. Ardila A (2014) Aphasia handbook. Florida International University, Miami
12. Geschwind N (1965) Disconnexion syndromes in animals and man. Brain 88:237–294. 585–644
13. Benson DF (1979) Aphasia, alexia, and agraphia. Churchill Livingstone, New York
14. Goodglass H, Kaplan E (1972) The assessment of aphasia and related disorders. Lea and Febiger, Philadelphia
15. Alexander MP, Benson DF (1992) The aphasias and related disturbances. In: Joynt RJ (ed) Clinical neurology. Lippincott, Philadelphia
16. Luria AR (1966/1980) Higher cortical functions in man, 2nd edn. Basic Books, New York
17. Hillis AE (2007) Aphasia: progress in the last quarter of a century. Neurology 69:200–213
18. Jakobson R, Halle M (1956) Fundamentals of language. Mouton, The Hague
19. Mesulam MM, Thompson CK, Weintraub S, Rogalski EJ (2015) The Wernicke conundrum and the anatomy of language comprehension in primary progressive aphasia. Brain 138(8):2423–2437
20. Alexander MP, Hiltbrunner B, Fischer RS (1989) Distributed anatomy of transcortical sensory aphasia. Arch Neurol 46(8):885–892
21. Luria AR, Tsvetkova LS (1968) The mechanism of 'dynamic aphasia'. Found Lang 4(3):296–307

22. Kleist K (1934) Gehirnpathologie. Barth, Leipzig
23. Vygotsky LS (1934/1982) Psychology and the theory of localization of psychic functions. In: Vygotsky LS (ed) Sobranie sochinenij. Tom 1. Voprosy teorii i istorii psikhologii. Pedagogika, Moscow (in Russian)
24. Ulatowska HK, North AJ, Macaluso-Haynes SM (1981) Production of narrative and procedural discourse in aphasia. Brain Lang 13:345–371
25. Bihrle AM, Brownell HH, Powelson JA, Gardner H (1986) Comprehension of humorous and non-humorous materials by left and right brain-damaged patients. Brain Cogn 5:399–411
26. Brownell HH, Simpson TL, Bihrle AM, Potter HH, Gardner H (1990) Appreciation of metaphoric alternative word meanings by left and right brain-damaged patients. Neuropsychologia 28(4):375–383
27. Joanette Y, Goulet P (1990) Narrative discourse in right-brain-damaged right-handers. In: Joanette Y, Brownell HH (eds) Discourse ability and brain damage – theoretical and empirical perspectives. Springer, New York, pp 131–153
28. Gagnon L, Goulet P, Giroux F, Joanette Y (2003) Processing of metaphoric and non-metaphoric alternative meanings of words after right- and left-hemispheric lesion. Brain Lang 87(2):217–226
29. Damasceno BP (1990) Neuropsychology of discursive activity and its disturbances. In: Cadernos de Estudos Linguísticos, vol 19, pp 147–157
30. Luria AR (1969) Frontal lobe syndromes. In: Vinken PJ, Bruyn GW (eds) Handbook of clinical neurology, vol 2. North-Holland, Amsterdam, pp 725–757
31. Luria AR (1973) The working brain: an introduction to neuropsychology. Basic Books, New York
32. de Beaugrande R, Dressler W (1981) Introduction to text linguistics. Longman, London
33. Van Dijk TA, Kintsch W (1983) Strategies of discourse comprehension. Academic Press, New York
34. Bernardez E (1982) Introdución a la linguistica del texto. Espasa Calpe, Madrid
35. Charolles M (1983) Coherence as a principle in the interpretation of discourse. Text 3:71–97

Chapter 6
Cognition as a Mediated, Self-Organized, and Dynamic Activity

6.1 Introduction

Cognition can be conceived as established knowledge registered in books, papers, and electronics, or as the process of acquiring knowledge and understanding about the world. This process is a complex, mediated, and dynamic mental activity functionally comprising sensation, perception, concept formation, language, and intellectual reasoning, as well as their corresponding brain networks. It is mediated by signs of language (words, symbols) for representing concepts about things, actions, relations, and ideas, which are learned (appropriated) by the individual in joint external activity with persons. Cognition is a self-organizing and dynamic neurofunctional system, seeing that it is self-sufficient, its own reason of existence, having its psychological structure determined by the way its components (mental operations) interact with each other as well as with the external conditions constituted by other neighboring systems; and it is dynamic to the extent that its mental operations and respective brain networks change from moment to moment as each action or operation goes on reversibly replacing one with another.

6.2 The Mediated Character of Cognition

The mediated character of the human mind is manifested in the fact that the individual relates himself with external things and phenomena not directly and immediately but indirectly, via sensations, that is, with the signals and signs that represent these things and phenomena. As seen by an external observer, it is evident that the bodily actions of the individual upon outside objects are direct, since he is just one among various other material things and forces which participate in his activity, but the individual's material actions are preceded and controlled by mental actions, images, symbolic representations, projects, and programs, which are kept online for

B. Damasceno, *Research on Cognition Disorders*,
https://doi.org/10.1007/978-3-030-57267-9_6

coordination, monitoring, and verification of the material actions involved in the activity and its results. The activity as a whole is, thus, unrolled in a mental and a material level.

During the development of the mind, from sensation to perception to thinking, the signals and signs become more and more generalized and abstracts, and in this way the individual mentally detaches himself more and more from the external reality at the same time that his unity with it becomes stronger [1]. The individual becomes able to reflect more and more perfectly the external reality as he evolves from the simple sensation of an isolated external stimulus to the perception of a whole object or situation and then to thinking, when he becomes able to recognize the mutual connections and relations of his own being. With the acquisition of the mind, the individual frees himself from his immediate natural environment and spreads the network of his being to an ever larger and deeper reality, which can then be creatively transformed by him to the extent that he knows its properties, interrelations, and laws.

6.3 Cognition as a Self-Organized Functional System

The term "system" may be conceived as a self-organizing and dynamic set of various components with their internal and external interactions and whose structure is determined by the way how their components interact with each other and are interconnected and integrated. Self-organizing systems are their own reason and cause of existence, being influenced by both their inner conditions and the boundary conditions from their environment constituted by neighboring external system(s). This concept can be applied to all forms of organization of matter, from the physical-chemical to the biological, social, and psychological level. According to Christian Fuchs [2], based on Friedrich Engels materialist dialectics [3], self-organizing systems produce themselves and have the following main characteristics: (1) *complexity*, which depends on the number of its elements and the connections between them, constituting a structure organized in a distributed manner; (2) *information production and exchange*; (3) *emergence of order*, with new qualities of the system emerging in critical phases of its evolution; and (4) *hierarchy*, with the emergent level being hierarchically higher and having new qualities that are not found in the lower levels or in any of the components, that is, the system as a whole is more than the sum of its parts. As illustrated, in a certain stage of the evolution of our planet, two hydrogen (H) atoms combined with one oxygen (O) to form a system – the water molecule (H2O), with new emergent properties different from those of its constituting elements (H, O) but resulting from the synergical interactions between these elements. Here, the term "synergical," as understood by Corning [4], refers in general to the combined or cooperative effects produced by things (parts, elements, or individuals) that operate together.

Here we apply these concepts to the analysis of the human mind. Any mental task (e.g., perceiving an object, understanding a discourse, or solving a problem) is carried out by a "complex functional system" [5, 6], which has also been conceived of as "neurofunctional network" [7], "distributed parallel processing" [8], or "multiple drafts model" [9]. This insight on the structure of mental functions was first articulated by Hughlings Jackson by conceiving them as organized in different levels of complexity and abstraction (the voluntary, conscious; and the involuntary, automatic, unconscious) [10].

The neurofunctional system comprises various basic operations (processes) organized in an assembly of interconnected brain regions, each region giving its specific contribution to the functioning of the system as a whole. As conceived of by Gazzaniga et al. [11], mental operations involve taking a representation as an input, performing some sort of process on the input, and then producing a new representation or output. Thus, mental operations are processes that generate, elaborate upon, or manipulate mental representations. The more abstract Piagetian formal operations [12] consist in dealing with concepts and ideas in a reversible and transitive way, as occurs, for example, when thinking deductively (e.g., "All metals are good conductors of heat. Titanium is a metal. Therefore, titanium is a good conductor of heat.") or solving the problem "If Antony is taller than John but shorter than Joe, who is the shortest?".

6.4 Cognition Conceived as a Kind of Activity

The neurofunctional system can be conceived of as both the psychic (abstract, virtual) and the cerebral (bodily) form of a real external activity (e.g., productive labor), with which it constitutes a functional unity. Leontyev [13, 14] termed this tripartite unity as "activity" for emphasizing the primary role of the real external activity in connecting the organism with its environment and in determining the development of mind, consciousness, and its components. This concept of activity was elaborated by Soviet psychologists following Vygotsky's earlier foundational works, particularly by Leontiev and his contemporary colleague Rubinstein [15], on the basis of Marx [16] and Engel's [3] thesis that human consciousness emerges in the dialectical interaction between man and nature, subject, and object, in which both are creatively molded. In the same line of reasoning, Bakhtin [17] had expressed that the psychic activity constitutes a semiotic expression of the contact between the individual and its external environment, which is understood as comprising other interacting individuals.

In his analysis of the psychological structure of the activity, Leontiev elaborated the concepts of "activity," "action," and "operation." As reminded by Wertsch [18], Soviet psychologists' conception of "structure of an activity" refers to its subunits defined on the basis of the function they fulfill rather than of any intrinsic properties they possess and should then not be confounded with a Western structuralist approach.

"Activity" is the whole set of tasks, for example, those of productive labor, which accomplish a vitally or socially relevant activity in the real external world in order to satisfy some need of the subject, and has as distinctive characteristic the coincidence of its motive (motivation, need, desire to achieve a result) with its objective (the object that satisfy that need or motivation). An activity comprises sequences of actions and operations. "Actions" are the intermediary conscious acts or processes subordinated to the consciously represented final result or objective. "Operations" are the methods and skills, usually habituated and automatized, used for performing an action.

The main elements of a human activity are both its objective and its motive. Its motive is understood not only as internal emotion, feeling, or the subject's need for something but particularly as an objectified need, that is, as an object that drives the subject to the action. Other essential characteristics are the desires, emotions, and feelings linked with the object, course, and result of the activity.

Any activity comprises a series of subordinate actions, each with their intermediary partial goals, sequentially and strategically organized on the basis of cause-effect relationships. The motive of each action, which gives sense to it, is that of the activity as a whole, linked to the final objective. Thus, the motive of every action does not coincide with its partial objective, which is to accomplish only part of the whole process that leads to the wished result. Illustratively, Leontiev applied these concepts to analyze the structure of the individual's activity in collective labor, for example, the collective hunting of mammoths in prehistorical times (Fig. 6.1).

A member of the hunting group, for instance, a beater, is motivated to participate due to his need for food or clothing, which could be furnished by the meat and skin of the dead animal. The specific procedure of the beater is to frighten the animal and drive it toward other hunters, namely, the killers. The frightening of the prey, pushing away something that would satisfy a vital need, is in itself biologically a nonsense but gets its sense for the individual beater and becomes possible only within a

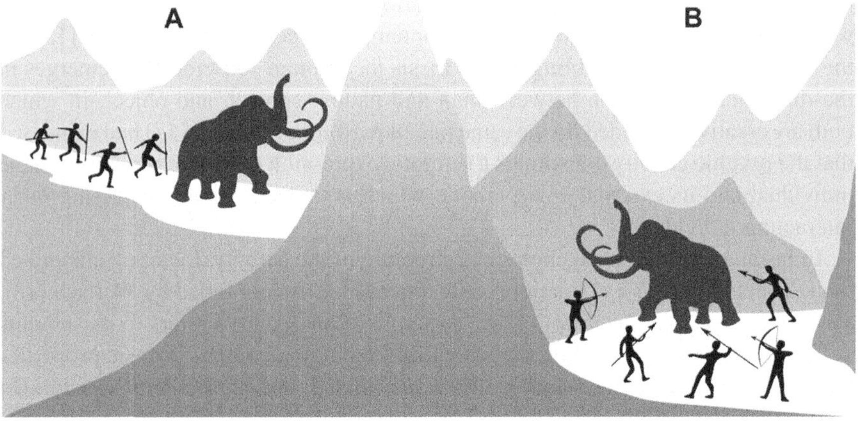

Fig. 6.1 Hunting collaborative labor. In (**a**), the beaters frighten the prey, driving it away toward the killers hidden in ambush down in the mountain gorge, in (**b**)

collective activity whose final product is distributed to the beaters, in this way satisfying their needs. The action of the beater, whose partial objective is to frighten the prey, does not coincide with his real motive. Therefore, for Leontiev, the hunting is the beater's "activity" and the frightening of the prey, his "action."

As a component of the psychological structure of the activity, "action" is a mental construct; it is an ideal action which operates with sensory-perceptive or conceptual images of its object and is consciously executed by the subject and cannot be reduced to (or confounded with) the external motor actions or movements performed with the object. There are movements without actions (e.g., the movements of innate reflexes) as there are actions without movements, for example, the mental actions of the immobile sentry guard at the entrance of the palace, which are necessary for inhibiting any movement and keeping him as a motionless statue.

These concepts may be illustrated with activities using tools and material objects. Consider, for example, the learning of car driving. The subject's objective is to become a skilful professional driver in order to obtain a driver's license and get a job. In the initial learning phase, the subject follows his tutor's verbal and nonverbal instructions at the same time that he interacts with the corresponding instruments and parts of the vehicle, executing consciously and in detail every act, such as looking at the rearview mirror and speedometer; stepping on the accelerator, brake, and clutch; paying attention to the sound of the motor; and manipulating the steering wheel and gears. In this phase of learning, each movement or procedure is a conscious action whose sense is given by the final objective of the whole activity, namely, to become a skilful driver, which in its turn will satisfy the motivation (motive) of obtaining a driver's license for getting an employment afterward. Social motivations are also implicated here, particularly the need to drive correctly, respecting traffic rules as well as the law and principles of moral, in order to get good reputation. Afterward, when the individual already masters completely the act of driving, his various actions have become more agile, automatic, and partially subconscious and converted into operations, which all together constitute the habit of driving. As pointed out by Rubinstein [1], when the subject's actions are converted into operations and habituated, the focus of his consciousness can be freed from the regulation of relatively elementary acts and be allocated to the solution of complex problems, for example, to the discussion of financial subjects with his tutor sitting beside him, but this change of the focus of consciousness does not exclude the possibility of the individual to consciously control the execution of the automatized act.

Later on, when the individual is employed in a company and works as traveling salesman, selling and distributing sodas to bars and grocery stores, the act of driving is no more an aim in itself but a means or habitual operation integrated in a more complex activity whose objective and motivation is, for the company, to increase its capital, and for the employee, to accumulate a reserve fund in order to buy a house for his family.

According to Rubinstein [1], automatization occurs with learning not only of motor actions but also of all other acts, methods, and procedures, including mental operations, which in the beginning are consciously elaborated and then, through exercise and training, become improved, automatic, and fixed in semantic and procedural memory, as occur with schemes and formulas used in solution of mathematical problems.

6.5 The Dynamic Structure of the Mental Activity

Every mental act (e.g., object perception, narrative production, decision-making, problem-solving) is dynamic regarding its psychological structure and cerebral organization, which change from moment to moment as each action or operation goes on replacing one with another, in a reversible and transitive way (transitivity here is understood as a kind of relation between magnitudes such that if one magnitude is equal to a second and this second is equal to a third, then the first magnitude is also equal to the third one). As suggested by Kiverstein and Miller [19], following arguments developed in Pessoa [20], "psychological function is better understood at the level of the whole brain-body-environment system" and "structure-function mappings are not fixed and static properties of networks; instead, structure-function relationships are dynamic, with the functions a given network performs varying over time in a highly flexible and context-dependent manner." As illustrated, consider the solution of the following problem presented orally to a subject: "Anthony has 11 horses and Mary has 6 horses less than he has. How many horses do they have together?" The solution of this problem requires various mental operations processed both sequentially and simultaneously, reversibly, in an assembly of brain regions crucial for their execution (Fig. 6.2): (1) processing of sounds in the auditory pathways and primary cortical area (Heschel's gyri); (2) extraction and synthesis of phonemes and words in adjacent secondary cortical auditory area of the dominant hemisphere; (3) semantic analysis with decoding of meaning of words, sentences, and logical-grammatical relationships (as "less than") (posterior and anterior tertiary multimodal cortical areas); (4) symbolic-spatial reasoning (subtracting 11 minus 6) (mainly inferior parietal cortex); (5) orientation in (and analysis of) the data and the final question (goal) of the problem, which are maintained in working memory; hypothesis testing; monitoring the solution and verifying the obtained final result, deciding whether or not it is in accordance with the data and the final question of the problem (prefrontal regions).

The whole process is both serial and parallel, since any one of these operations may require several neuron groups and pathways for dealing with the same information or its subtypes. In the problem presented above, consider just the understanding of the word "horse." A word comprises a network of phonological, morphological, semantic, and discursive-pragmatic relations. "A word designates a certain object, but at the same time it includes the object in a system of connections..." [21]. As regards the word "horse," as analyzed by Hillis [22], there must be (1) the construction of a phonological percept of it (/h/ /or/ /s/) and (2) the access to the meaning of horse by activating its visual percept and semantic representation, which consists in a complex co-activation of all the relevant features of the object (visual, motion, eat hay, neigh, can wear saddles, humans ride horses, etc.), including category

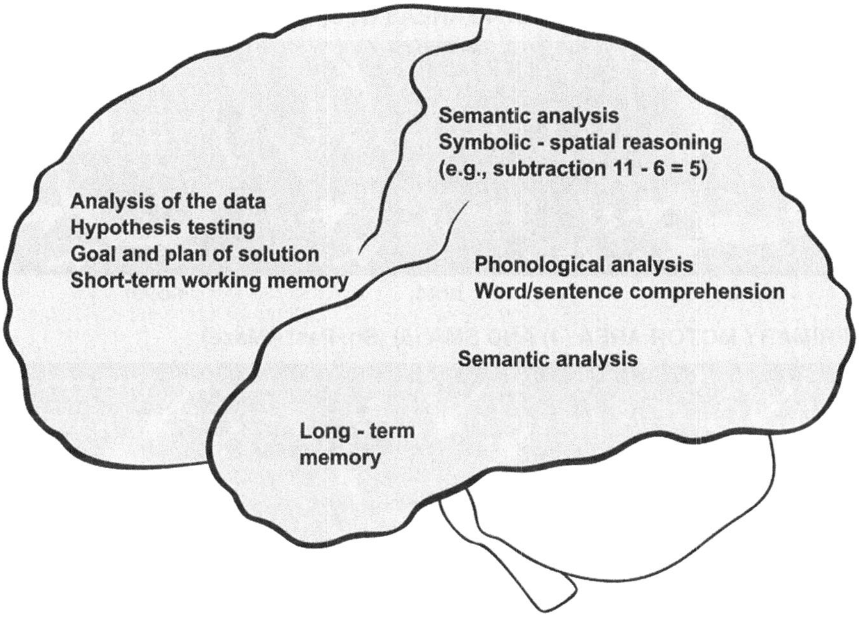

Fig. 6.2 Ensemble of most relevant mental operations and correlated crucial brain regions involved in the arithmetical problem-solving

membership (animate being, animal), all of these features bound together via a synchronized 30 Hz gamma rhythm neuronal firing in interconnected cortical regions, mediated by the thalamus [23].

The objective of an activity and its intended results have to be kept constant for a need to be fulfilled, while its actions and operations may vary depending on the concrete conditions or circumstances in which the object (objective) is situated [24]. The ensemble of chosen cognitive actions and operations, besides the motivational, volitional, and emotional components involved, constitute a highly dynamic and plastic functional system. This plasticity also occurs during the acquisition of any new ability, for example, car driving. The initial learning phase requires numerous mental components (visual-spatial, auditory, and motor-proprioceptive perception; attention; working memory) and various brain regions (sensory-perceptive, prefrontal, premotor, posterior parietal, basal ganglia, and others). Later on, when skilful mastery is achieved, the execution of the task becomes automatic, partly unconscious, as a kind of implicit knowledge (procedural memory) which then involves fewer brain regions (premotor, primary motor, parietal, and basal ganglia circuit). Such brain changes have been found in functional neuroimaging studies, as shown, for example, in a PET study by Petersen and van Mier [25] during maze learning (Fig. 6.3). Thus, the structure of the activity, initially expanded and made up of numerous essential aids (operations, actions, methods, instruments), becomes afterward condensed and converted into an automatic sensory-motor skill.

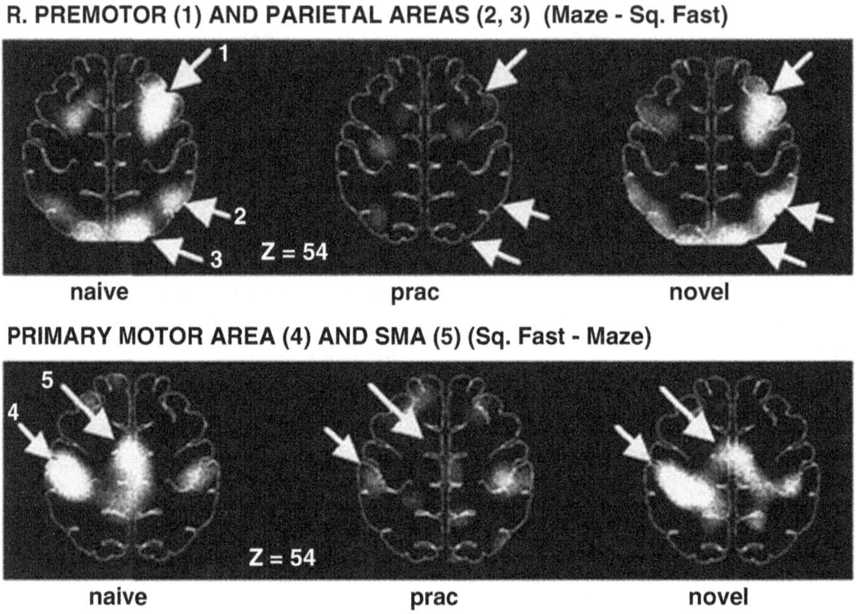

Fig. 6.3 PET difference (subtraction) images showing areas of increased (upper images) and decreased (lower images) blood flow when maze tracing (under naive, practiced, and novel conditions) is compared with fast square tracing. During naive (left images) and novel (right images) maze tracing, increased blood flow in right premotor and parietal areas was found compared with square tracing, whereas decreased blood flow was observed in primary and supplementary motor cortex. The center images show that blood flow in these areas changed to a level almost identical to that found during simple square tracing after the maze was practiced. A linear gray scale is used, with white representing maximal activation and black, minimal activation. The brain outlines were traced from the stereotaxic atlas of Talairach and Tournoux [26] and represent a transverse section 54 mm above the AC-PC line. (From Petersen et al. [25], with permission)

6.6 Conclusion

Cognition, the act of knowing the world, is mediated by signs that represent concepts about things, phenomena, actions, and relations. It comprises a complex, self-organizing, and dynamic system constituted by various mental functions such as perception, language, memory, intellectual-executive reasoning, and their respective brain networks. Its self-organization refers to the cooperative effects produced by its constitutive mental functions (and their corresponding cerebral networks) that operate together, many of them at an unconscious level. So, cognition is not an isolated a priori faculty but a kind of complex psychic, abstract activity interconnected with its two counterparts: the bodily (cerebral) functioning and the external practice in the world. As an activity, its psychological structure comprises the "activity" itself (e.g., productive labor), constituted by the whole set of tasks (actions and operations) that lead to satisfying some need; the "actions", which are ideal actions, that is, intermediary conscious acts subordinated to the consciously represented final objective, and "operations," the methods and skills, usually habituated and automatized, used for performing each action. Besides the objective, this psychological structure also includes the motive, understood not only as an internal feeling or the subject's need for something but as an objectified need (i.e., the object that drives the subject to action). In every mental act (e.g., problem-solving) the objective, the goal (e.g., the problem's final question), is kept constant for a need to be fulfilled, but the ensemble of chosen cognitive actions and operations is highly dynamic, changing from moment to moment as each action and operation go on replacing one with another in a reversible and transitive way.

References

1. Rubinstein SL (1972) Princípios de Psicologia Geral, 2nd edn. Estampa Editorial, Lisbon (translated from the original title in Russian: Osnovy Obschei Psijologuii)
2. Fuchs C. (2001) Dialectical philosophy and self-organization. In: Arshinov V, Fuchs C (eds) Causality, emergence, self-organization. International INTAS research project "Human Strategies in Complexity. Philosophical Foundations for a Theory of Evolutionary Systems". http://www.self-organization.org
3. Engels F (1976) Dialectics of nature. Progress Publishers, Moscow; original: *Dialektik der Natur*, 1886
4. Corning PA (1998) The synergism hypothesis. J Soc Evol Syst 21(2):133–172
5. Vygotsky LS (1934/1982) Psychology and the theory of localization of psychic functions. In: Vygotsky LS (ed) Sobranie sochinenij. Tom 1. Voprosy teorii i istorii psikhologii. Pedagogika, Moscow (in Russian)
6. Anokhin PK (1935). Problems of center and periphery in the physiology of nervous activity. Gozizdat, Gorki (in Russian)
7. Mesulam MM (1990) Large-scale neurocognitive networks and distributed processing for attention, language, and memory. Ann Neurol 28:597–613
8. Rummelhart DE, McClelland JL (1986) Parallel distributed processing: explorations in the microstructure of cognition. MIT Press, Cambridge, MA
9. Dennet DC (1991) Consciousness explained. Little, Brown and Co, Boston
10. Jackson JH (1958) On the nature of the duality of the brain. In: Selected writings of John Hughlings Jackson. Basic Books, New York
11. Gazzaniga MS, Ivry RB, Mangun GR (1998) Cognitive neuroscience: the biology of mind. W. W. Norton and Co, New York
12. Piaget J, Inhelder B (1958) The growth of logical thinking from childhood to adolescence. Basic Books, New York
13. Leontiev AN (1981a) Problems of the development of the mind. Progress Publishers, Moscow
14. Leontiev AN (1981b) The problem of activity in psychology. In: Wertsch JV (ed) The concept of activity in soviet psychology. M. E. Sharpe, New York
15. Rubinstein SL (1957) Being and consciousness (Bytie i soznanie). AN SSSR, Moscow
16. Marx K, Engels F (1976) The German ideology (1845–1846). Progress Publishers, Moscow
17. Bakhtin M (1929/1986) In: Voloshinov VN (ed) Marxism and the philosophy of language. Harvard University Press, Cambridge, MA
18. Wertsch JV (ed) (1981) The concept of activity in soviet psychology. M. E. Sharpe, New York
19. Kiverstein J, Miller M (2015) The embodied brain: towards a radical embodied cognitive neuroscience. Front Hum Neurosci, published 06 May 2015 9, article 237. https://doi.org/10.3389/fnhum.2015.00237

20. Pessoa L (2014) Understanding brain networks and brain organization. Phys Life Rev 11:400–435. https://doi.org/10.1016/j.plrev.2014.03.005
21. Luria AR (1973) Towards the mechanisms of naming disturbance. Neuropsychologia 11(4):417–421
22. Hillis AE (2007) Aphasia: progress in the last quarter of a century. Neurology 69:200–213
23. Hart J, Kraut M (2007) Neural hybrid model of semantic object memory. In: Hart J, Kraut M (eds) Neural basis of semantic memory. Cambridge University Press, New York
24. Luria AR (1973) The working brain: an introduction to neuropsychology. Penguin Books, London
25. Petersen SE, van Mier H, Fiez JA, Raichle ME (1998) The effects of practice on the functional anatomy of task performance. Proc Natl Acad Sci U S A 95:853–860
26. Talairach J, Tournoux P (1988) Co-planar stereotaxic atlas of the human brain. Thieme, New York

Part II
Historical-Cultural Origin of Cognition

Chapter 7
Evolutionary Perspective

7.1 Introduction

As with all things and phenomena, mind and cognition are better understood if we know their interrelatedness and temporal dimension, their origin, phylogenetic, ontogenetic, and historical-cultural development. Human cognition is conceived as the product of a long biological and social-cultural evolution starting with *sensation* and elementary forms of reactions to isolated properties of external objects, as seen even in unicellular organisms – the unconditioned and conditioned reflexes. Then, in the *perceptive* stage, associated with the development of the cerebral cortex, the animal detects the object as a whole (its abstract percept or image) as well as its context. In the *intellectual* stage, related to the development of the associative neocortex, the individual perceives things and their interrelationships and is able to solve problems and achieve goals by operating with and changing the conditions in which the goal (target object) is situated. Further on, in the stage of *self-consciousness*, accompanied by the development of a large-scale network engaging the associative prefrontal neocortex, temporal-parietal junction, and interconnected midline structures (the hippocampus, cingulate gyri, precuneus), the subject becomes aware of itself as detached from its own activity, as separated from itself as agent of this activity.

7.2 The Mind as the Product of a Biological and Social-Cultural Evolution

The human mental functions are product of a long biological and social evolution. The ability to detect and react to external stimuli is an essential property of all living organisms, having high adaptive value. According to Leontiev [1], its most primitive and elementary form is the irritability and tropism observed already in unicellular

B. Damasceno, *Research on Cognition Disorders*,
https://doi.org/10.1007/978-3-030-57267-9_7

organisms able to react to physical and chemical stimuli originated directly from external objects or phenomena which satisfy some need of these organisms or threaten their life. The so-called unconditioned or innate reflexes of multicellular organisms are of same nature. Departing from this level, organisms develop other more complex (psychic) forms of assimilation, reaction, and accommodation to the external world, becoming able to detect stimuli which are not directly linked to the vitally relevant objects, phenomena, or their properties but are temporally and/or spatially connected to them and signal their immediate presence. In the evolution of life, the main condition for sensation to arise in animals was their transition from a homogeneous (aquatic) medium to one formed of things (discrete objects): "the environment shaped as things operate (for the organism) not only by their properties capable of exerting some biological effect on it (e.g., as foodstuff substances), but also by those properties stably associated with them (the same foodstuff's form, color, etc.) which, though biologically neutral, at the same time objectively mediate the formed substance's properties essential for (the organism's) life", and in this way, "the capacity for sensation is genetically nothing other than irritability in relation to that kind of environmental influence that...orients it in the environment by performing a signaling function." [1]. Thus, sensation constitutes the first stage of psychic development, differing from irritability in that the now irritable qualities of external things are of no direct metabolic importance. The origin, first of receptors for chemical substances and, then, of visual and auditory sense organs constitute a decisive landmark in this process. The external reality is given to us by our sensations (visual, auditory, tactile, olfactory, gustatory, vibratory), but even at this level, the external, physical, and chemical stimuli are transduced in the sensory cells receptors and transformed into electric action potentials whose frequency and rhythm codify (as *signals*) the information we need to construct an abstract "virtual" reality, with which we can operate before starting to act and dwell with external real things for our survival.

The psychic phenomenon emerges with the conditioned reflexes, when the organism starts reacting to a stimulus which doesn't originate from and, in itself, has nothing to do with the vitally important external object or phenomenon but usually comes before and, therefore, announces its immediate occurrence, for example, when the dog salivates after hearing the sound of its owner opening the door (conditioned stimulus or "signal"), even before the food touches directly its mouth and stimulates taste receptors (innate, unconditioned stimulus).

Nature is rich in sequential and recurrent phenomena, with one of them signaling the occurrence of the other. The origin of mind and of life itself was conditioned by the temporal structure of the world in which we live, constituted by sequences of phenomena recurring rhythmically with the same components (day-night; cloud-lightning-thunder-rain; spring-summer-autumn-winter) [2]. From nature's signals (Pavlov's "first system of signals") on which the conditioned reflexes are based, to human linguistic signs ("second system of signals") that made possible more complex forms of mind and consciousness, there exist a huge distance and profound qualitative difference, but their essence is the same: both the first and second type of signals are, in themselves, not part of the object that is vitally important to the individual, but they announce, indicate, represent, and signify it. The psychic activity is thus mediated by internal, mental actions with signals or signs representative of real external things and phenomena, their properties, qualities, and interrelations, as well as the tacitly included (inter)actions of the subject with them.

A distinction between signal and sign is that the first is immediately interpreted by the organism ("interpreter") as actions to be performed, being chosen according to their usefulness, and the second, as concepts that are evaluated as true or false, not logically but pragmatically, and also on the basis of self-interest or usefulness [3, 4]. The whole set of signals and signs sensed, perceived, and acted upon by an organism constitute what Uexküll [5] called Umwelt ("environment," in German), understood as not just a set of any external objects but rather a system of signs meaning food, shelter, enemy, or anything vitally important from the point of view of the interpreter. According to Sass [6], based on Gibson [7], "we see the world primarily in terms of *affordances*, for instance, whether an object allows for (affords) walking on or jumping over; that is, in terms of self-affection, in accordance with our needs and wishes, thereby giving objects their significance for us as obstacles, tools, objects of desire, and the like."

7.3 Stages of the Phylogenetic Development of the Mind

According to Leontiev [1], the evolution of the mind in our planet has presented four main stages: elementary sensorial, perceptive, intellectual, and self-consciousness. This classification is not to be interpreted as a deterministic view of evolution occurring in a linear progression (*scala naturae*), from single-cell organisms extending ever upward to humans. It is compatible with the modern tree-like view of evolution, with new species evolving from older ancestral forms and showing a convergent adaptive development of cognition, not only in primates (monkeys, apes, and humans) but also in other vertebrates and even invertebrates.

In the *elementary sensory* stage, the individual (animal) reacts to one or more isolated stimuli from the external object, which is not perceived in its entirety. It occurs in invertebrates (worms, crustaceans, insects), for example, in a spider, when it reacts to the vibrations of an insect (or the experimenter's tuning fork) in its web. In this case, the biological meaning of the vibratory stimuli is food. What characterizes this stage is the animal's ability to "represent and react to some property (elementary stimulus) of the thing or phenomenon that affect the animal but which does not coincide with the properties that the animal's life directly depends on." More complex forms of representation and reaction may arise in this stage, with chains of reactions to isolated successive agents (as in the case of the ant lion in its funnel-shaped sand hole) and establishment of conditioned reflexes or instinctive behavior.

In the *perceptive* stage, the animal reflects the relations between the stimuli of the thing that constitutes the object of its activity (perception of forms) and the stimuli of other things that constitute the conditions or context in which that thing is situated. Here the animal creates and memorizes images of things and acquires the capacity to analyze and generalize information from the external environment, for example, with differentiation and generalization of different sounds that have same biological meaning for the animal. This perceptive stage became possible with the development of the cerebral cortex in our amphibious and reptiles ancestors, associated to the passage from the aquatic to the terrestrial life, that is, to a more unstable and changeable environment. Survival in such a milieu required the development of sense organs for detecting distant objects (olfaction, vision, audition) as well as of conditioned reflexes (even in chains) for predicting future events and acting beforehand accordingly.

The evolution of sensory-perceptive (visual, auditory) and sensory-motor cortex in primates is characterized by the relative reduction of the so-called "primary" or "projection" cortical areas (e.g., Brodmann´s area 17 for vision, and area 4 for motor function) and increase of "secondary" and "tertiary" areas (e.g., areas 18 and 19 for visual perception, and areas 6 and 8 for movement), as well as the increase of thickness of cortical layers II and III of association areas [8]. These two cell layers establish intercortical connections underlying simultaneous synthesis and generalization of information needed for construction of percepts and concepts and for elaboration of complex plans.

In the stage of *intellect*, the animal is able (a) to perceive not only things and phenomena but also their interrelationships; (b) to solve problems by operating with the elements of the conditions in which the goal or target object is situated, by changing and reorganizing these conditions (preparatory phase) in order to reach the goal (accomplishment phase) and satisfy biological or social needs; and (c) to quickly transfer to new problematic conditions the scheme of resolution successfully found for previous similar conditions. In this stage, the animal can generalize relations between natural phenomena, including relations with and between other animals, besides being able to memorize situations. This stage is typical of primates but arises already in superior mammals, related to the development of associative neocortex and its intra- and interhemispheric connections via corpus callosum, particularly in frontal regions. However, other animals without associative neocortex or corpus callosum, for example, corvids and octopuses, show problem-solving abilities superior to that of many mammals.

Other animals, from insects to primates, use objects as tools ("hammer," "anvil", "weapon," "bait"), but only anthropoid apes are able to understand cause-effect relationships which guide the use of objects as tools for solving problems, what suggests they have a symbolic representation of these objects [9]. Chimpanzees appear to have a mental representation of what would be the most appropriate instrument for determined task, at times producing it far away from the local of using it. Kanzi, a bonobo chimpanzee raised in captivity, learned to produce (without previous instruction or demonstration) cutting stone instruments similar to those of our hominid ancestors that lived in Olduvai (Africa) 1.5 million years ago [10].

Self-Consciousness Here, for the first time in the history of mind, the subject becomes conscious of itself and detaches itself mentally from its own activity, from itself as agent of this activity, which is now a process of reciprocal transformation of subject in object and vice versa. Accordingly, in this activity, especially in the productive collective labor, the object of the activity turns into its subjective form (mental image), and the subject's mental activity is converted into its objective outcomes or products (here the word "objective" means "being external, having independent existence apart from sensation, experience or thought").

Collective labor (e.g., hunting of big animals) offered appropriate conditions for emergence of self-consciousness in humans. As mentioned before regarding mammoth hunting, the action of the beaters (frightening the prey from themselves), which is biologically a nonsense, gets conscious sense because of its motive (to get part of the final product distributed to them, satisfying their need), which is fulfilled by the actions of the killers. To execute such a nonsense action, the beaters must conceive it as part of a chain of cause-effect relationships in the collective activity. It is necessary that the relationship between their (the beaters') action and that of the killers be subjectively perceived by them (beaters and killers) as existing objectively, in this way becoming conscious for them. In other words, as clearly put by Mikhailov [11], "man separates himself from his activity insofar as it is simultaneously also the activity of another, that is, insofar as it is activity performed together, intercourse. In this way a person looks upon his own action with the eyes of another and this is why he himself (as if seeing himself from the side) can check, correct, and guide his actions – guide them in accordance with a general plan, a joint plan, a goal."

Differently from what occurs in the remaining of the animal world, human conscious activity is mediated by production instruments (tools, for acting on nature) and by psychological instruments (linguistic signs, for acting on other individuals), both being products of the social-cultural history. In this way the relation of the individual with nature becomes mediated by the relation between himself and other individuals. Both the instrument of labor and the linguistic sign reify (make objective, concrete) the relationship man-nature and man-man, respectively; and both of them are social products regarding their origin (created and improved by countless generations of human beings) and their use (learned in the joint activity with other people); and with them the transmission of experience from one generation to the other stops being only biological (genetic) and becomes also social-cultural. This nongenetic transfer of skills and behaviors (for instance, by social learning and imitation) took place long before the appearance of humans (and even of mammals), since purely genetic processes are limited in their capacity to predict future environmental changes and cannot provide the individual with anticipatory responses for each contingency [12].

The brain structures responsible for the higher level conscious activity are the phylogenetically most recent parts of the associative neocortex, particularly prefrontal region and temporal-parietal junction, in connection with older temporal medial (hippocampus) and midline structures (posterior cingulate, precuneus), in a large-scale neurofunctional network. Here we refer to the most complex level of conscious functioning, called by Damasio [13] *extended* or *autonoetic consciousness*, which provides the organism with an autobiographical, narrative self, able to travel in time and revisit itself experiencing its past and future activities. As conceived by William James [14], this self is a continuous stream of experiences and thoughts, being at the same time the "observer," the thinker, the subject of experience (the "I"), and the "observed," the object, or content of the experience, with its emotions felt, things perceived (percepts), and ideas thought (the "Me").

A more simple and basic level, called *noetic consciousness*, *core consciousness* or *core self*, is the subjective experience of a self that catches itself in the act of knowing or simply perceiving something in the here-now, in a continuous present, devoid of past experiences and future plans. The core self has a sense of ownership, feeling the body is its own body (and not someone else's), and a sense of agency, feeling it is the actor of its own actions. This level of consciousness depends on semantic memory but not on autobiographical or working memory processes or language and seems to exist in other animals, such as anthropoid apes, dolphins, elephants, and even birds [13, 15, 16]. Well-designed experiments with scrub jays (*Aphelocoma californica*), for instance, have shown they have semantic and episodic-like memory, in a way that cannot be explained by operant conditioning [18, 19]. During unrewarded test trials, scrub jays remembered not only the location of their caches but also the diverse food types (the different perishability of mealworms, crickets, and peanuts) and the relative time since they were cached. Even elements of theory of mind (mental attribution) have been found in these corvids. They use to bury food far away from conspecifics, and if they must cache while being watched, they often return alone to the caches they had hidden and recache them in new places, being this behavior observed in jays with prior experience of pilfering another jay's caches, but not in jays without this experience of being thieves in the past [16, 19]. However, these authors recognize the need of an experimental approach for understanding the mechanisms underlying these behaviors, particularly in relation to so-called simulation theory of mind [20].

The most simple and basic level of the self is what Damasio [21] called *proto-self* or *primordial self*, which represents the unconscious basic state of the body, hypothetically processed in phylogenetically old paramedian brain regions, such as the cingulate, thalamus, hypothalamus, and superior colliculi, in connection with brain stem structures such as the periaqueductal gray, deep layers of superior colliculi, solitary tract, and parabrachial nuclei. The proto-self is considered by Panksepp [22] as a *primary* (anoetic) form of consciousness, as a primeval feeling of existing as a body, of its visceral, sensory-motor, and emotional functioning, but without knowledge or awareness of percepts, actions, emotions, or of itself. This primordial level appears to be the first manifestation of the self to emerge in newborn and infant babies before 1 year age, as was observed by Piaget [23], with feelings of pain, satisfaction, and anger and with emotional reactions to situations of boring waiting, unsatisfied effort, or failure, particularly when the subject's actions on the object meet obstacles or resistance. On the other hand, it seems also to be the last to disappear in advanced stages of Alzheimer's dementia, when the patient has already lost its episodic and semantic memory, its notion of objective time, its expanded autobiographical self, and even its core self, when, from the point of view of the individual (as a mental subject), the dissociation (distinction) between its own actions and the object of these actions is about to be dissolved, with the object turning into the mere extension of the subject's actions and the subject then becoming reduced to its own actions [24].

7.4 Conclusion

The mind is the product of a long biological and social-cultural evolution. Its primordial manifestation is the ability of living organisms to detect and react to external stimuli, as seen in the irritability, tropism, and unconditioned reactions of unicellular organisms. In the elementary *sensory* stage of cognition, the individual reacts to one isolated property of the external object, whose stimulation indicates food or threat. Further developments in this sensory stage is the ability to analyze and generalize stimuli as well as to form conditioned reflexes, with the detection and reaction to stimuli that have no immediate metabolic importance and are not directly linked to (or coming from) the vitally relevant object but signal its imminent presence. The following stage, the *perceptive*, starts with the development of the cerebral cortex in our amphibious and reptiles ancestors allowing the animal to detect sets of relevant properties of the external object and construct its abstract image by integrating the constant relationships between its parts and properties, besides also representing the conditions in which the relevant object is located. In the stage of *intellect*, paralleled by the development of the associative neocortex, the individual is able to (1) perceive things and their interrelationships; (2) solve problems by operating with the elements of the conditions in which the goal (target object) is situated (preparatory phase) in order to reach the goal (accomplishment phase); and (3) to quickly transfer the scheme of successful solution to new similar problematic situations. The intellectual stage is typical of superior animals (primates), but other animals (corvids, octopuses) also show problem solving abilities. Further on, in the stage of *self-consciousness*, the subject becomes aware of itself and detaches itself mentally from its own activity, from itself as agent of this activity. The collective productive labor (particularly the hunting of big animals) mediated by instruments (tools, for acting on nature, and signs, for acting on other individuals) created the conditions for the development of self-consciousness and its large-scale neurofunctional networks comprising the phylogenetically most recent parts of the associative neocortex, particularly prefrontal region and temporal-parietal junction, in connection with old midline structures (hippocampus, posterior cingulate, and precuneus).

References

1. Leontiev AN (1981) Problems of the development of the mind. Progress Publishers, Moscow
2. Anokhin PK (1974) Biology and neurophysiology of the conditioned reflex and its role in adaptive behavior. Pergamon Press, Oxford
3. Sharov AA (1999) The origin and evolution of signs. Semiotica 127(1–4):521–536
4. Sharov AA (2001) Umwelt-theory and pragmatism. Semiotica 134:211–228
5. von Uexküll J (1982) The theory of meaning (1940). Semiotica 42(1):25–82
6. Sass LA (2003) Self-disturbance in schizophrenia: hyperreflexivity and diminished self-affection. In: Kircher T, David A (eds) The self in neuroscience and psychiatry. Cambridge University Press, Cambridge
7. Gibson JJ (1979) The ecological approach to visual perception (Chapter 8: the theory of affordances). Houghton Mifflin, Boston
8. Luria AR (1973) The working brain: an introduction to neuropsychology. Penguin Books, London
9. Byrne R (1995) The thinking ape: evolutionary origins of intelligence. Oxford University Press, New York
10. Toth N, Schick KD, Savage-Rumbaugh ES, Sevcik RA, Rumbaugh DM (1993) Pan the tool-maker: investigations into the stone tool-making and tool-using capabilities of a bonobo (Pan paniscus). J Archaeol Sci 20:81–91
11. Mikhailov FT (1980) The riddle of the self. Progress Publishers, Moscow
12. Oakley DA (1979) Cerebral cortex and adaptive behavior. In: Oakley DA, Plotkin HC (eds) Brain, behavior and evolution. Londres, Methuen
13. Damasio AR (1999) The feeling of what happens: body and emotion in the making of consciousness. Harcourt Brace & Company, New York
14. James W (1890/1983) The principles of psychology. Harvard University Press, Cambridge, MA
15. Northoff G, Panksepp J (2008) The trans-species concept of self and the subcortical-cortical midline system. Trends Cogn Sci 12(7):259–264
16. Emery NJ (2006) Cognitive ornithology: the evolution of avian intelligence. Philos Trans R Soc B 361:23–43
17. Clayton NS, Dickinson A (1998) Episodic-like memory during cache recovery by scrub jays. Nature 395(6699):272–274
18. Clayton NS, Griffiths DP, Emery NJ, Dickinson A (2001) Elements of episodic-like memory in animals. Philos Trans R Soc Lond B 356:1483–1491
19. Emery NJ, Clayton NS (2001) Effects of experience and social context on prospective caching strategies by scrub jays. Nature 414(6862):443–446
20. Emery NJ (2005) The evolution of social cognition. In: Easton A, Emery NJ (eds) Cognitive neuroscience of social behavior. Psychology Press, Hove
21. Damasio A (2010) Self comes to mind: constructing the conscious brain. Vintage Books, New York
22. Panksepp J (1998) Affective neuroscience: the foundations of human and animal emotions. Oxford University Press, New York
23. Piaget J (1952) The origins of intelligence in children. International Universities Press, New York
24. Damasceno BP (1996) Time perception as a complex functional system: neuropsychological approach. Int J Neurosci 85:237–262

Chapter 8
Ontogenetic Perspective

8.1 Introduction

From birth on, the child acquires its sensory-motor schemas (Piaget's "circular reactions"). Perception and imitation give way to representation ("internalized imitation") and, through triadic interactions with adults, the first linguistic sign, the pointing gesture, is developed, followed by words. At 2–3 years of age, the first peak of rapid cortical growth, particularly of associative prefrontal and temporal-parietal cortices, makes possible intersensory connections and multimodal abstract syntheses, coordination of cognitive schemas, and mental construction of the object as existing outside the subject. At the same time, a functional hierarchy is established between the primary, secondary, and tertiary cortical regions, with decreasing modal specificity from the primary to the tertiary ones; and some higher mental functions as language and musical ability become lateralized.

8.2 Early Cognitive-Cerebral Development

The various forms of reception-reaction acquired by our animal ancestors during millions of years reappear in the embryonic and early phases of the development of the human organism, in which they are organized as different hierarchical and interdependent levels of information processing. Thus, we have receptor cells in the sensory organs with the ability to detect elementary stimuli; in the secondary zones of the associative cerebral cortex, the perception of forms of the corresponding sensory modality; and in the tertiary cortical regions, the multimodal perception of external things and their reciprocal relations (scenes, complex events) as well as the formation of concepts and the matrix of logical and discursive thinking.

An important characteristic of the development of primary, secondary, and tertiary cortical zones is the establishment of a functional hierarchy between them, in

B. Damasceno, *Research on Cognition Disorders*,
https://doi.org/10.1007/978-3-030-57267-9_8

such a way that the modal specificity decreases from the primary to the secondary and tertiary zones, that is, the neurons of a primary zone react only to a sensory modality of stimuli (e.g., visual), while the neurons of secondary and mainly tertiary zones also react to stimuli of multiple modalities (tactile, auditory, visual, etc.). Another feature of this functional hierarchy is the lateralization (hemispheric dominance) of some higher cortical functions as language and musical ability, the first being highly dependent on the left and the second on the right hemisphere. From the primary (projection) cortical zones to the associative secondary and tertiary ones, the receptive fields of their neurons become larger and larger at each level of processing, at the same time that the properties of the processed signals become more complex, making possible more and more abstract synthesis [1].

Furthermore, as the individual components of the higher mental functions change during the successive early stages of ontogenesis, the consequences of a local brain lesion will differ depending on the stage of functional development [2, 3]. In infancy, the normal development of a secondary zone would not occur without the integrity of the corresponding primary zone which furnishes the trophic stimuli originated from sensory-motor activities; and, in the same way, the formation of a tertiary zone depends on the normal functioning of the corresponding secondary zones with their information needed for more complex cognitive synthesis. In this phase of life, an early lesion of the primary zone would therefore lead to incomplete development of the other higher cortical regions. On the other hand, in the adult with its higher mental functions already established, the tertiary zones take over the dominant role and control the functioning of the subordinate secondary and primary zones. So, a lesion of the primary zone (e.g., visual) will not significantly affect the subject's activities (e.g., in household chores), since the afferent field of his functional brain systems (coordinated by the tertiary zones) includes other uninjured primary zones (auditory, tactile-proprioceptive-motor) which up to then constituted the "reserve fund" of all afferentations [4].

The diverse cortical regions reach their maturation in different periods depending on the environmental influences. By using electronic microscopy to compare the formation and elimination of synapses in diverse cerebral regions, Huttenlocher and Dabholkar [5] found maximal synaptogenesis in the primary visual cortex at the ages of 3–4 months and in the prefrontal cortex (middle frontal gyrus) at 4 years age. From this age on (from 4 through 20 years), this frontal region presents reduction of its synaptic density. Other studies using PET scan [6] attained similar results, showing rapid increase of cerebral metabolism during infancy (reflecting synaptogenesis), followed by its reduction later on, corresponding to the period of elimination (pruning) of synapses. This elimination of synapses is related not only to the chronologic age but also to the acquisition and development of language, which determine a cerebral reorganization, as established by event-related potentials studies [7]. At 13 months age, understanding of words requires the participation of both posterior and anterior parts of brain hemispheres, while at the age of 20 months, this effect occurs only in the left parietotemporal region. On the other hand, when comparing children with the same age (13 months), those with richer vocabulary showed a more localized effect, in the left parietotemporal regions. There is no definitive evidence for the left hemisphere specialization for language at birth, even though the left *planum temporale* (future "Wernicke's area" for language) is larger than the right one in most (67%) right-handed people and in chimpanzees, and this asymmetry is present already around 31 weeks gestation [8–10]. What is lateralized in the left hemisphere is the linguistic-communicative meaning of the sign, be it verbal (spoken) or visual (as in sign language).

The tertiary cortical regions are the last to become mature [11]. The prefrontal cortex, for example, presents two peaks in the speed of growth of its surface area: from birth to 2–3 years and around 6–7 years. This second peak is associated to the increasing role of language in the organization of complex programs and autoregulation of behavior.

The first peak of cortical prefrontal development corresponds to the period when the child acquires cognitive sensory-motor schemas (Piaget's "circular reactions") [12] and then starts to mentally construct the object as something with permanent existence and independent from himself and to learn symbolic representations and language. The neonate begins with repeated exercises of innate and conditioned reflexes, which become more complex in its interaction with the environment and originate primary isolated schemas and habits (e.g., sucking emptily, sucking the thumb or the mother's nipple), which become afterward (around 3–6 months age) coordinated with each other, so that everything that is looked at or sucked tend to be grasped and vice versa. For Piaget, this is an essential step in the mental construction of the object as existing outside (independent of the subject), since when an object is simultaneously looked at, grasped, and sucked, it becomes exterior from the viewpoint of and relatively to the subject; "the object tends to be simultaneously assimilated to multiple schemas, thus acquiring a set of meanings and, consequently, consistency" [12]. The cerebral counterpart of this coordination of cognitive schemas might be the establishment of intersensory connections in the multimodal associative cortices.

The further generalization of these schemas by applying them to new situations and to different objects makes possible for the child to solve problems: first (before 12 months), through the discovery of new means in the active experimentation with external objects, on the basis of trial and errors, and then (from around 12 months on), thanks to the invention of new means by mental combination in order to meet goals. The child makes use of any object as a tool with which to achieve another (objective) that satisfies its desire or need, for example, when it wants to grasp the toy bear that is placed outside the reach of its hands. These acquisitions may represent the prelinguistic development of our executive function, in which the prefrontal cortex, functionally connected to posterior associative parietal-temporal-occipital cortices, would play relevant role.

In the subsequent developmental stage, that of invention of new means by combination of mental schemas, the child predicts which operations will fail or be successful. The external experimentation with things present in the perceptive field of the child is substituted by the internal mental experimentation with the representations (symbolic sensory-motor images) of these things, also taking into account their interrelationships as well as the relations (actions) of the subject with them. If in the previous stage perception was enough, in this phase representation is needed, making possible to mentally operate on absent objects. For Piaget, imitation plays relevant role in the transition from the previous phase to this one. He considered imitation as a "representation in acts" and the representation, as an "internalized imitation", which the child employs immediately before acting externally on real objects.

The representative images are signs (the signifiers) whose meaning (the signified) is the sensory-motor schema itself or the objectified activity that unrolls in the external world; they are the "tools of the nascent thinking" [12], besides constituting sine qua non condition for the acquisition of language, as they begin to be represented by words (signifiers of signifiers).

8.3 Social-Cultural Learning

Vygotsky [2] calls attention for the moment of the intellectual development of the child when speech and practical activity, up to this time following two independent lines, converge giving origin to specifically human forms of practical and abstract intelligence. For him, this is the moment of internalization or internal (mental) reconstruction of external (material) operations, as occur with the linguistic sign. When the child wishes some object that is outside the reach of its hands, it stretches out its arms in the direction of the object and does unsuccessful grasping movements. These actions of the child are interpreted by its mother as a pointing gesture, indicative of the object. In reality, from the point of view of the child, it is simply a primary sensory-motor schema in action (grasping), provoked by the object. Later on, with the repetition of this experience, the child takes for its own use (appropriates) this meaning (indicative gesture) established from the outside, by its mother. At this time a change occurs in the function of its movement: initially oriented by (and to) the object, the movement becomes directed to another person, as a means to establish relations with other people (Tomasello's "triadic interaction") [13, 14]. Gradually, the grasping movement converts into the act of pointing, resulting in a true gesture, through its simplification (being now enough stretching the arm and forefinger). In fact, it becomes a true gesture after manifesting for the others all functions of the pointing indicative gesture and after being understood as such by the others. According to Tomasello [14], these moments of triadic social interactions mark a transition to true cultural learning, which should be distinguished from other forms of social noncultural learning also found in other animals, such as stimulus enhancement, observational conditioning, response facilitation, and emulation learning.

8.4 Social, Noncultural Learning

Stimulus enhancement is the focusing of attention and interest of the learner on a local or object with which another animal of the same species interacts, for example, by focusing on and approaching another conspecific getting a good meal in a branch laden with fruit, but also, in the case of "negative enhancement," by avoiding the place where other animals were seen to be hurt [15].The learning of the negative or aversive significance of places and things is also called *observational conditioning*, happening, for example, when young monkeys develop fear responses to stimuli that they saw frightened others [16]. Stimulus enhancement learning is social to the extent that the learner gets knowledge about places and things from others, just by observing how others interact with them.

Response facilitation is the enhanced probability of an animal responding in the same way as others of the same species, by observing them reacting to alarm or other signal from predators, as a kind of contagious response, for example, when a bird sees other conspecifics taking to the wing or turning in flight [15]. A similar reaction is *social facilitation*, characterized by increased activity of an individual when in the presence of nearby active conspecifics, so that the noticing of activity of other animals serves to increase motivation and activity level of the individual, for example, when a capuchin monkey increases its eating of novel foods just by feeding in the company of other monkeys [17]. Unlike imitation, in stimulus enhancement and response facilitation, nothing really new is learned, since the action (reaction) is already part of the animal's repertoires. On the other hand, these kinds of social learning have high survival value by allowing the animal to escape from predators and avoid dangerous foods in a more rapid and efficient way than would be with isolated, individual trial and error experience. Besides this, the individual trial-and-error learning itself becomes improved in the presence of similarly active conspecifics.

In *emulation learning*, the subject is attracted by and focuses on the result of the actions of another individual and attempts to devise its own idiosyncratic strategy to reproduce the same end result. For instance, the subject may learn from the others that hitting a fruit with a stick can cause it to fall or that twisting the bolt of a box with the hand can open it and find a piece of food inside it. In emulation, the subject learns some temporal-spatial causal relations, dynamic properties, and affordances (what can be yielded) of the objects manipulated by the others, but not the specific methods and behavioral strategies used [13, 15, 18–20].

8.5 Conclusion

From birth to 2–3 years, the child acquires its cognitive sensory-motor schemas (Piaget's "circular reactions") associated with the first peak of rapid cortical growth, particularly of the prefrontal and multimodal temporal-parietal associative cortices, making possible intersensory connections and abstract syntheses, coordination of cognitive schemas, and construction of the object as existing outside, independent of the subject. Here, in the triadic interaction child-object-adult, perception and imitation give way to representation (a kind of "internalized imitation") which the child uses immediately before acting on external objects, at the same time that it acquires the first linguistic sign – the pointing gesture – and then words. Similarly to words, the pointing gesture has the two main characteristics of a linguistic sign: the referential, for indicating something in the world, and the discursive-pragmatic, for acting on other individuals. The early stages of the child cognitive development is accompanied by the establishment of a functional hierarchy between the primary, secondary, and tertiary cortical zones, with the modal specificity decreasing from the primary to the tertiary (multimodal) zones, and by the lateralization (hemispheric dominance) of some higher mental functions as language (to the left) and musical ability (to the right). For instance, at 13 months age, understanding of words depends on anterior and posterior parts of both hemispheres, but at 20 months age, only left parietal-temporal region is recruited. In infancy, the normal development of secondary and tertiary cortical zones depends on the primary zone which furnishes the trophic stimuli originated from sensory-motor activities. For this reason, an early lesion of the primary zone would lead to incomplete development of the other higher cortical regions.

References

1. Gardner EP, Martin JH (2000) Coding of sensory information. In: Kandel ER, Schwartz JH, Jessell TM (eds) Principles of neural science, 4th edn. McGraw-Hill, New York
2. Vygotsky LS (1978) Mind in society: the development of higher psychological processes. Harvard University Press, Cambridge
3. Luria AR (1966/1980) Higher cortical functions in man, 2nd edn. Basic Books, New York
4. Tsvetkova LS (1998) Hacia una teoría de la enseñanza rehabilitatoria. In: Rojas LQ (ed) Problemas teóricos y metodológicos de la rehabilitación neuropsicológica. Universidad Autonoma, Tlaxcala
5. Huttenlocher PR, Dabholkar AS (1997) Regional differences in synaptogenesis in human cerebral cortex. J Comp Neurol 387:167–178
6. Chugani HT, Muller RA, Chugani DC (1996) Functional brain reorganization in children. Brain Dev 18:347–356
7. Neville HJ, Bevelier D (2000) Specificity and plasticity in neurocognitive development in humans. In: Gazzaniga MS (ed) The new cognitive neurosciences. The MIT Press, Cambridge, pp 83–98
8. Kuhl PK (2000) Language, mind, and brain: experience alters perception. In: Gazzaniga MS (ed) The new cognitive neurosciences. The MIT Press, Cambridge, pp 99–115
9. Gannon PJ, Holloway RL, Broadfield DC, Braun AR (1998) Asymmetry of chimpanzee planum temporale: humanlike pattern of Wernicke's brain language area homolog. Science 279(5348):220–222. https://doi.org/10.1126/science.279.5348.220
10. Dronkers NF, Pinker S, Damasio A (2000) Language and the aphasias. In: Kandel ER, Schwartz JH, Jessel TM (eds) Principles of neural sciencess, 4th edn. McGraw-Hill, New York, pp 1169–1187

11. Yakovlev PI, Lecours AR (1967) The myelogenetic cycles of regional maturation of the brain. In: Minkowski A (ed) Regional development of the brain in early life. Blackwell, Oxford
12. Piaget J (1952) The origins of intelligence in children. International Universities Press, New York
13. Tomasello M, Kruger A, Ratner H (1993) Cultural learning. Behav Brain Sci 16(03):495–511
14. Tomasello M (1999) The cultural origins of human cognition. Harvard University Press, Cambridge, MA
15. Byrne R (1995) The thinking ape: evolutionary origins of intelligence. Oxford University Press, New York
16. Cook M, Mineka S (1990) Selective associations in the observational conditioning of fear in rhesus monkeys. J Exp Psychol 16(4):372–389
17. Visalberghi E, Fragaszy D (1995) The behavior of capuchin monkeys, *Cebus apella*, with novel foods: the role of social context. Anim Behav 49:1089–1095
18. Whiten A, Custance DM, Gomez JC, Texidor P, Bard KA (1996) Imitative learning of artificial fruit processing in children (*Homo sapiens*) and chimpanzees (*Pan troglodytes*). J Comp Psychol 110:3–14
19. Boesch C, Tomasello M (1998) Chimpanzee and human cultures. Curr Anthropol 35(5):591–614
20. Huang CT, Charman T (2005) Gradations of emulation learning in infants' imitation of actions on objects. J Exp Child Psychol 92:276–302

Chapter 9
Role of Imitation and Appropriation in the Cognitive Development

9.1 Introduction

Different from the apparent "imitation" shown by animals (e.g., response facilitation) and human neonates (e.g., smiling, tongue protrusion), which are actions and behaviors already present in the individual's repertoire, in cultural learning, the copied actions are novel, belong to the culture, and are acquired and transmitted by true imitation, which consists in the learner reproducing the most relevant goal-directed actions, methods, and strategies of the adult in order to accomplish something together, recognizing the adult as an intentional agent and taking his/her perspective and viewpoint on the objects and actions involved. In the joint triadic activity (child-object-adult), the child acquires (appropriates) the culturally established ways of using objects and instruments and interacting with people, by means of tools and linguistic signs. Different from the concept of "internalization," that gives more importance to societal influences (from the outside), that of appropriation emphasizes the active, creative efforts of the child itself (from inside) for matching the adult's methods and opinions. More recent electrophysiological and functional neuroimaging studies in monkeys and humans have shown evidence of a network of mirror neurons in anterior parietal and lateral ventral premotor regions playing a relevant role in imitation.

9.2 Imitation Learning

Different from other forms of social learning shared with animals, in *imitation*, particularly in imitative learning of novel actions (nonexistent in the imitator's repertoire), the learner appropriates and reproduces ("copies") the most relevant goal-directed actions and methods of another individual, as well as the strategies and

B. Damasceno, *Research on Cognition Disorders*,
https://doi.org/10.1007/978-3-030-57267-9_9

hierarchical structure of its behavior, by combining and coordinating sequences of components and subgoals.

True imitation requires the subject to understand the other, first of all, as an intentional agent (what the other intends and knows), since the recognition of an action requires the recognition of a goal and of an agent's intentions. As stated before, actions are not to be confounded with simple movements. There are movements without actions (e.g., those of innate reflexes) and actions without movements (e.g., the motionless statue-like position of a sentry guard). The meaning of an action is grasped by perceiving and understanding the mutual relationship it has with its agent and with its object, that is, by recognizing the context in which it is performed.

True imitation also requires the imitator to take the perspective of the other individual in order to understand and adopt its viewpoint on the objects and on the social interaction involved. Otherwise, as asked by Byrne [1], how does an animal recognize that its behavior is "the same as" the actions of another? Particularly when the imitator does not see its own movements (e.g., in imitation of facial gestures), for true imitation is also required that the animal or human first store a visual representation of the pattern of movement exhibited by another, and then, the imitator must use its proprioceptive or kinesthetic senses to match its own movements to the stored visual representation [2]. This cross-modality and intersubject matching are a complex cognitive task that would require a certain degree of brain maturation, particularly of associative cortical areas of occipitoparietal and frontal regions. Accordingly, this seems to be the reason why true imitative learning begins later on, in the final quarter of the infant's first year of life, comprising both imitation of object-directed actions and use of conventional communicative symbols of language [3, 4].

A network of mirror neurons in anterior parietal and lateral ventral premotor regions have been found to play a relevant role in imitation. As shown by the pioneering studies of Rizzolatti et al. [5], neurons in these regions discharge when a monkey performs a specific movement with its hands, for example, picking up a piece of food, but also when the monkey watches the experimenter or another monkey executing the same action, what indicates these cells are involved in the sensory motor commutative transductions needed for the internal, abstract representation of the motor task. Mirror neurons have also been demonstrated in the same brain regions in humans by using magnetoencephalography [6], transcranial magnetic stimulation [7], brain imaging studies with positron emission tomography [8, 9], and functional magnetic resonance imaging [10]. In a study by Buccino et al. [11], using an event-related fMRI paradigm, musically naive participants (nonguitar players) were asked to observe complex, unfamiliar hand actions (guitar chords played by an expert guitarist) and, after an interval, to execute the observed chords as accurately as possible. The results showed a basic neural circuit underlying imitation learning of hand actions: inferior parietal lobule, posterior part of the inferior frontal gyrus, and adjacent premotor cortex. For Buccino et al. [11], the role played by mirror neurons would be by "resonating" in response to the elementary motor acts (e.g., finger lifting, precision grip) observed in the action to be imitated. On the other hand, when a novel motor pattern or motor sequence has to be learned by imitation (i.e., true imitation, not just the replication of acts already present in the imitator's repertoire), mirror neurons would code the elementary motor acts present in the action to be imitated and recombine these coded acts in the new motor pattern or motor sequence [11–13]. Moreover, there is evidence from fMRI studies that mirror neurons participate in the brain networks that underlie the understanding of the intention of another person's action. In the study by Iacoboni et al. [14], healthy participants watched three kinds of stimuli: (1) hand actions grasping a tea cup without a context; (2) context only: a scene containing objects (teapot, mug, cookies, jar, etc.) arranged either as just before having tea (the "drinking" context) or as just after having tea (the "cleaning" context); and (3) grasping hand actions performed in the two different contexts (with the intention to drink or to clean). They found that watching grasping actions embedded in both contexts yielded greater activation in the inferior frontal cortex (premotor mirror neuron area), as compared with observing only grasping actions or only contexts.

For most primatologists and comparative psychologists, in true imitation, the actions copied should be novel, not present in the individual's repertoire, different from stimulus enhancement, emulation, and every day "imitation" seen in human infants within the first weeks of life (e.g., tongue protrusion, smiling), in which nothing really new is learned. This novelty principle is a condition for imitative learning to be a form of cultural, nonbiological transmission of information. The concept of culture is very broad. Culture is understood here, first of all, as that which constitutes its material basis, comprising the mode of production of all means that a group of social beings need for feeding, sheltering, defending, and reproducing themselves; the various kinds of artifacts, including material and psychological instruments (tools and communicative signs); and the modes how the individuals organize and cooperate with each other in the work process. Secondarily, culture is all that constitute its spiritual superstructure, that is, beliefs, customs, arts, behavioral traditions, languages, and social, economic, political, juridical, and educational institutions. Cultural transmission, primordially through imitative learning within the same group or between different generations of individuals, is a sine qua non condition for the evolution of culture, which is based on the gradual accumulation of modifications ("ratchet effect") of artifacts and instruments across generations, typical of humans [3, 15]. Imitative learning assures cultural evolution to the extent that the learner succeeds in reproducing with fidelity all actions and behaviors that are relevant for the task at hand by attempting to see the whole task or activity the way the other sees it, from inside the other's perspective, as if the other were "himself-another".

Imitative learning requires triadic social interactions between child, adult, and outside objects and occurs at 9–12 months of age, when the infant begins to look where adults are looking (gaze following) and acts on objects in the way adults are acting on them. For Tomasello et al. [3], these interactions "are triadic in the sense that they involve the referential triangle of child, adult, and some outside object to which they are both attending" ("joint attention"), and they represent cultural learning in at least two senses: (1) the imitative learning is an attempt to reproduce cause-effect relationships and strategies used by other persons for achieving determined goal (but see Whiten [16]), and (2) in the imitative learning, "the child is not just learning things *from* other persons but is learning things *through* them, in the sense that he or she must know something of the adult's perspective on a situation in order to learn the same intentionally communicative act" [3]. Carpenter et al. [17] have found three main types of joint attentional interaction and their corresponding ages of emergence, with the child (1) *checking the adult's attention* by looking from the object up to the adult's face and back to the object to see if the adult is jointly engaged in looking to the same object; hence this behavior of the child be called "joint attentional engagement" (9–12 months); (2) *following the adult's attention* to more distal external objects by following the direction of the adult's visual gaze or manual pointing gesture and knowing precisely and fixing attention on the outside object the adult is focused on (11–14 months); and (3) *directing the adult's attention* to a distal object by gazing or pointing to it for the adult to do the same or, when desiring an object, attempting to direct the adult's behavior to help obtain that object, as a kind of imperative gesture, or simply desiring that the adult shares attention to an interesting object (declarative gesture) (13–15 months).

In this triadic social interaction, when the child points to an object, the adult usually also names it. In this way, the child learns two basic functions of the linguistic sign, be it as a primordial pointing gesture or as a word: (1) the *referential*, indicating or designating something in the world, as an attempt to draw or direct the adult's attention (attentive perception) to it and (2) the *discursive* or *pragmatic* function, as a means to act on other people, influencing their behavior so that they do what the child desires or wants they do.

9.3 The Process of Appropriation of Adult's Cognitive Functioning by the Child

Leontiev [18] introduced the term "appropriation" instead of "internalization" to designate the active character of learning, giving as an example the appropriation of the adequate use of the spoon by the child. Initially, the child handles the spoon in the same manner it uses to do with any other object, grasping it either way, beating it on the table, etc. In the situation of real everyday life, first the mother feeds the child with the spoon and then puts the spoon in the hand of the child for it to feed itself. At first, the child takes clumsy hold of the spoon, letting the food drop. However, the mother helps it by intervening in its actions, and in this joint activity, the child acquires (appropriates) the habitual way of using the spoon.

The concept of "internalization" gives more value to the role of society (from the outside) in the genesis of higher psychological functions, while that of "appropriation" emphasizes the active participation of the subject (from the inside) with his/her personality, motivational and emotional characteristics, which give him/her the fundamental reason, and mental energy necessary to engage actively in the tasks. Wertsch et al. [19] also highlight the value of this active and participant character of the appropriation, which involves the creative efforts of the subject for fitting in different opinions with the others in order to accomplish something together, and in this way, the appropriation being a process of transformation of the subject himself. For these authors, this dynamic approach to appropriation considers cognition not as a group of stored belongings (as thought, representation, memories) but as an active process or action of thinking, representing, and memorizing, which cannot be reduced to the possession of stored objects or faculties.

Thus, in the process of appropriation, the primary and decisive role is played by the practical actions of the subject with other people, tools, artifacts, and objects of the natural and cultural world, that is, by the objectified actions of the subject himself and not the actions of other people, since from the psychogenetic point of view, we are dealing here with the formation of the ideal *action* and not of the *image* of the action [20], neither are we dealing with the realization of a mental image or consciousness that exists a priori and gradually manifests itself as the brain attains its complete maturation on the basis of merely biologic determinations. In reality, as formulated by Marx and Engels [21], what exists is not the consciousness as a disembodied, isolated mental faculty (*das Bewusstsein*) but the conscious being (*das bewusste Sein*), and the being of man is its process of real life. The being of man is its activity, which presents itself simultaneously in three interdependent and interconnected forms: the material-social, the mental, and the bodily cerebral. From the psychogenetic point of view, the primordial, basic, and initial form is the material-social, external. Let's go into more details on these forms of the human activity.

The *material-social* activity is that of the everyday practices of man, particularly those of labor, in which the subjects, by using material instruments (tools), transform objects of nature making them useful for human life, at the same time that they interact with other people by means of psychological instruments (verbal and nonverbal signs). In the process of labor, at the same time that humans act upon external nature, transforming it, they modify their own nature, developing the potentialities that exist in themselves. As Marx [22] pointed out, "the eye has become a human eye, just as its object has become a social, human object, an object made by man for man... The forming of the five senses is a labor of the entire history of the world down to the present." Moreover, different from animals, humans not only transform the material upon which they operate but carve in this material the project they consciously had in their intention, and this project constitutes the determinant law of the way how they operate and to which they have to subordinate their will [23]. The instrument is a kind of external memory and represents in its form the labor processes employed in its production and use. According to Lektorsky [24], when children master the use of an instrument, they select in it the characteristics which are essential for the realization of determined activity as well as the general characteristics it shares with other similar instruments developed and used during the history of this activity. The instrument represents objective forms of expression of cognitive norms existing outside the individual and in society, and the mastering of these norms (socially mediated) makes possible that they function as structure-forming components of cognition.

In the *mental* or psychic form of the activity, external objects are replaced by their images (representations, concepts), and the practical actions, by mental actions, which have generalized, abbreviated, automatized, and abstract form, and this mental form has semiotic nature, being mediated by signs, be them verbal or nonverbal, conscious or unconscious.

The *bodily cerebral* form of the activity comprises the complex functional system responsible for its accomplishment, including both the brain (for formulating intentions, programs, coordination, monitoring and correction, by means of neural codes) and the corresponding interconnected parts of the nervous system and the body participating in it.

These three forms of the activity constitute a dialectical unity, the "being of humans." Reciprocal influences and interactions between them are necessary for acquisition of higher mental functions and their neural substrate, namely, the more recent and sophisticated formations of the associative cerebral cortex. Biological (genetic) factors yield only the possibility for their development, which will become impaired without the social-interactional practice of the individual, as has occurred in children and apes raised in isolation during the critical period for the development of the social behavior [25–28]. Dunbar [29] and Byrne [1] analyzed the brain of different primates (prosimians, apes, humans) and found that the increase of volume of the neocortex (relatively to body size) points to a social origin of intelligence in these species. The growth of neocortex, which attains its highest degree in anthropoid apes and humans, correlates with differences in the complexity of their social life, capacity to understand cause-effect relationships between instrument and task, and "Machiavellian intelligence." This last term was introduced by Byrne and Whiten [30] to designate the social intelligence used by the subject in its relations with other people, consisting in the ability to distinguish and imagine what other people think about the subject and other things, to intentionally deceive and manipulate others, as well as to predict and prepare beforehand for the deceptive intentions of others. Byrne [1] postulates that the anthropoid apes capacity of discernment seems not to be a mere function of brain size but instead reflects brain reorganization or reprogramming.

9.4 Conclusion

Different from other forms of social learning (e.g., stimulus enhancement, response facilitation), in true imitation, novel actions (nonexistent in the imitator's repertoire) are learned. This novelty principle is a condition for imitation to be a form of cultural (nonbiological) learning. The imitator appropriates and reproduces the most relevant goal-directed actions, methods, and strategies of another individual, recognizing this individual as an intentional agent and taking his/her perspective in order to understand and adopt his/her viewpoint on the objects and social interaction involved, as if the other were "himself-another." This requires the imitator to store a visual representation of the pattern of movements exhibited by another and then use its proprioceptive senses to match its own movements to the stored visual representation. This cross-modality and intersubject matching require a certain degree of maturation of anterior and posterior associative cortical regions, particularly of the network of mirror neurons in anterior parietal and lateral ventral premotor regions. This seems to be the reason why true imitation, comprising both imitation of object-directed actions and use of linguistic signs, begins later on (at 9–12 months of age). In the joint triadic activity (child-object-adult), the child acquires (appropriates) the habitual, culturally established, way of using objects (e.g., the spoon). Different from the concept of "internalization," that gives more value to the role of society (from the outside), that of appropriation emphasizes the active participation of the child itself (from inside), with its personality, motivation, and creative efforts in order to fit into the adult's methods and opinions for accomplishing something together. Thus, in its practical activity handling tools and artifacts jointly with the adult, the child's objectified actions are converted into ideal actions (not contemplative images of actions) to be used in the process of perceiving, representing, memorizing, and thinking. This is the origin of our higher psychological functions.

References

1. Byrne R (1995) The thinking ape: evolutionary origins of intelligence. Oxford University Press, New York
2. Galef BG (2001) Social learning and imitation in animals. In: Bateson PPG, Alleva E (eds) Frontiers of life (vol 4): biology of behavior. Academic, San Diego, pp 261–269
3. Tomasello M, Kruger A, Ratner H (1993) Cultural learning. Behav Brain Sci 16(03):495–511
4. Bates E (1979) The emergence of symbols: cognition and communication in infancy. Academic Press, New York
5. Rizzolatti G, Fadiga L, Fogassi L, Gallese V (1996) Premotor cortex and the recognition of motor actions. Cogn Brain Res 3:131–141
6. Hari R, Forss N, Avikainen S, Kirveskari E, Salenius S, Rizzolatti G (1998) Activation of human primary motor cortex during action observation: a neuromagnetic study. Proc Natl Acad Sci USA 95:15061–15065
7. Fadiga L, Fogassi L, Pavesi G, Rizzolatti G (1995) Motor facilitation during action observation: a magnetic stimulation study. J Neurophysiol 73:2608–2611
8. Rizzolatti G, Fadiga L, Matelli M, Bettinardi V, Paulesu E, Perani D, Fazio F (1996) Localization of grasp representation in humans by PET: 1. Observation versus execution. Exp Brain Res 111:246–252
9. Grézes J, Decety J (2001) Functional anatomy of execution, mental simulation, observation, and verb generation of actions: a meta-analysis. Hum Brain Mapp 12:1–19
10. Buccino G, Binkofski F, Fink GR, Fadiga L, Fogassi L, Gallese V, Seitz RJ, Zilles K, Rizzolatti G, Freund HJ (2001) Action observation activates premotor and parietal areas in a somatotopic manner: an fMRI study. Eur J Neurosci 13:400–404
11. Buccino G, Vogt S, Ritzl A, Fink GR, Zilles K, Freund H-J, Rizzolatti G (2004) Neural circuits underlying imitation learning of hand actions: an event-related fMRI study. Neuron 42:323–334
12. Byrne RW (2002) Seeing actions as hierarchically organized structures: great ape manual skills. In: Melzoff AN, Prinz W (eds) The imitative mind: development, evolution and brain bases. Cambridge University Press, Cambridge, pp 122–140

13. Rizzolatti G (2003) The mirror-neuron system and imitation. In: Hurley S, Chater N (eds) Perspectives on imitation: from mirror neurons to memes. The MIT Press, Cambridge, MA
14. Iacoboni M, Molnar-Szakacs I, Gallese V, Buccino G, Mazziotta JC, Rizzolatti G (2005) Grasping the intentions of others with one's own mirror neuron system. PLoS Biol 3:529–535
15. Tomasello M (1990) Cultural transmission in the tool use and communicatory signaling of chimpanzees? In: Parker S, Gibson K (eds) Language and intelligence in monkeys and apes: comparative developmental perspectives. Cambridge University Press, Cambridge
16. Whiten A (2000) Primate culture and social learning. Cogn Sci 24(3):477–508
17. Carpenter M, Nagell K, Tomasello M (1998) Social cognition, joint attention, and communicative competence from 9 to 15 months of age. Monogr Soc Res Child Dev 63(4):1–143
18. Leontiev AN (1981) Problems of the development of the mind. Progress Publishers, Moscow
19. Wertsch JV, Del Rio P, Alvarez A (eds) (1995) Sociocultural studies of mind. Cambridge University Press, Cambridge
20. Galperin PY (1976) An introduction to psychology. Moscow University Press, Moscow
21. Marx K, Engels F (1976) The German ideology (1845–1846). Progress Publishers, Moscow
22. Marx K (1959) Economic & philosophic manuscripts of 1844. Progress Publishers, Moscow
23. Marx K (1977) Capital: a critique of political economy, vol 1. Vintage Books, New York
24. Lektorsky VA (1980) Subject, object, cognition. Progress Publishers, Moscow
25. Spitz RA (1946) Anaclitic depression: an inquiry into the genesis of psychiatric conditions in early childhood. Psychoanal Study Child 2:313–342
26. Harlow HF (1958) The nature of love. Am Psychol 13:673–685
27. Kandel ER, Jessel TM, Sanes JR (2000) Sensory experience and the fine-tuning of synaptic connections. In: Kandel ER, Schwartz JH, Jessel TM (eds) Principles of neural science, 4th edn. McGraw-Hill, New York, pp 1115–1130
28. Nelson CA III, Bos K, Gunnar MR, Sonuga-Barke EJS (2011) The neurobiological toll of early human deprivation. Monogr Soc Res Child Dev 76(4):127–146
29. Dunbar RIM (1992) Neocortex size as a constraint on group size in primates. J Hum Evol 20:469–493
30. Byrne RW, Whiten A (1988) Machiavellian intelligence: social expertise and the evolution of intellect in monkeys, apes and humans. Clarendon Press, Oxford

Chapter 10
Acquisition of Theory of Mind, Language, and Social Cognition

10.1 Introduction

Humans are social beings that need to interact with each other for survival, and their success in such interactions is highly dependent on mental functions as language, theory of mind, empathy, and social cognition. "Social cognition" is a comprehensive term for a set of motivational, affective, and cognitive processes which allow us to manage complex social situations in relationship with other persons [1]. The terms "emotional intelligence," "social intelligence," and "Machiavellian intelligence" refer to the capacity to solve problems specifically in the social domain by manipulating or deceiving other people or cunningly cooperating with them in order to achieve individual benefits [2–4]. These higher mental functions have as prerequisite and most basic component the theory of mind (ToM), the ability to "read" the mind of others, attributing to them perceptions, desires, intentions, and thoughts. ToM and language are learned simultaneously by the child in joint practice with adults in tasks and plays. ToM is, in fact, a prerequisite for the child, later on, to deal with the reciprocal images or conceptions each interlocutor (speaker and listener) has of his/her own position (or intention) and of that of the other, to learn the conversational rules (e.g., to follow the topic, to respect the turn of the interlocutor), in this way mastering the discursive, particularly argumentative, use of language (e.g., in conversations). In this "language game" (concept introduced by Wittgenstein; [5]), with argumentations and counter-argumentations for defending its points of view against that of others, the child develops the logical and discursive matrix of its thinking and the capacity for reflection and decision-making. The acquisition of all these higher mental functions is accompanied by the development of the tertiary associative neocortex, particularly of prefrontal-temporal-parietal networks.

B. Damasceno, *Research on Cognition Disorders*,
https://doi.org/10.1007/978-3-030-57267-9_10

10.2 Development of Theory of Mind, Empathy, and Social Cognition

Theory of mind (ToM) is considered as a "theory" because it explains mental states that are not directly observable and can foresee what is going to happen in the future, particularly regarding behavior of other individuals. ToM, also called "mindreading" and "mentalizing," is our ability to interpret the behavior of other individuals, attribute mental states to them, make inferences about their intentions, desires, and beliefs and, based on this knowledge, predict their actions and interact with them accordingly. It is a complex mental function, crucial for social interactions between individuals, and comprises two components: the *cognitive*, for inferring the mental state of the counterpart, his/her perceptions, intentions, pretenses, thoughts, and beliefs; and the *affective* or *empathic*, for recognizing and sharing the feelings of another person. The empathic ToM requires the *emotional self-regulation* for control of shared explicit emotions, for inhibiting or facilitating expression of empathic reactions, thus allowing the individual to show a more socially appropriate and acceptable attitude toward other people in daily life functioning [6, 7]. The loss of empathic self-regulation may be illustrated with the case BLR. This 31-year-old female lawyer got an acute herpes simplex virus encephalitis in November 2013 with convulsions and coma, followed by disinhibited behavior and mild amnesia. MRI (January 2014) and SPECT tomography (February 2014) then showed lesion and hypoperfusion bilaterally (with left predominance) in temporal medial and frontal medial-posterior regions. At the last neuropsychological evaluation in November 2017, what remained as sequela was an exacerbated empathy and a very mild verbal amnesia. She had become more conscientious and affectionate with other people, trying to help them but in an exaggerated way that required her mother to control her.

In the ontogenetic development of ToM, the first step is the mental construction of the object as existing outside and independent of the subject (objectively) and the recognition of himself as separated from the others, which are conceived as distinct individuals. At the same time, the child perceives similarities in himself and others, thus recognizing himself and others as intentional beings. This is a precondition for the child, further on (after 9 months age), to engage himself in joint attention activities with others establishing a triadic relationship with the other individual (adult) and the object of their attention, and coordinating their interactions, for example, the child sees a toy and sees that his mother also sees it [8].

Next stage in the development of ToM (after 18 months age) is pretense play, which requires the ability to uncouple simulation from reality, for example, when the child holds a banana in the hand nearby its ear, pretending it is a telephone [9]. Then, between 3 and 4 years age, the child becomes able to understand that others can have beliefs or false beliefs [10]. In false belief tests, the subject (child) is able to infer that another person may have a wrong (false) belief, different from its own. For example, in Sally and Anne story, Sally puts an object in a place in the presence of Anne and goes out from the stage scenery. Anne changes the place of the object, while Sally was out. Sally comes back to the stage, and, then, the examiner asks the child "where Sally thinks the object is placed." This is called "*first-order ToM*."

Later on, between 6 and 7 years age, the child begins to understand that the other person can also represent the mental state of other persons [11]. In this stage, the child can make inferences not only on the belief a person has about an event in the world but also on the belief this person has about the belief of another person concerning this world event. This is the "*second-order ToM*."

The cerebral organization of ToM is not well established, but there is enough neuropsychological and functional neuroimaging evidence that it is carried out by a widespread brain network comprising as core regions the ventromedial prefrontal, orbitofrontal cortex, temporal poles, temporoparietal junction, and adjacent posterior part of superior temporal sulcus [12–16]. Even the amygdala [17] and basal ganglia [18] seem to be involved, particularly in the affective component of ToM. A brain network comprising the dorsolateral and ventromedial prefrontal cortex, including rostral anterior cingulate cortex, and amygdala has been shown to be crucial for regulation of emotion and modulation of the expression of empathy [7, 13, 19].

In most neuropsychological studies, patients with frontotemporal degeneration (FTD) or delimited frontal lesions are impaired on typical ToM tasks such as first- and second-order false belief and *faux pas* detection. However, (1) these studies are limited by lack of precise lesion location, and most patients suffered head trauma, which is often associated with a rather diffuse brain damage, and (2) there are well-documented cases with extensive bilateral prefrontal lesions which do not impair performance on ToM tasks, for example, case GT (with bilateral anterior artery infarction) reported by Bird et al. [20] and some of our bifrontal and FTD cases [16]. There could be some plausible explanations for these negative cases: (1) ToM, as a high-level mental function (consciousness of self and other) requires a so widespread brain network that others of its parts (in connection with the frontal regions) remained intact, being sufficient for its functional integrity; (2) a postlesional recovery of function could play a role; and (3) the ToM tasks employed do not evaluate what they are intended to do.

10.3 Acquisition of Language

According to Kuhl [21], the development of oral language (speech production) goes through five distinct phases, independently of the culture: *cooing*, with sounds similar to vowels (1–4 months); *babbling*, producing series of consonant-vowel syllables, such as "mamamama" (5–10 months); *first words* (10–15 months); *utterances of two words* meaningfully combined (18–24 months); and *meaningful speech* with sentences of three or more words (15 months and beyond). Early social and linguistic interaction with adults is necessary for the cooing (universally similar) to give rise to determined mother language.

In the acquisition of its cognitive functions and practical abilities, the child not only learns by imitation the actions of others but also appropriates their language ("verbal instructions") during plays and tasks. When the mother holds her child's hand, which is holding the spoon, and helps manipulate the spoon with the proper movements, she uses words to name objects and actions, such as "spoon," "catch," "food," "put," and "in the mouth." In this way, as the child learns to master the correct use of the spoon, the concept of spoon is constructed in its mind and brain and is semantically codified with the word "spoon" as a category of objects and as a practical schema which represents the interactions between subject, instrument, and object. Thanks to the word, purely relational and functional characteristics of abstract concepts (such as "corruption" and "treachery"), devoid of physical materiality, gain a kind of material life and have an effect on the individual with the same strength as that of real material things.

Luria [22] pointed out that "the word is a nucleus of a complex semantic system..." The word represents a network of relations and meanings which constitute the multivariate matrix of logical and discursive thought, allowing us to think in a dynamic, quasi-automatic, and relatively easy way. This could be illustrated with the word "buy," which in itself, as an isolated phonological entity (pronounced *bai*) has no sense, but gets its real meaning in the exchange of values between at least two persons, comprising the following main components: who buys (the subject, the buyer), what (the object), from whom (the seller), and for how much (the price). The sequential components of the linearly expressed sentence (e.g., "I buy a book from a friend for U$ 250"; Fig. 10.1) have dependency relationships between each other, as a kind of implicit syntactic memory [called "syntagmatic relations" by Saussure [23], and each component constitutes a class of elements which can occupy the same point of the syntagmatic chain (e.g., "a store," or "a smuggler," or "a friend") and commute or substitute one for another (Saussure's "paradigmatic correlations"), in this way changing the sense of the whole sentence or narrative and giving it different connotations, some of which with social and legal consequences.

The learning and understanding of these characteristics of the word and concept require a complex cooperation of various cognitive processes (perception, memory, social cognition, language, heuristics, etc.), which in the child parallels the development of the tertiary associative cerebral cortex.

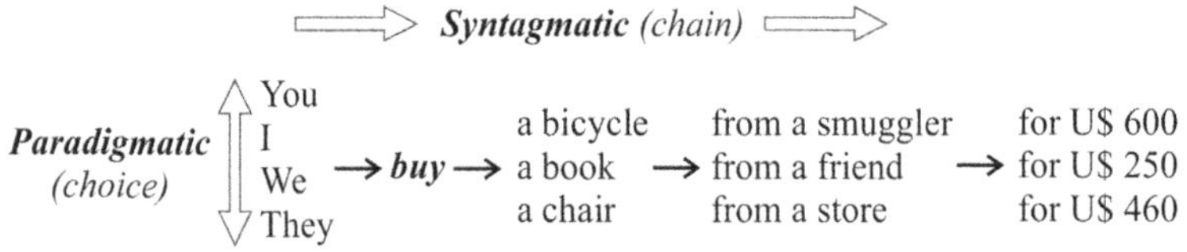

Fig. 10.1 Syntagmatic and paradigmatic relations between words

10.3.1 Development of the Regulatory Function of Language and of Logical and Discursive Reasoning

The second peak of cortical prefrontal development, around 6–7 years of age, is related to the increasing regulatory role of language in the organization of complex programs and in the autoregulation of behavior. From 3 years of age on, the child starts to master sentences of increasing complexity, which are pronounced out loud (external language), particularly in problematic situations (so-called egocentric speech). Vygotsky [24] showed how the use of external speech helps the child in its active effort to solve such situations. Initially, verbalization consists in the description and analysis of the situation, gradually acquiring the character of "planning," expressing possible ways for solving the problem.

As the child continues experiencing new situations from 4 through 6–7 years of age, its external speech starts internalizing more and more, becoming mental, internal speech, which is condensed in its form and predicative in its content. In this way, the child appropriates a powerful instrument that make possible for it to regulate (plan, monitor, correct) its own activity as well as that of others. On the other hand, by mediating the relations of the individual with other persons and with itself, language makes possible the control of the individual's point of view, actions, and behaviors by society's dominant mode of production, culture, and ideology.

In this period, with the acquisition of internal language, takes place the mental (re)construction of external objects, phenomena, and relationships according to an exclusively human system of values, as well as the transformation of natural psychological functions (which we share with other animals) into higher-level cultural psychological functions, whose cerebral counterpart is the development of the most recent, specifically human regions of the tertiary associative cortex (particularly prefrontal and parietotemporal junction) and its interconnections in both hemispheres.

After 6–7 years of age, the tertiary cortical zones continue their development until at least adolescence, probably by forming new interneuronal connections, which constitute the neural substrate of more complex cognitive processes, as the reasoning on the basis of logical-grammatical and logical-formal operations, reflection, and moral judgment. Language plays here a relevant and decisive role. When we interact with other people by means of language, we always have determined objectives, and we act on others in order to influence them so that they react and behave as we wish. In real- life situations, language use is essentially argumentative, especially in discussions in which the child has to defend its points of view against the opposition of others and have to adjust its arguments to theirs, and, in this way, the child learns to consciously use conjunctions (Ducrot's "argumentative operators" [25]), such as "but," "otherwise," "because," "if," "although," "however," "therefore," "since," etc. On the one hand, conjunctions contribute to the construction of the logical and discursive matrix of thinking, by establishing relations between propositions and ideas. On the other hand, the internalization (appropriation) of argumentations and counter-argumentations of the others by the child give rise to its capacity for reflection and decision-making. Reflection is actually an inner (mental) discussion, a chorus of internal "voices" and opinions of others.

In this manner, the child acquires new higher psychological functions and their corresponding brain functional systems. According to Leontiev [26], the formation of specifically human functional systems results from the mastering of instruments as well as of motor (external) and mental (internal) operations consolidated in the brain. Among the neurophysiological mechanisms making possible the dynamic consolidation of these operations in brain neural networks stand out the long-term potentiation and long-term depression, which promote the formation and disappearance of synapses in the pathways utilized in these operations [27, 28].

In the dialogs and discussions of everyday life, the child constitutes itself as a discursive and pragmatic subject, in spite of being in some way both heterogeneous and subjected. It is a heterogeneous subject, since its decision-making is not only its own but also results from the internalized opinions or "voices" of other subjects integrated in it, and it is subjected, to the extent that it is unconsciously influenced by the opinions, teachings, and advices of others and by the dominant ideology of the society in which it lives, having the delusion that it is the only source of what it says or decides, when in reality it assumes preexistent meanings and points of view of others [29–31]. For Orlandi [31], this delusion is not a "defect" but a necessity for the language to function in the subjects and in the production of meanings. When the subjects "forget" that what they say has already been said before them, they identify themselves with what they say, and in this way, they constitute themselves as the only subjects.

In the discursive "language game," with argumentations and counter-argumentations, the child learns the conversational rules (e.g., having to observe and follow the relevant topic and to respect the turn of the interlocutor, etc.) and how to establish own strategies and to handle "imaginary formations" [32], that is, the images or conceptions the speaker and the listener have of their own position and of the position of the other. A cognitive prerequisite for the child to learn and master these imaginary formations is the acquisition of a "theory of mind" or "mindreading" ability. Positions of speaker and listener may be symmetric, when they have equal social roles, as in everyday informal conversation among students of the same school degree, or asymmetric, when they have different social power, for example, as among employer and employee, factory director and laborer, teacher and pupil, and father and son.

Osakabe [33] has summarized the imaginary formations involved in discourse as follows: (1) *What conception do I have of the listener for me to talk to him the way I do?* (2) *What conception I think the listener has towards me, for me to talk to him the way I do?* (3) *What conception do I have of the referent for talking to him the way I do?* (4) *What conception I think the listener has about the referent for me to talk to him the way I do?* Based on the theory of "language game" [5] and "speech acts" [34, 35], Osakabe has added another fundamental imaginary formation, which refers to the influence ("performative" or "perlocutionary" act) that the speaker intend to have on the listener, namely, (5) *What effect do I intend to have on the listener for talking to him the way I do?* A perlocutionary speech act may have as aim, for example, to convince or persuade the interlocutor.

The reciprocal images and strategies involved in discourse, even in everyday conversation, require their online processing in working memory, with a sophisticated ability to activate and deactivate their underlying mental operations on the basis of a precise and rapid reversibility and commutation of excitatory and inhibitory brain processes. The cerebral counterpart of these higher mental functions should be the tertiary associative cortex, particularly that of prefrontal region. This region, in connection with the tertiary temporal-parietal cortices, seems to be the best equipped for performing these higher functions, since it has multimodal and pluripotential neurons playing key roles in working memory, planning and sequencing of actions and events [36–38], monitoring and correcting the task or activity as a whole, particularly in new or problematic situations [39], and in decision-making [40, 41]. Prefrontal regions are crucial in social-interactional and discursive-pragmatic contexts, in which the interpretative clues provided by the interlocutor and the presuppositions and implicatures change continually [42]. Thus, the acquisition of higher cortical functions depends on the activity of the subject, its social and linguistic-discursive interaction, both in the case of a child that learn to use a spoon or to say the first words, and of an adult (even elderly) that learns to drive a car or to speak a new idiom. The brain substrates of these abilities are complex neurofunctional systems, whose dynamics and flexibility correspond to the changeability of the "being of man," of its forms of material and social practices. These systems are characterized by the constancy of their objectives (final results that satisfy determined need and motivation) and by the variability (internal mobility) of their constituent methods and operations, permitting functional reorganizations both in the normal ontogenetic development and in the reconstruction of higher mental functions after brain damage.

10.4 Conclusion

Social cognition is a set of thought processes that make possible for the individual to understand itself, others, and the social environment. Its most basic component is the "theory of mind" (ToM) or "mindreading," the ability to interpret behavior of others, to make inferences about their intentions, desires, and beliefs (its cognitive component) as well as to recognize and share their feelings (its empathic component) and, based on this knowledge, to interact with them accordingly. One of its highest levels is Machiavellian intelligence, the ability to manipulate or deceive other people or cunningly cooperate with them for achieving individual benefits. Ontogenetically, ToM starts with the mental construction of the object, recognition of others as intentional beings (engaging with them in joint attention activities), pretense play, and then becoming aware that others have beliefs and false beliefs (first order ToM), and later on, understanding that another person can also represent the mental state of other persons (second order ToM). ToM is carried out by a large-scale brain network comprising as core regions the ventromedial and orbitofrontal cortex, temporal poles, temporoparietal junction, and adjacent posterior temporal sulcus. Another network interconnecting dorsolateral and ventromedial prefrontal cortex with amygdala seems to be crucial for regulation of emotion and modulation of the expression of empathy.

The development of ToM accompanies that of oral language, which starts with cooing and babbling (1–10 months), and then (10–15 months and beyond) with the first words and meaningful sentences. Language is acquired in the joint practice with adults in tasks and plays, in which the child imitates the actions of the adults and appropriates their words for naming and mentally constructing the concepts of those objects, instruments, and actions. First, from 3 years of age on, language is external, spoken out loud, especially in problematic situations. Then, from 4 to 7 years, corresponding to the second peak of cortical growth, it becomes internal, constituting a powerful instrument for the child to organize and regulate its own activity and behavior, as well as those of others. In discussions with adults, the child needs to argue for defending its points of view against those of others, in this way learning the conversational rules and the use of conjunctions. In this social interaction mediated by language, the child constructs the logical and discursive matrix of its thinking and, by internalizing argumentations and counter-argumentations, develops its capacity for reflection, moral judgment, and decision-making. The cerebral counterpart of these high-level mental acquisitions is the development of the specifically human regions of the tertiary associative cortex, particularly prefrontal and parietotemporal junction and their interconnections in both hemispheres.

References

1. Frith CD (2008) Social cognition. Philos Trans R Soc B 363:2033–2039
2. Humphrey NK (1976) The social function of intellect. In: Bateson PPG, Hinde RA (eds) Growing points in ethology. Cambridge University Press, Cambridge
3. Byrne R (1995) The thinking ape: evolutionary origins of intelligence. Oxford University Press, Oxford
4. Whiten A, Byrne RW (eds) (1997) Machiavellian intelligence II: extensions and evaluations. Cambridge University Press, Cambridge
5. Wittgenstein L (1958) Philosophical investigations. Macmillan, New York
6. Eres R, Molenberghes P (2013) The influence of group membership on the neural correlates involved in empathy. Front Hum Neurosci. https://doi.org/10.3389/fnhum.2013.00176
7. Decety J (2011) Dissecting the neural mechanisms mediating empathy. Emot Rev 3:92–108
8. Tomasello M (1999) The cultural origins of human cognition. Harvard University Press, Cambridge, MA
9. Leslie AM (1987) Pretense and representation: the origins of "theory of mind". Psychol Rev 94(4):412–426
10. Wimmer H, Perner J (1983) Beliefs about beliefs: representation and constraining function of wrong beliefs in young children's understanding of deception. Cognition 13:103–128
11. Perner J, Wimmer H (1985) "John thinks that Mary thinks that..." attribution of second-order beliefs by 5- to 10-year-old children. J Exp Child Psychol 39(3):437–471

12. Stuss DT, Gallup GG, Alexander MP (2001) The frontal lobes are necessary for 'theory of mind'. Brain 124:279–286
13. Amodio DM, Frith CD (2006) Meeting of minds: the medial frontal cortex and social cognition. Nat Rev Neurosci 7:268–277
14. Saxe R, Carey S, Kanwisher N (2004) Understanding other minds: linking developmental psychology and functional neuroimaging. Annu Rev Psychol 55:87–124
15. Carrington SJ, Bailey AJ (2009) Are there theory of mind regions in the brain? A review of the neuroimaging literature. Hum Brain Mapp 30:2313–2335
16. Igliori G, Damasceno BP (2006) Theory of mind and the frontal lobes. Arq Neuropsiquiatr 64:202–206
17. Fine C, Lumsden J, Blair RJR (2001) Dissociation between "theory of mind" and executive functions in a patient with early left amygdala damage. Brain 124:287–298
18. Bodden ME, Kübler D, Knake S, Menzler K, Heverhagen JT, Sommer J, Kalbe E, Krach S, Dodel R (2013) Comparing the neural correlates of affective and cognitive theory of mind using fMRI: involvement of the basal ganglia in affective theory of mind. Adv Cogn Psychol 9(1):32–43
19. Morawetz C, Bode S, Derntl B, Heekeren HR (2016) The effect of strategies, goals and stimulus material on the neural mechanisms of emotion regulation: a meta-analysis of fMRI studies. Neurosci Biobehav Rev 72:111–128. https://doi.org/10.1016/j.neubiorev.2016.11.014
20. Bird CM, Castelli F, Malik O, Frith U, Husain M (2004) The impact of extensive medial frontal lobe damage on "theory of mind" and cognition. Brain 127:914–928
21. Kuhl PK (2000) Language, mind, and brain: experience alters perception. In: Gazzaniga MS (ed) The new cognitive neurosciences. The MIT Press, Cambridge, pp 99–115
22. Luria AR (1973) Towards the mechanisms of naming disturbance. Neuropsychologia 11:417–421
23. Saussure F (1916) Cours de linguistique générale. Charles Bally & Albert Sechehaye Editors, Paris/Lausana
24. Vygotsky LS (1978) Mind in society: the development of higher psychological processes. Harvard University Press, Cambridge
25. Ducrot O (1972) Dire et ne pas dire: principes de sémantique linguistique. Hermann Editors, Paris
26. Leontiev AN (1981) Problems of the development of the mind. Progress Publishers, Moscow
27. Katz LC, Shatz CJ (1996) Synaptic activity and the construction of cortical circuits. Science 274:1133–1138
28. Beggs JM, Brown TH, Byrne JH, Crow T, LeDoux JE, LeBar K, Thompson RF (1999) Learning and memory: basic mechanisms. In: Zigmond MJ, Bloom FE, Landis SC, Roberts JL, Squire LR (eds) Fundamental neuroscience. Academic, San Diego, pp 1411–1454
29. Bakhtin MM (1986) Marxism and the philosophy of language. Harvard University Press, Cambridge, MA
30. Ducrot O (1984) Le Dire et le Dit. Les Éditiones de Minuit, Paris
31. Orlandi EP (2005) Análise de discurso: princípios e procedimentos. Pontes, São Paulo (in Portuguese)
32. Pêcheux M (1969) Analyse automatique du discours. Dunod, Paris
33. Osakabe H (1999) Argumentação e discurso político, 2nd edn. Martins Fontes, São Paulo (in Portuguese)
34. Austin JL (1975) How to do things with words. Urmson JO, Sbisà M (eds). Harvard University Press, Cambridge
35. Searle JR (1969) Speech acts: an essay in the philosophy of language. Cambridge University Press, Cambridge
36. Fuster JM (1989) The prefrontal cortex: anatomy, physiology, and neuropsychology of the frontal lobe, 2nd edn. Raven Press, New York

37. Baddeley A, Della Sala S (1998) Working memory and executive control. In: Roberts AC, Robbins TW, Weiskrantz L (eds) The prefrontal cortex: executive and cognitive function. Oxford University Press, New York, pp 9–21
38. Shallice T, Burgess P (1998) The domain of supervisory processes and the temporal organization of behavior. In: Roberts AC, Robbins TW, Weiskrantz L (eds) The prefrontal cortex: executive and cognitive function. Oxford University Press, New York, pp 22–35
39. Luria AR (1966/1980) Higher cortical functions in man, 2nd edn. Basic Books, New York
40. Damasio AR (1996) Human neuroanatomy relevant to decision-making. In: Damasio AR, Damasio H, Christen Y (eds) Neurobiology of decision-making. Springer, Berlin, pp 1–12
41. Adolphs R, Tranel D, Bechara A, Damasio H, Damasio AR (1996) Neuropsychological approaches to reasoning and decision-making. In: Damasio AR, Damasio H, Christen Y (eds) Neurobiology of decision-making. Springer, Berlin, pp 157–179
42. Damasceno BP (1995) Neuropsychology of discursive-pragmatic activity in subjects with frontal lesions. In: Damasceno BP, Coudry MIH (eds) Topics in neuropsychology and neurolinguistics, Neuropsychology series. Tec Art, São Paulo (in Portuguese)

Part III
Neuropsychological Investigation: Methodological Issues

Chapter 11
Systemic Approach and the Problem of Reciprocal Influences of Mental Functions on Each Other

11.1 Introduction

Neuropsycology, Neuropsychiatry, Behavioral Neurology, and Cognitive Neuroscience are interdisciplinary sciences whose object of study are the mental changes associated to brain dysfunctions. Their methods include psychological tests in combination with one or more of the following technical procedures: electroencephalography, event-related potentials, cortical electrical stimulation or transcranial magnetic stimulation, structural and functional neuroimaging with computerized tomography (CT), single-photon emission computerized tomography (SPECT), positron emission tomography (PET), and functional magnetic resonance (fMRI).

The main objectives of a neuropsychological investigation are (1) analysis of the patient's symptoms by means of a comprehensive and deepened interview complemented by appropriate psychological and cognitive tests searching for double dissociations which could contribute to detect the basic mechanism (mental operation) that is impaired and thus to diagnose the local or regional distribution of the brain dysfunction or lesion; (2) to yield a baseline and profile of psychological and cognitive disturbances for future comparisons, particularly in clinical trials (e.g., in testing new drugs, surgical interventions, or rehabilitation programs) or simply for following-up the evolution of the syndrome and come to a safer differential diagnosis of the disease; and (3) in forensic neuropsychology, to predict the functional relationship between the patient's performance in neuropsychological tests and his behavior in real-world settings, thus providing answers to legal matters (as requested by legal agents, judges, prosecutors, attorneys), for example, in issues such as suspect malingering (simulation), responsibility for a crime, and mental capacity to stand a trial. This last objective is outside the scope of this book. It is the most challenging, requiring the examiner has qualification and expertise in forensic psychology and clinical neuropsychology for determining whether or not there is a causal relation between the diagnosed brain dysfunction and the specific legal issue (e.g., misbehavior or criminal act). For attaining this goal, a thorough neuropsychological

B. Damasceno, *Research on Cognition Disorders*,
https://doi.org/10.1007/978-3-030-57267-9_11

assessment is needed, employing norm-based tests for covering a large range of cognitive functions, besides evaluating personality, emotional adjustment, and academic achievement and including multiple measures of a specific cognitive function in order to determine consistency of performance.

This book focuses mainly on the first objective, the clinical neuropsychological analysis. Although magnetic resonance imaging (MRI) may quickly and accurately localize the brain damage, conventional MRI may not show signs of lesion where the neuropsychological analysis indicates there is a dysfunction, for example, in the first hours of an acute ischemic stroke manifested as Wernicke's aphasia or in the early phase of Alzheimer's disease presenting evident impairment of retrieval and recognition of word list suggestive of an entorhinal-hippocampal degenerative lesion.

11.2 Systemic Approach

In the neurological examination, the analysis and interpretation of sensory-motor symptoms and signs are straightforward. The findings of hemiparesis, hemihypesthesia, hemianopsia, and hemispatial neglect indicate lesion in their respective contralateral projection pathways, primary cortical areas, or neighboring regions. Neuropsychological investigation, on the other hand, is always a challenge, since it deals with complex, mutually interrelated and inter-influencing mental and cognitive functions (perception, attention, visual-spatial-motor skills, memory, language, intellectual reasoning, motivation, mood), whose psychological structure and cerebral organization change continuously as each set of mental actions or operations goes on replacing one with another, in a reversible and transitive way, during the execution of any experimental or real-life task. At the symptom level, there can also be reciprocal influences between the patient's cognitive dysfunction and insomnia, fatigue, depression, and undesirable side effects of drugs (caused by antihistamines, anticholinergics, anticonvulsants, tricyclic antidepressants, or benzodiazepines). The clinical neuropsychological analysis has to disclose which of these symptoms or problems is primarily leading to the others. In this regard, a careful and thorough medical history of each of these problems would be needed. For example, insomnia and next day tiredness and drowsiness, due to bad sleep hygiene, chronic pain, restless legs, or drug side effect, can cause cognitive dysfunction and fatigue. The deleterious effect of depression and fatigue on cognitive performance is well-known. Cognitive dysfunction in its turn can cause social-occupational disability, which consequently leads to reactive depressive symptoms. The end result is a vicious circle that worsens the patient's quality of life.

Evaluation, analysis, and interpretation of mental and cognitive syndromes are based on at least three fundamental principles proposed by Luria [1] and Mesulam [2]:

1. Each brain region, particularly those in convergence zones or "hubs" (e.g., prefrontal, inferior parietal, medial temporal), contains the neural substratum (basic

operation) of different complex functions or tasks, thus contributing and belonging to the various partly overlapped neuronal networks that underlie each of these functions or tasks. The left inferior parietal region (Brodmann's area 39), for example, contributes with a basic operation, namely, "spatial reasoning," which is required for execution of different tasks, such as chess game, reproduction of a model by means of multicolored cubes (e.g., in Kohs block design test), construction of a chair by assembling its parts, orientation to right or left in a street or in the own body, subtraction of 14 from 41, and understanding of logical-grammatical structures as in sentences containing relational or comparative expressions (e.g., "the brother's father," "below," "between," "before," "taller than," "bigger than," "more than"), inverted grammatical constructions ("I had breakfast after I had sawed the wood – what did I do first?") or embedded relative clauses ("the woman who worked at the factory came to the school where Margaret studied to give her a birthday gift"). All these tasks require spatial reasoning either in the concrete-physical or in the abstract-symbolic level.

2. Consequently, lesion limited to a particular associative cortical brain region, as in the left inferior-posterior parietal region, leads to impairment of multiple complex functions or tasks, producing, not an isolated symptom, but a whole neuropsychological *syndrome* including right-left or geographical disorientation, constructive apraxia, acalculia, difficulties to understand sentences with complex logical-grammatical structure (Luria's semantic aphasia), and, secondarily, deficit of intellectual operations in space, as in checkers or chess game.
3. Different components or basic operations involved in a complex function or task (e.g., problem solving) can be impaired by lesions in their corresponding brain regions or interconnecting pathways. Problem-solving, for instance, requires understanding of the verbal statement of the problem (in left hemisphere language regions); short-term operational memory, planning, hypothesis testing, monitoring, and correcting (in prefrontal cortices); arithmetical and spatial reasoning (in inferior-posterior parietal zones); and long-term memory (in entorhinal-hippocampal structures). Damage to any of these regions may disturb problem-solving, but in different ways, with each local lesion leading to different syndrome profiles, depending on which basic operation is impaired. Thus, the problem-solving disorder may be due to a primary operational memory or intellectual-executive deficit or be secondary to an aphasia, poor spatial reasoning, or amnesia.

In order to disclose which basic component and, by inference, which brain region is dysfunctional, the neuropsychological evaluation has to employ a comprehensive battery of appropriate tests as well as control conditions and control tasks. The selection of the tests is based on their accuracy to evaluate and measure the hypothetical components involved in the complex task. A crucial *control condition* is the comparison of the patient's test performance with that of healthy individuals matched to the patient as for influential variables, such as age, sex, and educational level. This comparison is necessary for ascribing the patient's inferior performance to his brain lesion.

The problem is that the patient's inferior performance may be due to more widespread or diffuse disturbances (depression, fatigue, drowsiness) other than the supposedly malfunctioning basic component (be it spatial reasoning, memory recall, or recognition). The influence of these diffuse variables has to be controlled, minimized, or eliminated. If not possible doing this, the magnitude of their influence on the results of the research has to be statistically analyzed as covariants. Besides this, the poor scores on a task of episodic verbal or visual-spatial memory (using word list, series of figures, or spatial positions of items) could be due to impairment of some other component relevant to the learning task (e.g., auditory or visual perception, attention, verbal fluency) and not to a primary disorder of episodic memory. Therefore, all other variables that are relevant to the execution of the memory task have to be assessed by means of appropriate *control tests* (counterproofs), for instance, Poppelreuter's overlapping figs [1] or form discrimination test [3] for visual perception; "A" Random Letter Test [4] or WAIS-R digit span [5] for attention; FAS or category (animals) for verbal fluency [6]; Beck's Depression Inventory [7] for mood; and Fatigue Severity Scale [8] for fatigue. The use of multiple tests may yield a pattern of multiple dissociations between tests, thus contributing to disclose the nature of cognitive deficits in brain lesion patients [9].

11.3 Single and Double Dissociations

In neuropsychology, the term "dissociation" means that a function X and another function Y are in some way functionally dissociated, independent, or separated, without referring to any loss of association between two brain regions. As an example, a lesion in brain region A (e.g., left posterior-inferior frontal cortex) can disrupt function X (speech production) but not function Y (language comprehension). In this case, we have a *single dissociation* between these two functions. This single dissociation is, for instance, found in patients with lesion in the left posterior-inferior frontal cortex (Broca's area) and Broca's aphasia, presenting difficult, effortful, stuttering, telegraphic spontaneous speech, with a grammatical errors, but normal comprehension. In the single dissociation, it cannot be inferred that functions X and Y depend on different basic operations or brain regions, since it may simply be that function X is more difficult than function Y, requiring more "cognitive resources" [10]. In order to draw safer conclusions on brain localization of syndromes or basic operations, it is necessary to find another patient with brain lesion in another region B with the reverse condition, that is, impaired function Y (language comprehension) but normal function X (speech production). This was what Karl Wernicke [11] found in patients with lesions in the left posterior-superior temporal gyrus (Wernicke's area), showing normal, fluent, loquacious speech (though paraphasic), but very abnormal comprehension. Here we have the pioneering cases of *double dissociation* between brain functions, a concept introduced by Hans-Lukas Teuber [12] with the meaning that lesion to one brain area causes function X to be impaired, while function Y is normal, and lesion to another area causes function Y to be impaired, while function X is normal. The demonstration of double dissociation requires the evaluation of at least two individuals, one of them presenting a lesion in brain region A, and the other one, in region B, provided that they are matched for age, educational level, sex, and other influential variables.

Double dissociations can also be demonstrated in normal individuals by means of functional MRI studies using a paradigm with two different tasks, X and Y. In these subjects, execution of task X activates brain region A but not B, the reverse occurring during the execution of task Y. Based on this finding, we can conclude that these two brain regions (A and B) and the two tasks (X and Y) are functionally different and in some way dissociated [13]. Here the degree and distribution of activation are also influenced by age, education, sex, polyglotism, and other variables, depending on the cognitive function tested.

The demonstration of double dissociations is a difficult task, be it in cases with brain damage or normal subjects. For example, in patients with medial temporal lobe epilepsy submitted to a pre-surgical evaluation of his/her epileptogenic focus, the detection of a double dissociation may contribute to a surgical decision. The challenge is to establish the side and local of the temporal lobe dysfunction based only on the results of the neuropsychological tests which are chosen based on the functional difference between the two temporal lobes, according to the so-called material-specific memory model, with the left one (dominant) mediating memory for verbal and the right one for nonverbal material. The problem is that there are cases with impairment of nonverbal memory after left hippocampal sclerosis and left anterior temporal resection [14] and of verbal memory after right temporal lobe resection [15].

11.4 Conclusion

A neuropsychological investigation may aim (1) to analyze the patient's symptoms and performance by means of a thorough interview and comprehensive cognitive and behavioral testing in order to detect impaired basic mental mechanisms and their underlying brain lesions; (2) to yield a baseline or profile of psychological and cognitive disturbances for future comparisons; and (3) in forensic neuropsychology, to predict the patient's behavior in real-world situations based on his/her performance in neuropsychological tests. Here we focus on the first objective. Neuropsychological investigation adopts a systemic approach considering that the mental functions (perception, attention, memory, language, intellectual reasoning, motivation, mood) influence on each other during the execution of any task and that symptoms such as drowsiness, fatigue, anxiety, and depression also have an effect on cognitive performance. Neuropsychological inferences about localization or distribution of brain lesions are based on the following principles: (1) each associative cortical brain region, particularly the "hubs" (e.g., left inferior parietal), processes some basic mental operation (e.g., spatial reasoning) that is needed for accomplishing different complex functions or tasks (e.g., puzzle completion, construction with

Kohs blocks, subtraction of 14 from 41, chess game, and understanding of relational expressions as "brother's father", "less than"); (2) consequently, focal lesion in a particular associative cortical area (e.g., left inferior parietal) causes, not an isolated symptom, but a whole syndrome (e.g., constructive apraxia, acalculia, semantic aphasia, etc.); and (3) diverse basic operations involved in a complex function or task (e.g., problem solving) can be impaired by lesion in any of their corresponding brain regions or interconnected pathways. Therefore, the diagnosis of a dysfunctional basic operation and respective brain lesion requires both control conditions (comparison of the patient's test performance with that of healthy matched individuals) and a comprehensive battery that includes control tests for task relevant functions (e.g., perception, attention, and language) in order to verify whether a patient's low scores in, for example, a word list learning task are due to deficit of attention, language, or to a primary impairment of episodic memory (hippocampal lesion).

References

1. Luria AR (1966/1980) Higher cortical functions in man, 2nd edn. Basic Books, New York
2. Mesulam M-M (1990) Large-scale neurocognitive networks and distributed processing for attention, language, and memory. Ann Neurol 28:597–613
3. Benton AL, Hamsher KS, Varney NR, Spreen O (1983) Contributions to neuropsychological assessment. Oxford University Press, New York
4. Strub RL, Black FW (2000) The mental status examination in neurology, 4th edn. F. A. Davis Company, Philadelphia
5. Wechsler D (1981) Wechsler adult intelligence scale – revised: manual. The Psychological Corporation, New York
6. Lezak MD (1995) Neuropsychological assessment, 3rd edn. Oxford University Press, New York
7. Beck AT (1987) Beck depression inventory. The Psychological Corporation, San Antonio
8. Krupp LB, LaRocca NG, Muir-Nash J, Steinberg AD (1989) The fatigue severity scale. Application to patients with multiple sclerosis and systemic lupus erythematosus. Arch Neurol 46:1121–1123
9. Russel EW (1984) Theory and developments of pattern analysis methods related to the Halstead-Reitan battery. In: Logue PE, Shear JM (eds) Clinical neuropsychology: a multidisciplinary approach. Charles C Thomas, Springfield, pp 50–98
10. Shallice T (1988) From neuropsychology to mental structure. Cambridge University Press, New York
11. Wernicke K (1874) Das Aphasiche Symptomenkomplex. Cohn & Weigart, Breslau
12. Teuber HL (1955) Physiological psychology. Annu Rev Psychol 6:267–296
13. Huettel SA, Song AW, McCarthy G (2004) Functional magnetic resonance imaging. Sinauer Associates, Inc, Sunderland
14. Glikmann-Johnston Y, Saling MM, Chen J, Cooper KA, Beare RJ, Reutens DC (2008) Structural and functional correlates of unilateral mesial temporal lobe spatial memory impairment. Brain 131:3006–3018
15. Gleissner U, Helmstaedter C, Schramm J, Elger CE (2002) Memory outcome after selective amygdalohippocampectomy: a study in 140 patients with temporal lobe epilepsy. Epilepsia 43(1):87–95

Chapter 12
Brain-Behavior Correlations

12.1 Introduction

Neuropsychological researches of lesion-behavior correlations commonly use a case-control design. In this framework, all cases should be homogeneous as regards the kind of lesion (e.g., all having an infarction in left inferior parietal region), and all cases and controls should be identical in all influential variables (e.g., age, gender, education) except in that which is being studied (the lesion). As regards the brain damage, it is very difficult to keep this homogeneity principle in the groups, since lesions caused by natural diseases, even in cases with the most well delimited ones (ischemic stroke), are never exactly alike in all subjects, since they vary from patient to patient concerning size, distribution, and mental-behavioral manifestations.

12.2 The Challenge of Disclosing and "Localizing" the Basic Defect Underlying a Syndrome

The interpretation of possible brain-behavior correlations is a challenging task. In Neurology, Neuropsychology, and Neuropsychiatry, a mental-cognitive-behavioral syndrome should not be interpreted straightforwardly as produced exclusively by the loss of the function supposedly performed by the damaged structure (by a "subtractive maneuver," in Fuster's terms [1], since the syndrome results from the interaction and combination of many other factors (Fig. 12.1): (1) *biological* (age, brain reserve, concomitant comorbidities, and possible side effect of drugs); (2) *psychosocial* (patient's current life circumstances regarding family relations, employment status, and work satisfaction; previous life history); (3) *psychological* (motivation, interest, humor state, and degree of preservation of the subject's personality); (4) *neuropsychological* (the systemic, dynamic and self-organizing character of

B. Damasceno, *Research on Cognition Disorders*,
https://doi.org/10.1007/978-3-030-57267-9_12

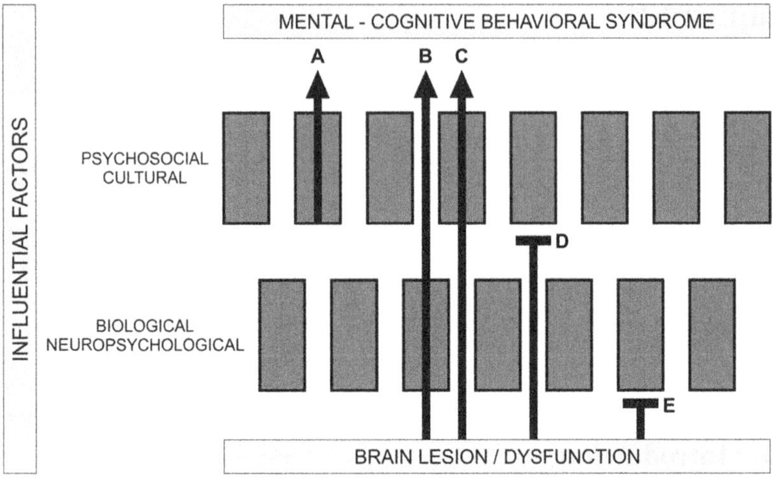

Fig. 12.1 Multifactorial genesis of mental-cognitive-behavioral syndromes (MCBS) in cases of brain lesion. Acute intense psychosocial stress alone (financial bankruptcy, family conflict, loss of a loved one) may cause MCBS, for example, a psychogenic amnesia (*A*). Psychosocial, cultural, biological, and neuropsychological factors may decrease, increase, or modulate the effect of a brain lesion (*B* and *C*) or even prevent it to manifest (*D* and *E*). [Modified from Damasceno BP. Basic neurological evaluation of organic psychosyndromes. In: Botega NJ (organizer), *Psychiatric practice in a general hospital*. Porto Alegre: Artmed, 2012, with permission] [4]

mental-cerebral functions; type and severity of the cognitive disturbance; degree of preservation of the regulatory function of language; and cognitive reserve, which depends on the educational and social-cultural level); and (5) *dysfunctions of other intact areas* interconnected with the damaged one, caused by immediate changes in neurotransmission, excitation-inhibition balance ("diaschisis" phenomenon of von Monakow [2], as well as changes in regional blood flow and cerebrospinal fluid dynamics, secondary axonal degeneration, possible septic complications, and mass effect of the lesion or non-intentional damage in neighboring structures [3].

Changes of excitation-inhibition balance and functional reorganization in other non-damaged structures also contribute to the resultant syndrome, since some of these structures normally activated or inhibited by the injured one are denervated, become respectively hypo- or hyperactive, and can in this way also produce symptoms. Another complicated issue is the continuous postlesional transformation of the clinical syndrome (Leischner's "syndromenwandel") [5] as a result of brain functional reorganization and recovery (plasticity), which depend on various factors, such as the individual's age and degree of handedness; nature, local, and size of the lesion; reduction of diaschisis and edema; revascularization; and functional rearrangement of neighboring, ipsilateral and contralateral non-damaged regions. For this reason, the age (duration) of the brain lesion has to be taken into account in research on cognitive disorders. Therefore, to localize a lesion even with high-resolution MRI does not imply in localizing in the same region the syndrome or, even less, the impaired or lost function.

In spite of the heterogeneity of the subjects in multiple cases or group studies and the complex nature of the neuropsychological syndrome, it is possible to disclose the basic or primary defect of a syndrome and to "localize" an isolated symptom. With this aim, we have at our disposal at least three methods:

1. A thorough neuropsychological assessment by means of a comprehensive battery of tests and appropriate counterproofs, with qualitative and quantitative analysis of the data. Illustratively, consider the task of detecting the primary defect of a patient's incapacity in solving the following arithmetic problem presented orally: "Anthony has 11 horses and Mary has 6 horses less than he has. How many horses do they have together?" (see in Fig. 6.2, the main cognitive components involved in its solution). The evaluation could use appropriate subtests of Luria's Neuropsychological Investigation (LNI) [6] and other batteries for testing the main mental-cognitive components, such as (1) level of attention and short-term memory [WMS digit span (verbal) and Corsi blocks (visual)]; (2) visual-spatial perception (LNI's subtests, Ratcliff's manikin test, and tests for mental rotation of figures); (3) receptive language (LNI's subtests for phonemic hearing, word comprehension, understanding of simple sentences, and logical-grammatical structures) and expressive language (word and sentence repetition, naming of objects and figures, verbal fluency, and narrative speech); (4) arithmetical skills (comprehension of number structure, arithmetical operations, including subtractions as 31 − 7, 41 − 14); (5) learning and memory (Rey auditory-verbal learning test comprising short-term or immediate recall, delayed recall and recognition; immediate and delayed recognition of series of abstract figures); (6) intellectual-executive functions (Kohs'multicolored cubes and/or Tower of London for intellectual operations in space; and verbal-discursive solving of arithmetical and non-arithmetical problems as, for example, "Antony is taller than John but shorter than Joe. Who is the shortest?" and "A man had to cross a river in a small canoe in order to carry to the other side a hen, a basket of corn and a fox. The canoe was only big enough to cross one thing at a time. If he carried the fox first, the hen would be with the corn and eat it all. If he carried the basket of corn first, the fox would be with the hen and eat it. How would the man bring all three things across the river?"

In the Kohs'test, the subject's performance is carefully observed in order to see whether he/she has difficulties with the spatial arrangement of the cubes (as often occur in cases of parietal-occipital lesions) or with the consecutive programming of the necessary steps, with monitoring of the execution or with verifying and comparing the end result with the model (frequent in cases of prefrontal lesions). As suggested by Luria [7], helping the subject in the execution of this test (with spatial or programming aids) will disclose which of the two difficulties predominates.

In the verbal-discursive solution of the arithmetical problem mentioned earlier, the subject is asked to say out loud how he/she is solving it (the steps and methods used), and the examiner takes note or record his/her answer. If the task is performed with difficulties, on the basis of trials and errors, he/she is asked concerning his/her understanding of the oral text ("Could you please repeat the problem I told you?",

"How many horses has Antony?", "How many horses has Mary?", "What does "less than" mean?", "What was the final question?"). If the subject has difficulties in memorizing or keeping online (in short-term working memory) all the data including the final question, the problem text is read to him/her again up to 3–5 times for him/her to repeat and solve. If yet unable, a written version of the problem is given to him/her to read out loud and solve. The use of this written form furnishes the subject a way to bypass difficulties with attention, short-term, and long-term (episodic) memory, and so he/she can tackle the problem with his/her intellectual-executive strategies and methods of solving it by orientating in the data, testing hypothesis, monitoring, and verifying the solution. With all these procedures, we have possibilities to disclose the subject's basic or primary defect.

2. "Localization" of an isolated symptom or specific deficit may be achieved by including in a group all patients with a specific symptom or deficit, superimposing the positions of their lesions as shown by neuroimaging, and looking for a "hot spot," that is, a local where all lesions overlap [8, 9]. The attempt to localize a lesion by means of MRI searching for a "hot spot" in a group of patients with determined cognitive deficit may result in error if they are not compared with control patients. A control group of patients with similar lesions but without that deficit is needed, since the overlay spot may be due to increased vulnerability of certain regions to the injury (e.g., due to their vasculature), without having any direct relation with the deficit of interest [10]. Dronkers' study of patients with apraxia of speech may illustrate this procedure [11, 12]. Twenty-five native English-speaking, right-handed and previously healthy patients had apraxia of speech after a single cerebral infarction in the left hemisphere. A reconstruction software could identify an area in the superior tip of the precentral gyrus of the insula where the lesions of all patients overlapped. In 19 control patients with nearly as large single infarctions in the left hemisphere but without apraxia of speech, the reconstruction software showed their lesions had spared that part of the insula (precentral gyrus) which was damaged in all patients with this syndrome (Fig. 12.2).

3. In group studies, statistical multivariate analysis after the data have been collected may determine the specific (independent) contribution of different variables to a single outcome. As previously discussed, a single outcome as, for instance, low episodic memory scores in patients with unilateral medial temporal lobe epilepsy and hippocampal atrophy may be influenced or caused by diverse factors (confounders) other than the epileptogenic focus or lesion, such as older age, educational level, depression, and attentional deficit. These confounding variables could have been eliminated in the planning phase of the study through randomization and matching, but after the data have been collected, in the analysis phase, a multivariate analysis reveals its strength in showing that, after adjusting for these confounders, the unilateral medial temporal lobe dysfunction has an independent contribution to the low memory scores. Thus, in this situation, by using a multivariate analysis (such as backward stepwise regression

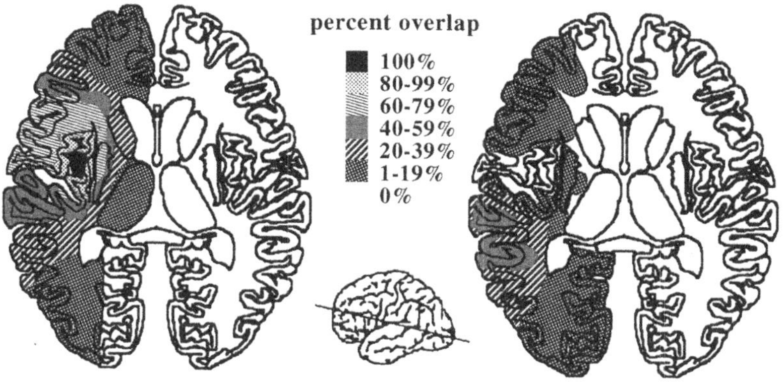

Fig. 12.2 Lesion overlapping in 25 patients with apraxia of speech (left) and 19 patients without this disorder (right). All of the 25 patients with apraxia of speech have a lesion encompassing a small section of the insula, as shown in black, while the lesions of the 19 patients without apraxia of speech completely spare the same area. (From Dronkers et al. 2000. In: M. S. Gazzaniga, editor, The New cognitive neurosciences, The MIT Press, with permission) [12]

or ANCOVA), we can demonstrate a primary, memory-specific impairment associated to that focal brain dysfunction.

12.3 Choosing Appropriate Neuropathological Cases and Methods for Valid Brain-Behavior Correlations

Brain lesions caused by natural diseases (infectious, neoplastic, degenerative, demyelinating, hypoxic, ischemic, traumatic) vary according to the degree of nervous tissue destruction and are often not well demarcated or limited to a precise region whose specific functional role one would like to investigate. Damasio and Damasio [13, 14] suggest following prerequisites for a valid brain-behavior correlation:

(1) To select and include appropriate neuropathological cases, the most suitable lesion types being ischemic strokes in chronic phase (more than 3 months old), followed by resolved herpes simplex virus encephalitis and neurosurgical ablation of tumor or epileptic focus
(2) To perform in the same period (with interval of days or week) the neuropsychological assessment and neuroimaging, gathering sufficient images for anatomical diagnosis
(3) To interpret the group data taking into account individual variations in neural-cognitive organization, age, gender, educational level, and other relevant characteristics of the subjects

In the chronic phase of a cerebral infarction (four or more months old), the area of abnormal signal seen on CT or MRI corresponds to actual (complete or partial) destruction of brain parenchyma, and the resultant syndrome has already evolved to a more stable phase, thus allowing safer brain-behavior correlations. Such correlations are difficult to establish in space-occupying lesions as hemorrhage and infiltrating tumors, in which the abnormal imaging area does contain functionally competent neurons and fibers.

In cases with surgical resection of an epileptic focus, brain-behavior correlations may be more problematic, particularly in those with bilateral or multifocal epileptogenic activity and long-standing seizures and in those with disorders of neuronal migration (cortical dysplasia, polymicrogyria). Preference should be given to cases with a consistently localized, unilateral medial temporal lobe epilepsy before the surgery and that have become seizure free after a well-delimited resection of the epileptogenic focus (medial temporal lobe removal or amygdalohippocampectomy).

Lesion-behavior mapping (LBM) by means of MRI has used two main methods: (1) by focusing on regions of interest (ROI method), which can only identify patterns within predefined brain regions and (2) by performing a voxel-by-voxel mapping of the entire brain, with an independent statistical test conducted for each voxel, thus revealing critical brain regions associated with determined deficit. Various voxelwise mapping methods have been developed, including Brain Vox [15], MRIcro [16], NPM [17], Anatomo-Clinical Overlapping Maps [18], and cortical surface-based analysis (FreeSurfer) [19]. In our laboratories of Neuropsychology and Neuroimaging (UNICAMP Clinics Hospital), we have used voxel-based morphometry (VBM) to correlate areas of brain atrophy to episodic and semantic memory performance in patients with amnestic mild cognitive impairment (aMCI), mild Alzheimer's disease, and normal controls [20–22] and FreeSurfer v5.1 for correlations between cognition, fatigue, and brain atrophy in multiple sclerosis patients [23, 24].

Structural MRI for lesion-behavior mapping presents at least two main limitations: (1) the modularity assumption that cognition is based on functional modules which have the same locations in different individuals, neglecting that they change their function in reaction to damage to one area and that in most cases the brain lesion is not limited to the boundaries of the underlying functional modules [25] and (2) the low temporal resolution of these structural mappings, without detecting the functional (plastic) changes in other intact brain regions, which accompany the "syndromenwandel" that follows the acute lesion. This last limitation has been partly overcome with the combination of structural and perfusion imaging [26] as well as with the introduction of new functional neuroimaging techniques, especially with functional MRI (fMRI). In the study by Shahid et al. [26], 191 patients with acute left hemisphere stroke were evaluated with MRI and language tests focusing on spoken word comprehension. After controlling for lesion volume and other covariants, they found that only the combination of structural and perfusion imaging within 48 h of onset could identify areas where more abnormal voxels were associated with more severe acute deficits. This study confirmed the left posterior superior temporal gyrus as a critical area for spoken word comprehension and indicated the need of choosing and timing the cognitive behavioral measurement and the appropriate imaging modality according to the acute or chronic phase of the brain damage.

fMRI consists in the activation of brain regions by stimuli or tasks presented in blocked or event-related design, resulting in vasodilation and increase in blood flow and in the ratio of oxygenated to deoxygenated hemoglobin, in this way creating the BOLD (blood-oxygenation-level dependent) contrast, which constitutes the basis for image construction [28]. This image is a statistical map overlaid on a normalized anatomical MRI image, whose colors indicate the probability that the findings could occur under the null hypothesis. fMRI allow us to look at the brain activity of healthy individuals and see every part of a neural network involved in a task or behavior and can thus eliminate the problems of differential vulnerability, plasticity, and disconnection associated with the lesion method [10].

In spite of these advantages, fMRI has limitations that should be taken into account when drawing conclusions about brain function on the basis of its results [27–30]:

(1) fMRI "normalization" process can lead to errors, particularly in elderly patients, since individual brains vary in their patterns of folds, size, overall shape, and ventricle size, and all their images have to be matched to a common (normalized) template image.
(2) It remains a limitation of time resolution, since cortical neuronal responses occur within tens of milliseconds following a stimulus, while the first observable hemodynamic changes do not occur until 1–2 s later.
(3) It may present artifacts related mainly to magnetic susceptibility changes in the frontal and temporal lobes, which are areas of greater interest in fMRI studies, as in cases with medial temporal lobe epilepsy.
(4) It provides a lot of activated areas some of which may not have direct role in information processing, thus making difficult their interpretation.
(5) As an activation method, fMRI shows brain regions *involved* with a task, but does not determine which of them are *necessary* or *critical* for performing the task, and for this reason, a more informative approach would be to combine brain activation techniques (such as fMRI) with brain disruption technique such as lesion-behavior mapping, as proposed by Rorden et al. [29].

12.4 Conclusion

Brain-behavior correlations are challenging even employing well-designed case-control studies, because it is very difficult to keep the homogeneity principle in all cases as regards the nature, size, and distribution of their brain lesions, besides the controls having to be matched to the cases in all influential variables. Moreover, a cognitive behavioral syndrome is explained not only by the loss of function of a damaged brain region but also by reciprocal influences of many other variables (biological, psychological, psychosocial, and neuropsychological) as well as by dysfunction of other intact brain regions caused by changes in neurotransmission, regional blood flow, excitation-inhibition balance (diaschisis) and secondary axonal degeneration. In spite of this, a comprehensive neuropsychological assessment may disclose the basic defect underlying a syndrome and, by inference, "localize" it by (1) using appropriate tests and counterproofs (2) including in a group all patients with a specific syndrome, superimposing the positions of their MRI lesions in order to find a local where all lesions overlap ("hot spot") and by comparing this group with a control group of patients with similar lesions but without that syndrome. Additionally, in group studies, the influence of confounder variables other than the lesion (e.g., older age, depression, attentional deficit) may be verified by running a statistical multivariate analysis, in case this influence was not reduced or eliminated before data collection by means of randomization and matching. A valid brain-behavior correlation requires appropriate neuropathological cases (e.g., ischemic strokes in chronic phase, neurosurgical ablation of tumor). Additionally, the neuro-imaging and neuropsychological assessment should be performed in the same period (with interval of days or weeks), and, due to the limitations of structural and functional MRI, the best approach would be to combine these techniques.

References

1. Fuster JM (1989) The prefrontal cortex: anatomy, physiology, and neuropsychology of the frontal lobe, 2nd edn. Raven Press, New York
2. Von Monakow C (1910) Über Lokalisation der Hirnfunktionen. Von Bergmann, Wiesbaden
3. Damasceno BP (2008) Research on cognition disorder: methodological issues. In: James PT (ed) Leading-edge cognitive disorders research. Nova Science Publishers, Inc, New York, pp 131–154
4. Damasceno BP (2012) Basic neurological evaluation of organic psychosyndromes. In: Botega NJ (org) Psychiatric practice in a general hospital. Artmed, Porto Alegre (in Portuguese, with permission)
5. Leischner A (1972) Über den Verlauf und die Einteilung der aphasischen Syndrome. Arch Psychiatr Nervenkr 216:219–231
6. Christensen A-L (1979) Luria's neuropsychological investigation. Text. Munksgaard Förlaget, Copenhagen
7. Luria AR (1966/1980) Higher cortical functions in man, 2nd edn. Basic Books, New York
8. Shallice T (1988) From neuropsychology to mental structure. Cambridge University Press, Cambridge
9. Gazzaniga MS, Ivry RB, Mangun GR (2002) Cognitive neuroscience: the biology of the mind, 2nd edn. W. W. Norton and Co, New York
10. Rorden C, Karnath HO (2004) Using human brain lesions to infer function: a relic from a past era in the fMRI age? Nat Rev Neurosci 5:813–819
11. Dronkers NF (1996) A new brain region for coordinating speech articulation. Nature 384:159–161
12. Dronkers NF, Redfern BB, Knight RT (2000) The neural architecture of language disorders. In: Gazzaniga MS (ed) The new cognitive neurosciences, 2nd edn. The MIT Press, Cambridge, MA, pp 949–958

13. Damasio H, Damasio AR (1989) Lesion analysis in neuropsychology. Oxford University Press, New York
14. Damasio H, Damasio AR (1997) The lesion method in behavioral neurology and neuropsychology. In: Feinberg TE, Farah MJ (eds) Behavioral neurology and neuropsychology. McGraw-Hill Co, New York, pp 69–82
15. Frank RJ, Damasio H, Grabowski TJ (1997) Brainvox: an interactive, multimodal visualization and analysis system for neuroanatomical imaging. NeuroImage 5:13–30
16. Rorden C, Brett M (2000) Stereotaxic display of brain lesions. Behav Neurol 12:191–200
17. Rorden C, Karnath HO, Bonilha L (2007) Improving lesion-symptom mapping. J Cogn Neurosci 19:1081–1088
18. Kinkingnéhun S, Volle E, Pélégrini-Issac M, Golmard J-L, Lehéricy S, du Boisguéheneuc F, Zhang-Nunes S, Sosson D, Duffau H, Samson Y, Levy R, Dubois B (2007) A novel approach to clinical-radiological correlations: Anatomo-Clinical Overlapping Maps (AnaCOM): method and validation. NeuroImage 37:1237–1249
19. Fischl B, Dale AM (2000) Measuring the thickness of the human cerebral cortex from magnetic resonance images. Proc Natl Acad Sci U. S. A. 97:11050–11055
20. Balthazar MLF, Yasuda CL, Cendes F, Damasceno BP (2010) Learning, retrieval, and recognition are compromised in aMCI and mild AD: are distinct episodic memory processes mediated by the same anatomical structures? J Int Neuropsychol Soc 16:205–209
21. Balthazar MLF, De Campos BM, Franco AR, Damasceno BP, Cendes F (2013) Whole cortical and default mode network mean functional connectivity as potential biomarkers for mild Alzheimer's disease. Psychiatry Res Neuroimaging 221:37–42
22. Weiler M, Teixeira CVL, Nogueira MH, Campos BM, Damasceno BP, Cendes F, Balthazar MLF (2014) Differences and the relationship in DMN intrinsic activity and functional connectivity in mild AD and aMCI. Brain Connect 4(8):567–574
23. Damasceno A, Damasceno BP, Cendes F (2016) Atrophy of reward-related striatal structures in fatigued MS patients independent of physical disability. Mult Scler J 22(6):822–829
24. Damasceno A, Damasceno BP, Cendes F (2016) No evidence of disease actitivy in multiple sclerosis: implications on cognition and brain atrophy. Mult Scler J 22(1):64–72
25. Raineteau O, Schwab ME (2001) Plasticity of motor systems after incomplete spinal cord injury. Nat Rev Neurosci 2(4):263–273
26. Shahid H, Sebastian R, Schmur TT, Nanayik T, Hillis AE (2017) Important considerations in lesion-symptom mapping: illustrations from studies of word comprehension: lesion symptom mapping. Hum Brain Mapp 38(6):2990–3000
27. Jezzard P, Matthews PM, Smith SM (2001) Functional MRI: an introduction to methods. Oxford University Press, Oxford
28. Huettel SA, Song AW, McCarthy G (2004) Functional magnetic resonance imaging. Sinauer Associates, Inc, Sunderland
29. Rorden C, Fridrikson J, Karnath H-O (2009) An evaluation of traditional and novel tools for lesion behavior mapping. NeuroImage 44(4):1355–1362
30. Karnath H-O, Sperber C, Rorden C (2018) Mapping human brain lesions and their functional consequences. NeuroImage 165:180–189

Chapter 13
Research Methods and Designs

13.1 Introduction

Method is a set of procedures, means, or ideas organized in such a way that lead to the achievement of determined objective or result. In research, the method has to be described in detail, in such a way that other investigators can examine it carefully and reproduce the findings.

The type of research design chosen is determined by the specific problem to be tackled and by the predictions and propositions of the investigator but also by taking into account feasibility, costs, and risks to study participants. Study design may be (1) *observational*, in which the researcher assesses a population by watching people's behavior, without intervening, manipulating, or altering the conditions of the participants or (2) *experimental* design, by manipulating the situation of the participants, and establishing how to control or eliminate extraneous factors (other than the independent variable) that may affect the results, especially by specifying an experimental (treatment) group and a control group, besides having the advantage of controlling influential confounding variables and minimizing bias by means of randomization, matching, and large enough sample sizes, when selecting and assigning people to the groups.

13.2 Experimental Method

An *experiment* is a procedure to collect proofs to verify associations between variables, particularly the effect of one variable on another, being the best test for verifying cause and effect relationship or, at least, associations between events. In this context, the term *variable* is defined as any characteristic of people, things, and situations which can vary and present different types, levels, or values. A variable (e.g., age), called *independent variable* (IV), can affect another one (e.g., logical thinking),

B. Damasceno, *Research on Cognition Disorders*,
https://doi.org/10.1007/978-3-030-57267-9_13

called *dependent variable* (DV). Usually, the experimenter, based on some hypothesis (predictions), manipulates an IV and look for changes in a DV, maintaining constant all other potentially influential variables. Thus, the experimenter intentionally changes the IV, be it quantitative (e.g., amount of night sleep time) or categorical (race, sex) and observe its effect on the DV (e.g., visual attention or reaction time or some other cognitive behavioral function). Hypothetically, any change in the DV should be caused by manipulations in the IV. The power of a neuropsychological experiment is based on its ability to ensure that only the IV is permitted to vary across the conditions of the testing. However, neuropsychological investigation is a challenging task due to the complexity of the functions being evaluated and to the great number of variables involved. The main problem here is that almost always there are other influential variables, even though they may be irrelevant from the point of view of the cause-effect relationship one is searching for, and these variables must be controlled or kept constant; otherwise they result in *confounding* and make the findings difficult to be interpreted or inconclusive. The confounding variables may be related to the subjects, to the tests, or to the situation of the experiment.

Psychological studies also deal with *latent* (hidden) variables, which cannot be directly observed (e.g., the concepts or constructs of "intelligence" or "quality of life") but can be inferred from other variables that can be directly observed and measured by using a series of questions or tests ("multi-item scale") and mathematical models (e.g., principal component analysis), thus giving an estimate of that latent variable. The "quality of life" construct, for instance, may be measured on the basis of the individual's wealth, education, physical and mental health, employment status, leisure time, etc.

Experiments involve some action, manipulation, or intervention by the investigators on at least part of study subjects, thus posing *ethical issues*. The investigator must be convinced that what he/she proposes to do with the subjects will probably help them directly or indirectly. This proposal should be clearly communicated and discussed with the subject, including information on the confidentiality of the subject's data, the potential risks and benefits involved, as well as the need of a control group which will not receive the proposed action or therapeutic intervention. After adequate understanding of the potential risks and benefits, the subject should decide whether or not to participate in the study and give his/her informed consent. Subsequent submission and approval by local and external (national) ethics committee is needed.

13.3 Influential Confounding Variables

13.3.1 Subject Variables

Human beings (even the homozygous twins) differ in many biological, social-cultural, and psychological characteristics that influence test performance. Age and education are among the most influential and should always be taken into account when interpreting the test results of a patient or comparing groups of subjects.

Age variations have well-known effects on cognitive abilities, which may not be fully developed in children and adolescents, or have suffered changes in normal aging. The effect of age on the cognitive-cerebral organization is partly mediated by *education* and *cultural* experience in such a way that the influence of these two factors may be greater than that of age itself. We have observed this in a comprehensive neuropsychological study of time perception in a sample of the Brazilian population comprising 92 brain-damaged patients and 111 normal control subjects with ages from 16 to 85 years [1]. The rate of illiteracy and low educational level were higher (>50%) among the elderly, which also carried the social-cultural and spiritual marks of the dominant ideology ("Zeitgeist") of the time when they were younger. The difference in cognitive abilities between our elderly and younger subjects could, at least in part, be explained by the huge social-economical and cultural transformations Brazil has undergone in the last eight decades. The subjects with low educational level had more difficulties with metacognitive and metalinguistic tests, showing an attitude of suspicion or aversion toward these tests. In a study of uneducated minorities in Central Asia, under the supervision of Vygotsky, Luria showed how changes in educationally and culturally organized activity may influence differences in cognitive functions (perception, memory, problem solving, and others) [2]. Thus, the influence of age, education, and cultural experience on cognition has to be taken into account before straightforwardly attributing differences in the performance of groups of subjects to a single difference between these groups, particularly in transcultural and cognitive developmental studies [3].

Handedness or unilateral hand preference is not unique to humans, being found in apes, which also prefer using their right hand for fine manipulation and their left hand for a more supportive function, and this hand preference influences cognitive function, especially language, as well as brain organization [4]. For example, chimpanzee's left planum temporale, a component of human Wernicke's receptive language area, is significantly larger in the left compared to the right hemisphere [5, 6]. Handedness can influence and change the hemispheric representation of tools and other artifacts, for example, in left handers living in a right-handed environment and forced to use their right hand [7].

Sex differences in cognitive functioning have been well demonstrated in human and animal studies, with the most consistent finding being a better performance of women in verbal fluency and of men in visual-spatial reasoning tasks. Men outperform women in spatial rotation (spatial working memory) and spatial visualization (route navigation), but this male advantage does not apply to object location, in which there is a female advantage [8–10]. Women excels men throughout the life span in verbal fluency (in phonemic more than in semantic) and in verbal learning and memory, as demonstrated in the Controlled Oral Word Association Task (COWAT), Rey Auditory Verbal Learning Test (RAVLT), and California Verbal Learning Test (CVLT) [11–13].

Polyglotism influences cognition and the brain representation of language, since every idiom vary according to their specific characteristics, such as syntactic/grammatical rules, phonologic versus ideographic type, and right-left versus left-right or up-down handwriting, which require specific cognitive-cerebral processing mechanisms. Functional imaging studies using MRI or PET scan have found differential activations in left posterior-inferior frontal region (Broca's area) and in posterior-superior temporal and angular/supramarginal gyri (Wernicke's area) [14–16]. Within Broca's area, second languages acquired in adulthood ("late" bilingual subjects) are spatially separated from native languages (e.g., English as native and French as second or German as native and English as second), while they tend to be represented in common frontal cortical areas when both are acquired in the early stages of language development ("early" bilinguals). On the other hand, in both early and late bilinguals, Wernicke's area shows little or no separation of activity based on the age of language acquisition. As a consequence of these differences between idioms, a focal brain lesion in language areas causes different aphasic syndromes in each idiom mastered by the same subject.

Other influential variables are *personality, affective behavioral patterns, autobiography, intelligence, and previous experience with the proposed testing task* or with cognitively similar tasks or hobbies, such as checkers and chess playing, puzzle solving, hunting, and professional skills. These experiences have an effect on test performance as well as on plastic brain reactions. Brain lesion, particularly those in basal medial prefrontal regions, often leads to personality changes and to different degrees of preservation of the subject as a self-conscious and accountable mental agent and consequently to differences in the outcome of the cognitive rehabilitation.

The execution of a test is also highly influenced by *motivation, interest, anxiety, depression, side effect of drugs*, and *circadian rhythm.*

Circadian variations of cognitive performance occur mainly with attention, reaction time, working memory, and executive functions [17, 18]. Studies measuring time-of-day variation of sustained attention show that accuracy and attentional stability peak between 9:00 and 11:00 a.m. and then decline progressively throughout the day [19]. The time-of-day variations of cognitive performance depend on the individual's chronotype, that is, if morning type (wake up early and are more active in the morning), evening type (wake up late and are more active in the evening), or intermediate type (usually sleep from 23:00 to 07:00). In the majority of adults with intermediate chronotype, performance is lowest at dawn and first hours in the morning (partly due to "sleep inertia"; [20]), improves toward noon, show a post-lunch dip, improves again in the afternoon, and then decreases later on in the evening, especially after 22:00 [21]. Sleep deprivation, insomnia, aging, and medications (antiepileptic, stimulants, anxiolytic, hypnotic, antidepressant, or antipsychotic drugs) further worsen cognitive performance under daytime. Thus, for the results of a neuropsychological evaluation to be reliable, particularly when comparing groups of individuals, the investigator should take into account circadian variations of cognitive performance and the factors that may influence it. Accordingly, as recommended by Valdez et al. [18], before starting the neuropsychological evaluation itself, the investigator should assess (1) the patient's sleep-wake cycle, scheduling the testing session at least 3 hours after his/her regular wake up time; (2) the patient's chronotype, for testing him/her in his/her best time (morning or afternoon); (3) the quality of sleep in the night before the planned evaluation, postponing the session if the patient did not sleep well; and (4) the patient's medications, if needed or possible scheduling the testing sessions in medication-free days.

13.3.2 Test Characteristics

Tests themselves have characteristics that influence their execution, such as type of stimulus, previous instructions, ecological validity, and degree of metacognition required.

Performance on cognitive tests may vary according to the *type of stimulus* used, its intensity, complexity, and emotional significance. For example, performance on discrimination of durations in the milliseconds range is more accurate for auditory than for visual stimuli. Sounds are judged longer than lights despite they have same duration [22]. More complex or emotionally significant stimuli are perceived as longer. For instance, in the visual perception of two stimuli of same objective duration – a shrub alone and a snake under the shrub, the last one has an emotional impact on the individual, triggering bodily changes (breathing and heart rate), which in turn increase sentience and thus perception of time [23].

Accomplishment of a test also depends on the presence (or not) of *previous instructions*, which facilitate its execution to the extent that they are clearly understood by the subject. In neuropsychological testing, the subject should not be allowed to start executing a task without having clearly understood what it is to be done. Lezak [24] has called attention to the fact that standardized test instructions (as in Wechsler Intelligence Scale tests) may be not well understood or even be misleading, especially in brain-damaged patients and elderly individuals. She further adds that "a little more flexibility and looseness in interpreting the standard procedures are required on the examiner's part…to elicit the patient's best performance," and quoting Williams [25], she reminds that "the same words do not necessarily mean the same thing to different people and it is the meaning of the instructions which should be the same for all people rather than the wording."

Psychometric characteristics of neuropsychological tests such as reliability (test-retest, inter-rater, internal consistency, standard error of measurement) and validity (internal, external, ecological) have to be taken into account when interpreting the subject's performance and scores (more on this topic in Sect. 13.5 on psychometric tests).

Many cognitive tests, due to their *metacognitive or metalinguistic character*, are very challenging and apprehension-producing, particularly for low education or illiterate people. As examples of such tests, the examiner (e.g., when testing for ideomotor apraxia) may ask the subject to "mime the movements of cutting slices of a bread with a knife" (without the actual objects) or to repeat a list of unrelated words (in a memory test) or decontextualized senseless sentences (e.g., "the ant is bigger than the elefant") or to solve syllogistic problems of the kind "All metals are good heat conductors. Silver is a metal. Is silver a good heat conductor?". As shown by Luria in his study on cognitive development [2], illiterate people do not understand or accept the first two sentences of this syllogism, which has an established general judgment derived from the historical-social experience, comprising a major premise ("All metals are good heat conductors") and a minor premise ("Silver is a metal"), whose logical interrelation imply the conclusion ("silver is a good heat conductor"). In Luria's study, illiterate people interpreted such syllogisms on the basis of their own practical individual experience and refused to draw inferences (conclusions) based on propositions on things with which they did not have practical experience. However, after enough schooling, they learned to draw such inferences. The term "metacognition" refers to the conscious knowledge of own cognitive abilities and self-regulation processes, as in thinking about one's own mental processes ("thinking about thinking"), for example, when employing strategies during problem solving or using mnemonic methods in memory tasks (metamemory). Metalinguistic knowledge (metalanguage) is the awareness of language, its structure and functions, phonemes, morphology, connectors, syntactic, and grammatical rules. Metacognitive and metalinguistic knowledge is acquired above all in school, especially by means of reading and writing practices, being a crucial component of successful learning, reasoning efficiency and fluid intelligence [26]. While the acquisition of a native (mother's) language by the child takes place naturally, implicitly and almost automaticallly, the learning of a second language by the adult is based on and facilitated by metalinguistic knowledge, with the learner becoming aware of phonemes (articulemes), morphological, and grammatical rules of that idiom. It is this conscious detachment or "abstract attitude" (in Goldstein and Scheerer terms; [27]) in relation to their own language (or cognitive function) that people with low education (or illiterate) have not acquired, what makes metacognitive and metalinguistic tests inappropriate for them. In these cases, transculturally and ecologically adapted tests should be used for evaluation of cognitive functions.

Another issue related to degree of difficulty of the neuropsychological tests is the floor and ceiling effects, which may make inconclusive the measurement of the dependent variable. The floor effect occurs when the task is too difficult, and the ceiling effect occurs when the task is too easy, with all participants scoring at the bottom or at the top of the scale, respectively. Due to these effects, differences between the participant individuals cannot be detected. A way to avoid these effects is to carry out pilot studies, conducted on smaller samples, to check the appropriateness of the subject pool and variables before carrying out the experiment proper, as proposed by Breakwell et al. [28].

13.3.3 Testing Situation

Various factors related to the local and conditions of the testing may influence and confound the effect of the independent variable that is being investigated, such as the presence of disturbing light, temperature, or noise; the experimenter's appearance, attitude, behavior, and lack of experience with the test; and the examiner's lack of acquaintance or closer rapport with the patient, hence the need for an initial interview before the testing. Other "noises" that can distract the attention of the patient may be, for example, appealing objects or pictures that can be seen by the patient; the examiner's improper dress, hair style, or ill-humored look; and the testing table with too many things in disarray. The table should have only what is needed for the examination. Variations of the examiner's voice (intonation, accent, intensity) from one patient to another may influence their performance, particularly in memory tests using list of words spoken by the examiner for the patient to repeat and memorize. This influence of voice variations could be avoided by using recorded instructions and list of words. Lezak [24] and Sbordone [29] remind us that this quiet testing environment with control of most influential local variables is necessary for establishing brain-behavior relationships, but this "sterile environment" and the tests used may be inadequate for predicting (generalizing to) the patient's behavior in noisy real-world situations. In these cases, better prediction could be achieved by developing ecologically valid tests and testing conditions.

13.4 Study Design and Control of Subject Variables

An experiment is accomplished through a *research design*, which is a general plan of investigation with detailed outline of how data are to be collected, analyzed, and interpreted, particularly regarding inferences about causal relations or associations among variables. Data collection for detecting change may be cross-sectional or longitudinal. In a *cross-sectional design*, information is collected from subjects (belonging to two or more groups) at a single point in time in a number of different conditions, while in a *longitudinal design* (also called "prospective", "within-subject" or "repeated measures" design), data are collected from the same sample of subjects on two or more occasions and has the advantage of providing stronger evidence supporting causality.

Control in research consists in removing the influence of any extraneous variables (other than the independent variable) that might have an effect on the dependent variable. The influence of subject variables can be controlled or minimized by means of (1) a within-subject design, using the same subjects in each of the experimental conditions of the study or (2) a between-subject design, allocating different people in each group through randomization and matching.

In the *within-subject* (*repeated measures*) *design*, the same group of subjects perform each of the experimental conditions. Illustratively, let us suppose an investigator wants to know whether or not the concrete versus abstract character of words has an effect on the learning of word lists, and for this purpose, he/she evaluates the same group of subjects with test A (10 abstract words) and test B (10 concrete words). This design has the advantages of balancing the subjects variables in the two conditions and of requiring fewer participants than the between-subjects design, but it has the disadvantage of occurring *order effect*, with subject's performance on the second test (B) being influenced by his/her performance on the first one (A), be it by the effect of practice, boredom, or fatigue, which tend to increase over time and confound study results. The effect of these confounding variables can be overcome by randomizing the order of the tests among all subjects of the group, with half the subjects following an order (A → B) and the other half the inverse order (B → A). Another problem that may occur with the repeated measures design is the *carryover effect*, that is, when the same participants are tested on two occasions with the same version of a test (e.g., memorization of the same list of words), they may in the second occasion remember some words of the list. Even when tested in the second occasion with a different word list, words of the first list may be remembered and introduced intrusively. A way of avoiding carryover effect is to use a longer delay between the two evaluations.

The *between-subject (independent groups) design* consists in allocating consecutively different subjects to different conditions (experimental tests or treatment interventions). A main problem that makes this design relatively inefficient is that the different subjects in each group and the groups themselves have different characteristics (subject variables) which influence their performance, particularly when many of the subjects share some advantageous characteristics that facilitate their performance on the dependent variable, for example, when former checkers or chess players execute a test of visual-spatial learning. A way around these problems is the use of randomization and matching.

Randomization is achieved by attributing to each subject a number or code, which is then randomly selected (*random assignment*) for allocation in each group. This procedure will not eliminate individual differences (subject variables) but will distribute them randomly between the groups, thus reducing their effect on the performance of each group as a whole. In this way, the randomized groups will be equal concerning confounders. The influence of subject variables may also be reduced by increasing sample size, since these variables become equally distributed the larger the sizes of the groups. However, randomization alone cannot increase the sensitivity of an experiment, that is, its power in detecting any effect of the independent variable on the dependent variable, particularly when this effect is small. This insufficiency may be overcome by means of matching, which can increase experiment sensitivity and its probability of revealing a cause-effect relationship between the independent and the dependent variable.

Matching consists in selecting pairs of subjects with similar characteristics that can influence test performance or have an effect on the dependent variable and then allocating randomly each subject of the pair in each group. Accordingly, for each subject in one group, there will be a similar subject in the other group as regards those subject variables considered to be relevant for the specific experiment, such as age, sex, intelligence (IQ), educational level, or others. The strength (sensitivity) of the design of independent groups depends on matching the subjects on the basis of characteristics that have great effect on the dependent variable or test performance. A difficulty with this design is to know before starting the experiment what subject characteristics potentially influence the dependent variable and to find and recruit enough number of participants that present all these characteristics for pairing one with the other. For instance, in a case-control study where age, sex, education, and intelligence are the influential individual characteristics, if the group of cases has a

38 years old male, with 10 years schooling and IQ 95, then the control group should have another male with identical characteristics. Non-matched independent group designs do not have these difficulties (nor the order effect or carryover effect of the within-subject design), but they cannot eliminate the influence of extraneous subject variables (other than the independent variable) on the dependent variable; hence they being insensitive, despite having larger groups sizes and randomization.

13.5 Psychometric Tests

Measurement of mental functions is a challenging endeavor. The mental constructs (intelligence, memory, personality traits, mood states) we want to measure are not directly accessible as, for instance, when measuring length with a ruler. In spite of this, these functions can be objectified in the form of speech, emotional bodily expressions, and external actions and behaviors with things and people, in this way making them possible to be operationally defined and "measured." Besides qualitative psychological research, which has given enormous contribution to our knowledge of the processes occurring in the dynamic architecture of the mind, quantitative research is also needed, particularly in clinical trials, with accurate measurement and treatment of the data, in order to demonstrate any scientific evidence of intervention efficacy. Such quantitative researches have to give an operational definition of the mental constructs investigated, with detailed description of the measures used; otherwise they cannot be replicated. In this regard, measures have to be reliable (consistently measuring a construct across time, subjects, and situations) and valid (measuring what it is intended to measure).

Reliability is the degree to which the test yields the same results (data) over repeated testing of the same people in different occasions (*test-retest reliability*), both when applied by the same researcher (*intra-rater* reliability) and when applied by different researchers (*inter-rater* reliability). The inter-rater reliability may be estimated by the percentage of agreement between two (or more) raters (by tabulating their scores on a contingency table) or by a correlation coefficient, but a more accurate estimate is the *Cohen's kappa* (κ) [30].

The reliability of a test may also be estimated by its *internal consistency*, which is based on the correlations between different items of a test or between one subtest (subscale) and the test battery as a whole, where higher correlations between the items indicate greater internal consistency. A way of determining internal consistency is by administering the whole test to a large sample and then dividing it in half (split-half approach) by taking all the even-numbered items as one half of the test and the odd-numbered items as the other half and calculating the correlation (Pearson's r) between the two halves. Another way is by calculating the *Cronbach's alpha* [31], based on pairwise correlations between the test items (for more information on calculating Cohen's kappa and Cronbach's alpha, see Clark-Carter [32]).

A test's reliability is also expressed in the *standard error of measurement* (SEM), related to the fact that the score obtained by a person in a testing occasion is usually not the same obtained in another occasion. SEM estimates how repeated measures ("observed" scores) of a person on the same test tend to be distributed around his/her "true" score. Since all measurements, particularly of psychological constructs, contain some error, the true score is unknown, but may be established in terms of a confidence interval (CI) comprising a range of scores with high probability of including the subject's true score, e.g., a 68% or 95% probability or confidence level (CL) that the subject's true score is found between the lowest and highest scores in the range.

Validity of a test is the extent to which its measurement is true, corresponding accurately to real-world facts, measuring what it claims to measure (the test's *construct* validity), and indicating how much the results are attributable to the independent variable and not to some other variable (its *internal* validity) as well as the extent to which the findings can be generalized to other people or to other conditions (*external* validity). The validity of a test that measure a theoretical construct, for instance, intellectual-executive function (e.g., the Tower of London test) is best estimated by using two or more tests supposed to measure this same construct (e.g., solution of problems, Trail Making version B, construction with multicolored Kohs cubes), by showing that they are highly correlated and measure the same construct (so-called *convergent* validity), while other tests supposed not to measure this construct (e.g., Boston Naming and visual perception test) are not related to it (*discriminant* validity). Convergent and discriminant validities together provide evidence of the construct validity of that test (Tower of London).

The generalization of the subject's performance or test results to other conditions in the real world, outside the artificial laboratory conditions, is the *ecological validity* (EV) of the test [29, 33]. EV requires an adaptation of the test to the subject's sociolinguistic and cultural milieu, with the maximum control of extraneous variables, minimum artificiality, and use of methods, materials, setting, and task demands similar to those of the real-life situation that is being investigated. These requirements may pose difficulties and limitations in the EV of the test, but the only way of definitively answering cause-effect relationship questions is by gathering data generated in laboratory conditions [28].

The EV of tests has become increasingly relevant, particularly in the planning of a rehabilitative program as well as in forensic neuropsychology, when the court requires information about how the changes in the patient's cognition and behavior (as detected by the neuropsychological assessment) affect his capacity or behavior in an everyday real-life situation [34].

13.6 Case Studies (Single-Case, Multiple Cases) Versus Group Studies

Case studies focus on a person (single-case) or more people (multiple case study) with comprehensive and detailed collection of data from diverse sources of information, using various methods or experiments. As compared to the single-case study, the multiple case study is more expensive and time-consuming but allows the investigator to detect differences and similarities between the cases and, by analyzing the data across them, can collect empirical evidence supporting a more reliable and convincing interpretation or theory [35, 36]. Case studies may contribute to a better understanding of cognitive processes by analyzing in detail the performance of individual brain-damaged patients and making comparisons across multiple cases, in this way getting in-depth insights into the functional mechanisms and components of cognition, particularly when using sophisticated theoretical cognitive constructs and high-resolution neuroimaging techniques [37–39]. Caramazza's studies [38] of single cases with category-specific anomia are quite illustrative in this regard. One of his patients was unable to generate names of fruits and vegetables but had no impairment in naming tools and furniture, thus supporting a category-specific organization of the mental lexicon and suggesting independence of the processing pathways involved in naming and name recognition [40]. Warrington and Shallice had previously (1984) reported four cases in recovery phase of herpes simplex encephalitis, which identified inanimate objects significantly better than living things and foods [41].

Multiple case studies made possible for Luria to further develop Vygotsky's concept of "complex functional system" by evaluating individual cases with comprehensive batteries of tests and counterproofs and by interpreting the data on the basis of which components constituted the dynamic psychological structure of the tasks used. Luria's main endeavor with his testing of higher cortical functions was neither the "where" (localization) nor the "how much" (psychometrics) but "how" these functions were impaired by the lesion, "how" their complex, internal, and dynamic functional structure was changed, that is, his prime aim was the qualitative analysis of symptoms, syndromes, and their interrelationships, searching for which of them were primary or secondary, and attempting to disclose which basic mechanism or cognitive operation was dysfunctional and which were preserved, thereby furnishing relevant information for appropriate programs of rehabilitative reorganization of these functions. Luria's procedure has been criticized by Western neuropsychologists for not having used validated psychometric tests with reliability and validity based on group studies, but group studies could hardly give the kind of contribution he gave with his method, since many potentially interesting findings would not be reckoned in the statistical analysis of the data. Indeed, single-case studies have difficulties and limitations for linking cognitive operations to neural structures, even in patients with unique cognitive deficits associated to a focal cortical lesion [39]. It is difficult to know which affected region is correlated to the deficit, since the lesion usually involve different cortical regions plus the underlying white matter (i.e., intercortical connecting pathways), besides patients' idiosyncrasies in their cognitive-cerebral organization, so that a lesion of same nature, local, and size in different subjects can produce different syndromes. When the objective is a psychometric study of a single case, the patient's performance and scores have to be compared to those of a control or normative group in order to avoid type I errors (i.e., rejecting the null hypothesis when it is true). For this purpose, Crawford and Garthwaite [42] suggest a control sample size of at least 20–30 subjects to achieve a marked effect on power and reduction of type I errors.

Group studies may have one group (using within-subject design) or more groups (between-group design). The simplest and most used between-group design is the case-control design, with two subgroups: the *cases* that receive the new intervention or treatment being tested and the *controls*, which don't receive the new treatment but can be given a placebo, a traditional or old treatment, or no treatment at all. In order to prevent observer-expectancy and subject-expectancy biases and consequently false conclusions, a case-control study must have *double-blinding*, that is, neither the participant subjects nor the tester, the treating researcher, or those performing statistical analysis know which subjects are receiving the new treatment and which are receiving placebo or no treatment at all. Group researches are more powered than case studies in detecting weak effects of a treatment, which may contribute to a further development of the treatment tested.

Group studies are more complex and expensive, requiring larger samples of participants and more resources, besides presenting practical difficulties. For example, due to the strict selection criteria, it may take a long time to recruit and include enough cases, and even when the participants fulfill the selection criteria, they may not be in condition of being tested or willing to be so at the appropriate time [43]. In spite of these disadvantages as compared to multiple case studies, group studies are the best method to increase intragroup homogeneity by balancing individual variability, and they can yield more reliable data, being particularly useful in clinical trials with new drugs and in brain-behavioral correlation studies.

Sometimes it is useful to run a *pilot work* with a smaller group of participants before conducting a group study with larger sample which could reveal itself unfeasible due to its expensiveness, practical difficulties, and lack of enough number of individuals to be included in the time required. Moreover, such a pilot study could test the adequacy and feasibility of the methods, procedures, instructions, equipment, and materials used, besides gathering invaluable information that could contribute to changes in the original research project, making it more viable.

13.7 Conclusion

Designs and methods are determined by the objectives of the research. They must be carefully described so that other researchers can replicate the findings. Study design may be observational or experimental. The experimental design manipulates the conditions of the participants in order to verify whether an independent variable (IV) can affect a dependent variable (DV). In any experiment, there are often subject-related variables other than the IV – the "confounders," which also can influence the DV. Subject variables may be controlled by means of an appropriate study design, be it cross-sectional "between-subjects" (gathering information from subjects at a single point in time) or longitudinal "within-subjects" (by collecting data from the same sample of subjects on different occasions). In the between-subject design, individuals are allocated to different groups of experimental tests or interventions, and both the subjects and the groups have different characteristics that can influence their performance. This influence can be reduced by means of randomization, matching, and large enough sample size. The within-subject design has the advantage of requiring smaller sample size but with the disadvantage of the subject's performance on the second testing being influenced by that on the first one due to the effect of practice or fatigue ("order effect") or the subjects may in the second occasion remember some items of the first testing ("carryover effect"). We can avoid the order effect by randomizing the order of the tests in each half of the group of subjects and the carryover effect by using longer delay between the evaluations. In case-control double-blinding clinical trials, there must be clear operational definition of the mental constructs and detailed description of the measuring tests, which should have high psychometric qualities (i.e., intra-rater, inter-rater, and test-retest reliability; internal consistency; and internal, external, and ecological validity). Group studies are the best method for brain-behavior correlations and case-control clinical trials. Single-case or multiple case studies, on the other hand, have limitations for linking cognitive operations to brain structures, but depending on their mental constructs and methods, they can get deep understanding about the functioning of the mind.

References

1. Damasceno BP (1996) Time perception as a complex functional system: neuropsychological approach. Int J Neurosci 85:237–262
2. Luria AR (1976) The cognitive development: its cultural and social foundations. Harvard University Press, Cambridge
3. Cole M, Means B (1981) Comparative studies of how people think: an introduction. Harvard University Press, Cambridge
4. MacNeilage PF (1987) The evolution of hemispheric specialization for manual function and language. In: Wise SP (ed) Higher brain functions. Wiley, New York
5. Gannon PJ, Holloway RL, Broadfield DC, Braun AR (1998) Asymmetry of chimpanzee planum temporale: humanlike pattern of Wernicke's brain language area homolog. Science 279(5348):220–222
6. Hopkins WD, Marino L, Rilling JK, MacGregor LA (1998) Planum temporale asymmetries in great apes as revealed by magnetic resonance imaging (MRI). Neuroreport 9(12):2913–2918
7. Gainotti G (2015) The influence of handedness on hemispheric representation of tools: a survey. Brain Cogn 94:10–16. https://doi.org/10.1016/j.bandc.2014.12.005
8. Linn MC, Petersen AC (1985) Emergence and characterization of sex differences in spatial ability: a meta-analysis. Child Dev 56:1479–1498
9. Andreano JM, Cahill L (2009) Sex influences on the neurobiology of learning and memory. Learn Mem 16:248–266
10. Li R, Singh M (2014) Sex differences in cognitive impairment and Alzheimer's disease. Front Neuroendocrinol 35(3):385–403
11. Rodriguez-Aranda C, Martinussen M (2006) Age related differences in performance of phonemic verbal fluency measured by Controlled Oral Word Association Task (COWAT): a meta-analytic study. Dev Neuropsychol 30:697–717
12. Gale SD, Baxter L, Connor DJ, Herring A, Comer J (2007) Sex differences on the Rey Auditory Verbal Learning Test and the Brief Visuospatial Memory Test-Revised in the elderly: normative data in 172 participants. J Clin Exp Neuropsychol 29:561–567

13. de Frias CM, Nilsson LG, Herlitz A (2006) Sex differences in cognition are stable over a 10-year period in adulthood and old age. Neuropsychol Dev Cogn B Aging Neuropsychol Cogn 13:574–587
14. Kim KH, Relkin NR, Lee KM, Hirsch J (1997) Distinct cortical areas associated with native and second languages. Nature 388(6638):171–174
15. Halsband U (2006) Bilingual and multilingual language processing. J Physiol Paris 99(4–6):355–369
16. Sakai KL (2005) Language acquisition and brain development. Science 310(5749):815–819
17. Gerstner JR, Yin JCP (2010) Circadian rhythms and memory formation. Nat Rev Neurosci 11:577–588. https://doi.org/10.1038/nrn2881
18. Valdez P, Ramirez C, Garcia A (2012) Circadian rhythms in cognitive performance: implications for neuropsychological assessment. ChronoPhysiology Therapy 2:81–92
19. Riley E, Esterman M, Fortenbaugh FC, DeGutis J (2017) Time-of-day variation in sustained attentional control. Chronobiol Int 34(7):993–1001
20. Tassi P, Muzet A (2000) Sleep inertia. Sleep Med Rev 4(4):341–353
21. Wright KP, Lowry CA, LeBourgeois MK (2012) Circadian and wakefulness-sleep modulation of cognition in humans. Front Mol Neurosci 5:50. https://doi.org/10.3389/fnmol.2012.00050
22. Goldstone S, Lhamon WT (1974) Studies of auditory-visual differences in human time judgement:1. Sounds are judged longer than lights. Percept Mot Skills 39:63–82
23. Shirmer A (2011) How emotions change time. Front Integr Neurosci 5(58):58. https://doi.org/10.3389/fnint.2011.00058
24. Lezak MD (1995) Neuropsychological assessment, 3rd edn. Oxford University Press, New York
25. Williams M (1965) Mental testing in clinical practice. Pergamon, Oxford
26. Demetriou A, Kazi S (2006) Self-awareness in g (with processing efficiency and reasoning). Intelligence 34(3):297–317. https://doi.org/10.1016/j.intell.2005.10.002
27. Goldstein K, Scheerer M (1941) Abstract and concrete behavior: an experimental study with special tests. In Dashell JF (ed.). Psychol Monogr 53(2):1–151
28. Breakwell GM, Hammond S, Fife-Schaw C, Smith JA (eds) (2006) Research methods in psychology, 3rd edn. SAGE Publications, London, pp 36–37
29. Sbordone RJ (1996) Ecological validity: some critical issues for the neuropsychologist. In: Sbordone RJ, Long CJ (eds) The ecological validity of neuropsychological testing. GR/St. Lucie Press, Orlando, pp 15–41
30. Cohen J (1960) A coefficient of agreement for nominal scales. Educ Psychol Meas 20:37–46
31. Cronbach LJ (1951) Coefficient alpha and the internal structure of tests. Psychometrika 16:297–334
32. Clark-Carter D (1997) Doing quantitative psychological research: from design to report. Psychology Press Ltd, Hove
33. Spooner DM, Pachana NA (2006) Ecological validity in neuropsychological assessment: a case for greater consideration in research with neurologically intact populations. Arch Clin Neuropsychol 21:327–337
34. Long CJ, Collins LF (1997) Ecological validity and forensic neuropsychological assessment. In: McCaffrey RJ, Williams AD, Fisher JM, Laing LC (eds) The practice of forensic neuropsychology: meeting challenges in the courtroom. Plenum Press, New York
35. Yin RK (2003) Case study research: design and methods, 3rd edn. SAGE, Thousand Oaks
36. Baxter P, Jack S (2008) Qualitative case study methodology: study design and implementation for novice researchers. Qual Rep 13(4):544–559
37. Damasio H, Damasio AR (1989) Lesion analysis in neuropsychology. Oxford University Press, New York
38. Caramazza A (1992) Is cognitive psychology possible? J Cogn Neurosci 4:80–95
39. Gazzaniga MS, Ivry RB, Mangun GR (2002) Cognitive neuroscience: the biology of the mind, 2nd edn. W. W. Norton and Co., New York

40. Hart J, Berndt RS, Caramazza A (1985) Category-specific naming deficit following cerebral infarction. Nature 316:439–440
41. Warrington EK, Shallice T (1984) Category specific semantic impairments. Brain 107:829–854
42. Crawford JR, Garthwaite PH (2006) Detecting dissociations in single case studies: type I errors, statistical power and the classical versus strong distinction. Neuropsychologia 44:2249–2258
43. Shallice T (1988) From neuropsychology to mental structure. Cambridge University Press, Cambridge

Part IV
Fundamentals of Statistics Applied to Biomedical and Psychological Research

Chapter 14
Elements of Statistics: Basic Concepts

14.1 Introduction

Any scientific research is a limited cut in the reality, but the endeavor of science is to abstract from concrete facts and generalize the findings in order to know the universal properties and laws that govern the functioning of the real world in its different levels (physical-chemical, biological, economic-social-cultural, and psychological). What makes this endeavor more challenging is the fact that science deals with a world that is dynamically ever changing, with every object, phenomenon, or behavior being weaved by innumerable internal and external relationships and interactions of its components, a world that includes not only necessary, law-regulated, and causal processes but also accidental, unpredictable, casual events or influences. The casual is dialectically interconnected with the causal and constitutes the circumstances or conditions in which a causal process occurs. The casual and unpredictable is the rule in the microcosm and in the biological, social-cultural, and psychological level, having put pressure and led to the development of mathematics probability theory, quantum physics (uncertainty principle), and statistics. Today statistics is applied even in such a stochastic area as stock market prediction, giving investors valuable information on a company's stock probable future price.

Biological and psychological researches often deal with observations that may be quantifiable as data. Here, a decisive role is played by statistics, the science that deals with the collection, classification, analysis, and interpretation of numerical data by using mathematics probability theory for drawing general conclusions about a whole population data on the basis of a sample of it. Statistics can aid in different phases of a study: (1) when planning and designing the experiment; (2) when organizing and summarizing apparently chaotic data in terms of mean, variance, standard deviation, and so on (*descriptive statistics*); and (3) then when generalizing and making inferences about the whole (population) based on characteristics of its parts (samples) (*inferential statistics*).

B. Damasceno, *Research on Cognition Disorders*,
https://doi.org/10.1007/978-3-030-57267-9_14

14.2 Definition of Basic Concepts

In statistics, *population* is a whole set of real-world objects or individuals (persons, animals, plants, houses, institutions) that share at least one common characteristic, which we are interested in studying. Population is not the simple collection of people and objects in themselves but the set of measurements or counts made on these people or objects, according to the interest of an investigator [1]. Since the population is usually very large or theoretically infinite, it is not feasible to test or measure every of its individuals. For this reason, we draw a *sample* from it, that is, we select a group of individuals representative of the wider population and their measurements, with the aim to make inferences and generalize the findings to the whole population. The main reason for drawing a sample is not to study the sample itself but its parent population. For the sample to be representative, its elements have to be randomly selected from the population (*simple random sampling*) in such a way that every individual has equal (quantifiable) probability of being chosen, without any influence from the part of the researcher. For this purpose, the researcher's first step is to choose the population of interest and calculate the sample size on the basis of the accuracy he/she wants for generalizing from the sample to the population, taking into account that the larger the sample, the more accurate the generalizations. As second step, each population element is identified and given a code or number. Then, these numbers are selected randomly by means of a computer program or a table of random numbers or simply by being written on separate identical pieces of paper and drawn from a hat.

When the population consists of different mutually exclusive subgroups or strata which the researcher aims to study, a better option may be a *stratified random sampling* comprising elements of all strata of the population (e.g., male and female; Protestants, Jews, and Catholics; lower, middle, and upper socioeconomic class). The so-called *proportional sampling* is essentially the same as the stratified random sampling, but the number of participants from each subgroup is determined by their number (percentage) relative to the entire population. The random sampling (even for gathering participants in each subgroup of the stratified and proportional ones) is a sine qua non condition for drawing correct inferences and making generalizations to the population based on findings of only one sample. Non-random sampling (e.g., *convenience sampling* of a hospital's cases) is likely to introduce biases in the estimate of population parameters. Even using a well-planned and carefully executed random sampling for extracting a representative sample from the population, there will be some difference between sample statistics (mean $\bar{X}$, standard deviation s) and population parameters (mean μ, standard deviation σ). This difference, called *sampling error*, is intrinsic to the random process of sampling and diminishes as the sample size increases. The larger the errors associated to sampling and to measurement of psychological constructs (*measurement error*), the less accurate the generalizations of results from the sample to the population. With non-random sampling, these generalizations are not possible.

14.3 Levels of Measurement

Measurement of mental constructs and behaviors is crucial for an accurate evaluation of how changes in the independent variable relate to changes in the dependent variable. In this regard, the measurement of the dependent variable needs to be quantitative and objective, yielding the same result independently of who is measuring it. For this purpose, the measurement (testing) should use standardized instructions, procedures, and conditions, but particularly in cases of brain lesion patients, the examiner should adopt "a little flexibility and looseness… (in order to) elicit the patient's best performance… (and considering that) it is the meaning of the instructions which should be the same for all people rather than the wording" [2, 3].

According to Steven's classification [4], which is the best-known and most used in psychological research, there are four main levels or scales of measurement (categorical or nominal, ordinal, interval, and ratio scales). The quantification or degree of information obtained increases from the nominal to the ratio measures, with more information allowing more robust statistical tests to be used for their analysis.

Categorical or *nominal* level concerns mutually exclusive qualitative differences (not quantitative ones) which may have two (dichotomous) or more categories, such as "yes or no"; "male or female" gender; "Caucasoid, mongoloid, or negroid" race; "conservative, liberal, or radical" political party; and "brown, black, blonde, gray, or other" hair color.

Ordinal scale is the rank-ordered arrangement of a category according to some of its qualities, with the rankings indicating more or less (but not how much) of something, for example, when measuring non-numeric concepts as satisfaction (1-"very unsatisfied," 2-"somewhat unsatisfied," 3-"neutral," 4-"somewhat satisfied," 5-"very satisfied"); happiness (1-"very unhappy," 2-"unhappy," 3-"OK," 4-"happy," 5-"very happy"); and opinion (1-"completely disagree," 2-"disagree," 3-"indifferent," 4-"agree," 5-"completely agree"). At the ordinal level, it is possible to use a measure of central tendency, the median (i.e., the middle-ranked, item 3 of the examples above), but not the mean.

Interval scales indicate not only the order but also the numeric values and degree of difference between the items, with equal interval between them. For instance, when measuring temperature with the Celsius scale, we can say that there is the same difference (10 °C) between 20 °C and 30 °C and between 40 °C and 50 °C. On the other hand, as there is no fixed starting point (true zero) for the scale (0 °C does not mean there is no quantity of temperature), we cannot say that 20 °C is half of 40 °C.

Ratio scales, on the contrary, have a numeric scale with an absolute (true) zero, and this makes it meaningful to affirm that one object has "twice the length" or "triple the weight" of another. Thus, these scales not only indicate the order and the exact values between units, but they also allow additions, subtractions, multiplications, and divisions (ratios) to be done with their values, besides calculating measures of central tendency (mode, median, mean) and dispersion (standard deviation, coefficient of variation). For this reason, they make possible to carry out more complex and robust statistical analyses with their data.

Numerical scales can also be classified, particularly by statisticians and mathematicians, in *discrete* and *continuous*. Discrete data are whole numbers (integers, such as 2, 7, or 5, but not their subdivisions as 2.5 or 4.3), for example, scores in a cognitive test or number of persons in a meeting. Continuous data, on the other hand, can have infinite subdivisions between their units, which can be subdivided in ever smaller units, as happens with time, age, weight, height, and length. For example, if you say you are 40 years old now, your actual age could be 40 years, 12 days, 3 h, 35 min, 20 s, 1 ms, and so on. As suggested by statisticians, this classification of data is relevant, since if your data is ratio and continuous and fulfills the requirements of a parametric test (e.g., *t*-test, ANOVA), this should be used instead of a non-parametric test (Mann-Whitney test, Kruskal-Wallis test); otherwise you could lose precious information and even commit Type II error (i.e., by concluding that does not exist any difference or correlation when it in fact exists).

14.4 Describing and Summarizing the Data

The raw data collected in observational or experimental research usually present random variations associated to uncontrolled factors. In order to make the data more meaningful and to verify whether or not the variations and differences observed inherently belong to the variables studied, the researcher has to analyze the data, firstly by summarizing them by means of measures of central tendency (average) and dispersion, frequency distributions, contingency tables, and graphical methods.

Measures of central tendency (mean, median, mode) may be applied to ordinal, interval, or ratio data. *Mean* is obtained by adding the scores together and dividing the total by the number of scores. The population mean is represented by μ and the sample mean by $\overline{X}$. *Median* is the central value, located in the middle of all the values after these have been put in order of magnitude, as happens when the number of values is odd (e.g., 15). When the number of values is even (e.g., 8), for example, the scores 2, 4, 4, 8, 10, 12, 15, and 20, the median is the middle point between the 4th and 5th value, calculated by adding $8 + 10 = 18$ and dividing 18 by $2 = 9$. If the 4th and 5th values were 8 and 9, the median would be 8.5. *Mode* is the most frequent value in a set or series of values put in order of magnitude (in the example above, the mode is 4). In psychological research, the mean is the most used, probably because in its construction (calculation) participate all the values of the data, and it can be used in the most complex statistical analyses. A problem with the mean is the possible occurrence of *outliers* (i.e., values that are much smaller or larger than most of the other values in the data set). In this case, the researcher either adopt the median, since it is not affected by the extreme values, or remove the outliers from the analysis and keep reporting the mean.

Measures of dispersion (maxima and minima, range, interquartile range, variance, standard deviation) are also highly relevant for describing the characteristics of a population. The mean alone is insufficient in this regard, since two populations may have the same mean but differ in the degree of variation of their values. A deeper knowledge of the populations is achieved by determining at least the variance and standard deviation.

Variance represents the degree to which the values of each individual differ from the mean of the group. The population variance is represented by σ^2 and the sample variance by s^2, which may be defined as the average of the squared differences of each value from the group mean. It is calculated by first finding the mean, then subtracting the mean from each value in the data set, then squaring the result of the subtractions in order to make the negative differences positive, and then averaging the squared differences. In the set of scores already mentioned (2, 4, 4, 8, 10, 12, 15, 20), the mean is 75 ÷ 8 = 9.37, and the variance can be calculated as follows:

	Scores	Deviation from the mean (d)	Squared deviation (d^2)
	2	−7.37	54.31
	4	−5.37	28.83
	4	−5.37	28.83
	8	−1.37	1.87
	10	0.63	0.39
	12	2.63	6.91
	15	5.63	31.69
	20	10.63	112.99
Total	75		$\Sigma d^2 = 265.82$
Mean	9.37		

Then, dividing the sum of squared deviations (265.82) by the number of scores (8), we obtain the variance (s^2) of 33.22. However, we can obtain a more accurate estimate of the variance for the population (from which the data came) by dividing the sum of squared deviations (Σd^2) by one fewer than the number of scores in the sample. Therefore, the most commonly used formula in computer programs for statistical tests (see Clark-Carter [5]) is $s^2 = \Sigma d^2/n{-}1$. In this case, for the scores given above, the variance would be $s^2 = 265.82/7 = 37.97$.

The *standard deviation* (σ for the population and SD or s for the sample) is the square root of the variance: $s = \sqrt{s^2}$. So, in the set of scores above, $s = \sqrt{37.97} = 6.16$. The standard deviation has the advantage of being expressed in the same units of the original data. When these data have normal distribution in the population, the standard deviation (σ) indicates the proportion of individuals which fall within a given range of values, for example, $\mu \pm 1\sigma = 68\%$; $\mu \pm 2\sigma = 95\%$; and $\mu \pm 3\sigma = 99.7\%$ of the distribution. The lower the standard deviation, the closer the data values to the mean.

Besides these measures of central tendency and dispersion, another way to organize the raw data and make them more meaningful, particularly when they are in great amount, is by distributing them in *frequency tables*, as illustrated in Table 14.1 for the ages of a sample of 90 people.

Table 14.1 Distribution of number of people according to age range

Age (in years)	Number of people (frequency)
20–29	10
30–39	40
40–49	25
50–59	10
60–69	5

Table 14.2 Distribution of opinions of supporters of different political parties regarding income tax increase

Political groups	Agree	Disagree	Total
Conservative	20	32	52
Liberal	10	26	36
Social democrats	14	29	43
Total	44	87	131

This frequency distribution may be better understood when represented by a *histogram*, a *pie chart*, or another graphical method.

The data can also be organized in a more informative way by means of *contingency tables*, particularly when we want to know whether or not the proportion of certain characteristics are equally (homogenously) distributed among groups of individuals or variables that are classified at the nominal or ordinal level. As exemplified in Table 14.2, the contingency table shows the distribution of opinions of supporters of different political parties agreeing or disagreeing with the increase of income tax proposed by the government. An advantage with contingency tables is that the data can be shown in terms of percentages. In the table, for instance, 38% (i.e., $20 \times 100/52 = 38$) of conservatives, 28% of liberals, and 33% of social democrats agree with income tax increase. Besides this, contingency tables allow us to verify whether or not the differences between frequencies (proportions) are statistically significant, by using the chi-squared test (χ^2) (How to calculate the χ^2, see Chap. 17, Sect. 17.3.1).

14.5 Conclusion

In our world, causal, law-regulated processes are intertwined with casual, accidental, and unpredictable events or influences. This unpredictability put pressure for the development of mathematics probability theory and statistics. Statistics deals with analyses and inferences about a whole (population) on the basis of samples (counts, measurements) collected from it. Population is a whole set of things that share some common characteristics we want to study. Since the population is commonly very large, it is not feasible to measure all of its individuals, hence the need to draw a sample from it. For the sample to be representative of the whole population, its elements have to be randomly selected ("simple random sampling"); even so, there will be some difference (called "sampling error") between sample statistics (mean $\bar{X}$, standard deviation s) and population parameters (mean μ, standard deviation σ). For minimizing the errors associated to sampling and to measurement of psychological constructs ("measurement error"), a large enough sample size is needed. There are four main levels or scales of measurement: *categorical* or *nominal*; *ordinal*, with rank-ordered classification of a category; *interval scale*, numerical values with equal interval between them, but without subdivisions or true zero; and *ratio scale*, numerical values with subdivisions and true zero. Numerical values are also classified in *discrete* (whole numbers without subdivisions, e.g., test scores 2, 5, 8, 9) and *continuous* (numbers with subdivisions between their units, e.g., an individual's weight: 32 kg, 4 g, and 57 mg). Discrete and continuous data allow the use of more complex and robust statistical parametric analyses. After collection of the raw data, they need to be described and summarized by means of measures of central tendency (mean, median, mode), dispersion (maxima and minima, range, interquartile range, variance, standard deviation), frequency distribution, contingency tables, and graphical methods.

References

1. Rebecca GK (1978) Basic statistics for nurses. Wiley, New York
2. Lezak MD (1995) *Neuropsychological* assessment, 3rd edn. Oxford University Press, New York
3. Williams M (1965) Mental testing in clinical practice. Pergamon, Oxford
4. Stevens SS (1946) On the theory of scales of measurement. Science 103:677–680
5. Clark-Carter D (1997) Doing quantitative psychological research: from design to report. Psychology Press Ltd, Hove

Chapter 15
Fundamentals of Statistical Analysis

15.1 Introduction

After the data have been randomly sampled from the population, they are described, organized, summarized (descriptive statistics), and then analyzed for making inferences and drawing conclusions (inferential statistics) about characteristics of the entire population (mean μ, standard deviation σ) or concerning possible associations between variables. The first step is to verify whether or not the frequency distribution of the data follows a normal curve, whose properties make possible to determine probabilities of occurrence of observations in specific intervals of the distribution, which is facilitated by calculating the standard Z score or the t score. We can come near to population parameters (μ, σ) by calculating the mean of the means of different samples of the same size drawn from the same population and the standard deviation of all these means (standard error of the mean) or by finding in the observed data of a sample a range of values, called confidence interval, within which we can assume, with a certain confidence level, that the parameter is located.

15.2 Data Frequency Distribution

The majority of measurable physical, biological, social, and mental phenomena present values that are more frequent around the mean (reaching the maximal frequency in the mean), with extreme values becoming gradually more rare to the extent they differ from the mean. This is considered as a *normal* (also called *Gaussian*) *distribution*, represented by the *normal curve* (Fig. 15.1), a theoretical (mathematical) construct for frequency distribution of measurements in the population of interest, particularly for variables with interval or ratio (continuous) scales.

A frequency distribution may be assumed to be normal when it is already known to be normal (as with temperature, weight, length, time, and other ratio continuous

B. Damasceno, *Research on Cognition Disorders*,
https://doi.org/10.1007/978-3-030-57267-9_15

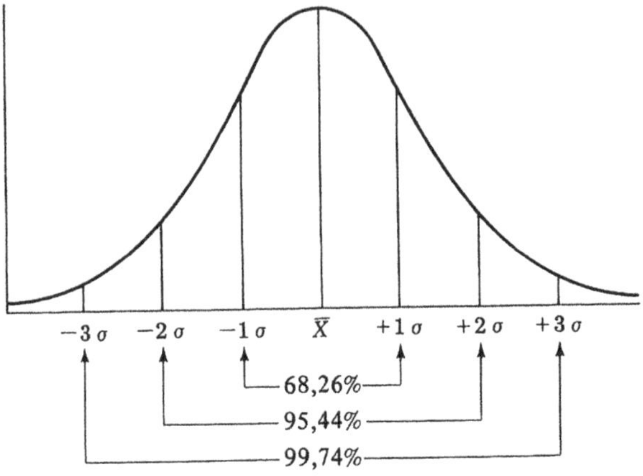

Fig. 15.1 Normal curve with the percentages of frequency distribution under it

variables) or when the distribution of the variable in the population is not normal but the number of observations or participants is large (admittedly at least 100). According to the *central limit theorem* [1], as the sample size increases, the sampling distribution of the mean becomes approximately normal.

For a normal distribution, the frequency (*f*) of an observed value of size X is calculated on the basis of the equation:

$$f(\mathrm{X}) = \frac{1}{\sigma\sqrt{2\pi}} e^{-(\mathrm{X}-\mu)^2/2\sigma^2}$$

In this formula, there are two mathematical constants: π (lower case Greek *pi*) = 3.1416 and *e* (the base of Naperian logarithms) = 2.7183. Additionally, we have the empirically observed values (X) and their distribution parameters (the mean μ or $\bar{x}$ and the standard deviation σ or *s*) that constitute the exponent $-(\mathrm{X}-\mu)^2/2\sigma^2$, which is the changeable and most important component of the formula.

In the normal curve, the vertical (ordinate) axis represents frequency, and the horizontal (abscissa) axis indicates the intervals of measurements or variations (dispersions) between individual observations, depending on the values of the standard deviations. The curve is characteristically *bell-shaped*, *symmetrical* (with two halves from each side of the mean), *unimodal* (it has only one peak of maximal frequency, where mean, median, and mode coincide), and *asymptotic* (it endlessly approaches the horizontal straight line without ever touching it). The form of the curve may be tall and thin when the values of σ are small, or it may be short and fat when the values of σ are large. When the distribution is not symmetrical around the mean (median or mode), the curve is said to be *skewed*, for example, the distribution of per capita income in Brazil and other countries presenting a majority of people with very low and a minority with very high incomes.

The whole area between the curve and the horizontal straight line below it contains 100% of all observations. Due to the curve's symmetric nature, each half in each side of the mean has an equal number of observations, comprising 68.26% (34.13% + 34 0.13%) of all data between 1σ above (+1σ) and 1σ below (−1σ) the mean ($\bar{x}$); 95.44% (47.72% + 47.72%) between +2σ and −2σ; and 99.74% (49.87% + 49.87%) between +3σ and −3σ. This is the same as saying that 68% of all measurements are located within 1σ above and below the mean; 95% lie within 1.96σ above and below the mean; and 99% of all measurements locate within 2.58σ above and below the mean.

These properties of the normal curve make possible to determine probabilities of occurrence of observations in specific intervals of the distribution and to draw statistical inferences. This is further facilitated by *standardizing* the normal distribution, by calculating a *standard score* (*Z*), also called *normal deviate*. For any value of the empirical single score X extracted from a normal population that has mean μ and standard deviation σ, the value of *Z* is calculated as

$$Z = \frac{X - \mu}{\sigma}$$

Since the population standard deviation (σ) is rarely known, we can use the sample statistics, and operate with its estimate (*s*), provided that the sample size is equal to or larger than 30. In this case,

$$Z = \frac{X - \bar{x}}{s}$$

When we compare a sample mean with a population mean and the sample size is smaller than 30 observations, *Z* is substituted by the *t* distribution, and we use *s* instead of *σ*, as follows:

$$t = \frac{\text{sample mean} - \text{population mean}}{\dfrac{\text{sample standard deviation}}{\sqrt{\text{sample size}}}} = \frac{\bar{x} - \mu}{s / \sqrt{n}}$$

Any empirical raw score (X) can be converted into units of standard deviation (*σ* or *s*) by taking the distance (difference) between this raw score (X) and the mean (μ or $\bar{x}$) and dividing it by the standard deviation of the distribution. For instance, if the raw score (X) is 12 and the distribution of data has mean 8 and standard deviation 2, then the score difference (12–8 = 4) divided by 2 shows that the raw score 12 is 2 standard deviations above the mean. Thus, the *Z* score is the number of standard deviations that an observed value or score X locates away from the mean of the population from which that score is drawn (*μ* or $\bar{x}$). Scores above the mean are positive, and those below the mean are negative.

The standardized normal distribution has always mean 0 and variance 1, independent of the scale of measurement used. This facilitates the determination of what proportion (percentage) of a normal distribution lies beyond (i.e., is more extreme than) a given value of Z, by using the Z table (Table 15.1).

For instance, the proportion of a normal distribution for which $Z \geq 1.68$ is 0.0465, represented by the shaded area under the curve in the Fig. 15.2.

The areas under the one-tailed standard normal curve help us to determine probabilities of occurrence of observations in specific intervals of the distribution. For example, in a normal distribution of scores on the delayed recall of 12 words of the Selective Reminding Test (SRT-DR), where $\mu = 9$, $\sigma = 2$, range 2–12, and $N = 237$ healthy subjects, we can calculate proportions of score distributions.

1. What is the proportion of the population of SRT-DR scores larger than 10?
   First, Z has to be calculated:

$$Z = \frac{X - \mu}{\sigma} = \frac{10 - 9}{2} = 0.5$$

Then, the probability $P(X > 10) = P(Z > 0.5) = 0.3085$ (given by the Table) = 30.85%

Table 15.1 *Z* table with proportions of the standard normal curve (one tailed) that are more extreme than a given *Z* score. In the first column are the *Z* scores with their first decimals, and in the first row are their second decimals

Z	0	1	2	3	4	5	6	7	8	9
0.0	0.5000	0.4960	0.4920	0.4880	0.4840	0.4801	0.4761	0.4721	0.4681	0.4641
0.1	0.4602	0.4562	0.4522	0.4483	0.4443	0.4404	0.4364	0.4325	0.4286	0.4247
0.2	0.4207	0.4168	0.4129	0.4090	0.4052	0.4013	0.3974	0.3936	0.3897	0.3859
0.3	0.3821	0.3783	0.3745	0.3707	0.3669	0.3632	0.3594	0.3557	0.3520	0.3483
0.4	0.3446	0.3409	0.3372	0.3336	0.3300	0.3264	0.3228	0.3192	0.3156	0.3121
0.5	0.3085	0.3050	0.3015	0.2981	0.2946	0.2912	0.2877	0.2843	0.2810	0.2776
0.6	0.2743	0.2709	0.2676	0.2643	0.2611	0.2578	0.2546	0.2514	0.2483	0.2451
0.7	0.2420	0.2389	0.2358	0.2327	0.2296	0.2266	0.2236	0.2206	0.2177	0.2149
0.8	0.2119	0.2090	0.2061	0.2033	0.2005	0.1977	0.1949	0.1922	0.1894	0.1867
0.9	0.1841	0.1814	0.1788	0.1762	0.1736	0.1711	0.1685	0.1660	0.1635	0.1611
1.0	0.1587	0.1562	0.1539	0.1515	0.1492	0.1469	0.1446	0.1423	0.1401	0.1379
1.1	0.1357	0.1335	0.1314	0.1292	0.1271	0.1251	0.1230	0.1210	0.1190	0.1170
1.2	0.1151	0.1131	0.1112	0.1093	0.1075	0.1056	0.1038	0.1020	0.1003	0.0985
1.3	0.0968	0.0951	0.0934	0.0918	0.0901	0.0885	0.0869	0.0853	0.0838	0.0823
1.4	0.0808	0.0793	0.0778	0.0764	0.0749	0.0735	0.0721	0.0708	0.0694	0.0681
1.5	0.0668	0.0655	0.0643	0.0630	0.0618	0.0606	0.0594	0.0582	0.0571	0.0559
1.6	0.0548	0.0537	0.0526	0.0516	0.0505	0.0495	0.0485	0.0475	0.0465	0.0455
1.7	0.0446	0.0436	0.0427	0.0418	0.0409	0.0401	0.0392	0.0384	0.0375	0.0367

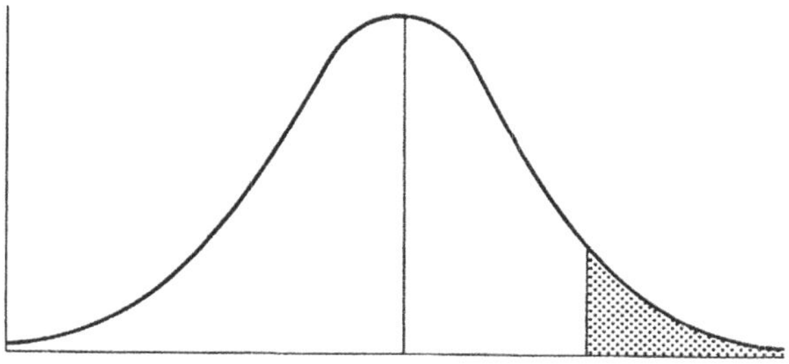

Fig. 15.2 Proportion of a normal distribution for which $Z \geq 1.68$

2. What proportion of scores is smaller than 6?

$$Z = \frac{X - \mu}{\sigma} = \frac{6-9}{2} = \frac{-3}{2} = -1.5$$
$$P(X < 6) = P(Z < -1.5) = 0.0668\,(\text{or}\,6.68\%).$$

3. What proportion of the population of SRT-DR scores locates between 9 (the mean) and 10?

Of the total population of scores, 0.5000 (or 50%) is larger than 9, and 0.3085 (or 30.85%) is larger than 10. Thus, $P(9 < X < 10) = 0.5000 - 0.3085 = 0.1915$. That is to say that 19.15% of scores lie between 9 and 10.

4. How many scores in this population are larger than 10?

$$(0.3085)(237) = 73$$

15.3 Distribution of Sample Means and Their Properties

Different samples of the same size drawn from the same population commonly present different means. As we did with raw scores obtained from a single sample, we can also construct a distribution of means of samples that were randomly extracted from the same population. We can determine the mean of all these means as well as the variation (dispersion) between them, that is, the standard deviation of the means, called *standard error of the mean* (abbreviated as SEM; $s\bar{x}$ or $\sigma\bar{x}$). The SEM is found by dividing the sample standard deviation (s) by the square root of the sample size (n): $s\bar{x} = s/\sqrt{n}$. The sampling distribution of means has the following properties, provided that all samples have the same size and were extracted from the same population: (1) the mean of the sampling distribution of all means ("mean of means", $\mu\bar{x}$) is equal to the population mean (μ); (2) the distribution of the means of all samples has the shape of a normal curve; but even when the parent population is not normal, the sampling distribution is approximately normal; and (3) the standard deviation of the sampling distribution of all means is smaller than the standard deviation of the parent population, because we take into account the mean scores of every sample and not their raw scores (with their extreme values).

15.4 Confidence Intervals

In experiments, when we draw samples, our aim is to make inferences and generalize the findings to the whole population. For this reason, we need firstly to have an estimate of the population parameters (mean μ and standard deviation σ). One simple and straightforward procedure could be to take the sample mean ($\overline{x}$) as an unbiased estimate (called *point estimate*) of the population mean (μ), provided that (1) the sample was randomly drawn, (2) the sample size is enough large (greater than 100), (3) the measurements were done without bias or random error, and (4) the variance of the measured characteristic in the population is not large, since the more variable the characteristic of the object we are measuring, the less accurate the estimate of the population parameter. However, even when satisfying all these requirements, there will be some difference (sampling error) between sample statistics ($\overline{x}$, s) and population parameters (μ, σ). So, we can never be absolutely confident that our sample mean ($\overline{x}$) is equal to the true population mean (μ). Therefore, another alternative for estimating the population parameter is to find in the observed data a range of values within which we can assume the parameter must locate. This range of values, called *confidence interval* (CI), is established by the researcher with a certain *confidence level* (CL) or degree of certainty that the population parameter lies in that range.

The CL chosen by the researcher is expressed in percentage, most commonly 95%, which indicates that if he drew 100 samples of same size, he would be confident that 95% of all these sample means ($\overline{x}$) would lie within a distance of $1.96\sigma/\sqrt{n}$ on either side of μ. This level of confidence also assumes that 5% of all sample means would fall outside this range of the sample mean ± 1.96 standard errors and that the researcher's sample mean could have been one of those 5% that fell outside the given interval. For this reason, in hypothesis testing, a CL of 95% is the complement of the level of significance, in such a way that a 95% CL corresponds to a significance level of 0.05.

In the example given before, in a sample of 237 healthy individuals drawn from the Brazilian population [2], we found mean score of 9 in the delayed recall of 12 words of the SRT memory test, with standard deviation of 2. In this case, we can be 95% confident that the true population mean score is $9 \pm 1.96 \times 2/\sqrt{237} = 9 \pm 0.25$. Therefore, the population mean lies between 8.75 and 9.25 (i.e., $\text{CI } 95\% = 8.75 < \mu < 9.25$). If the CL was 99%, the mean population score would be $9 \pm 2.58 \times 2/\sqrt{237} = 9 \pm 0.34$, that is, $\text{CI } 99\% = 8.66 < \mu < 9.34$, thus wider than the CI 95%. The higher the percentage of confidence level chosen, the larger the interval and the less precise the estimate, but with this higher confidence level, we can be more confident that the population parameter is located in that interval. A smaller CL (e.g., 68%) could be adopted for increasing precision, provided that we have a sufficiently large sample size and less variance in the population.

15.5 Conclusion

Most measurable phenomena present values distributed more frequently around the mean, as represented by the *normal curve*, with 68% of all data between 1σ above ($+1\sigma$) and 1σ below (-1σ) the mean; 95% between $+2\sigma$ and -2σ; and 99% between $+3\sigma$ and -3σ. These properties of the normal curve allow to determine probabilities of occurrence of observations in specific intervals of the distribution, which is facilitated by calculating the standard Z score or t score. In order to generalize research results to the whole population, first we estimate the population parameters (μ and σ) by finding in the observed data a range of values within which we assume the parameter must locate – the so-called confidence interval (CI), established with a definite degree of certainty – the *confidence level* (CL, commonly 95%).

References

1. Clark-Carter D (1997) Doing quantitative psychological research: from design to report. Psychology Press Ltd, Hove
2. Damasceno A, Amaral JMSDS, Barreira AA, Becker J, Callegaro D, Campanholo KR, Damasceno LA, Diniz DS, Fragoso YD, Franco PS, Finkelsztejn A, Jorge FMH, Lana-Peixoto MA, Matta APDC, Mendonça ACR, Noal J, Paes RA, Papais-Alvarenga RM, Spedo CT, Damasceno BP (2018) Normative values of the brief repeatable battery of neuropsychological tests in a Brazilian population sample: discrete and regression-based norms. Arq Neuropsiquiatr 76(3):163–169

Chapter 16
Hypothesis Testing

16.1 Introduction

Hypothesis is a theory or tentative explanation of certain phenomena, relationships, or behaviors and constitutes the first step before running an experiment that is designed to test whether it is true. After the description of the sample data, the findings are analyzed and tested regarding their generalization to the whole population or whether or not (and how) an independent variable would affect a dependent variable. This is done by means of inferential statistical testing of two main hypotheses about facts in the population or real world: (1) the *null hypothesis* (also called *Ho*), stating that there is no effect of an independent variable on a dependent variable or any relationship (correlation) between variables in the population, and (2) the *alternative* or *experimental* hypothesis (called *H1*), that the independent variable indeed affects the dependent variable or that there is real correlation between variables in the population. *Ho* is the working hypothesis. Here you can commit a Type I error, concluding that *Ho* is wrong and rejecting it when it is true, or Type II error, rejecting *H1* when it is true. Research on mental functions usually starts with a bidirectional two-tailed testing of these hypotheses, for avoiding Type I error, but can run a unidirectional one-tailed testing if there is a strong hypothesis that the variables are positively or negatively correlated.

16.2 Hypothesis Testing

The challenge here is to establish whether or not any differences between means or correlations observed in samples are explained by real differences or correlations in the population, or are mere product of sampling errors. It is not possible to definitively prove that an experimental hypothesis (*H1*) is true, but it can be accepted to the extent that the null hypothesis (*Ho*) is rejected on the basis of a predefined level

B. Damasceno, *Research on Cognition Disorders*,
https://doi.org/10.1007/978-3-030-57267-9_16

Table 16.1 The two types of errors in hypothesis testing

Hypothesis testing	*Ho* is true	*Ho* is false
Rejection of *Ho*	Type I error	Correct decision
Acceptance of *Ho*	Correct decision	Type II error

of confidence or significance. For instance, if the probability (p) of a sampling difference being due to sampling error is equal to or smaller than a critical level of significance (e.g., $p \leq 0.05$, i.e., only 5 or less cases due to sampling error occurring in 100 cases), then we can reject *Ho*. In hypothesis testing, we always risk committing one of two types of errors.

A *Type I error* occurs when we reject the null hypothesis (*Ho*) even though it is true, for example, concluding that the independent variable has an effect on the dependent variable when, in fact, it does not have or that two variables are correlated when, in reality, they are not. This kind of error may have dangerous consequences in clinical trials, for example, when concluding that a new drug with serious side effects has efficacy against a disease which is not life-threatening, besides misleading other researchers into doing further studies with this inefficacious drug.

A *Type II error* occurs when we reject our research hypothesis (*H1*) when it is true, for instance, concluding that an independent variable has no influence on or no correlation with a dependent variable when it actually has. In clinical trials, a common error is to accept the null hypothesis when the study power is low and the sample size is insufficient, with the serious consequences of abandoning a drug that could be efficacious. A common cause of Type II error is the very small size of the treatment effect. The smaller the size of the expected treatment effect, the larger the size of the sample required for verifying it. On the other hand, a clinical trial with high power and large enough sample size may have as its investigational hypothesis the null hypothesis of no difference between the new treatment and the conventional one or placebo, in order to discourage other researchers from further investigating this inefficacious new treatment [1]. Table 16.1 summarizes possible types of errors involved in the decision-making when using null hypothesis significance testing.

The probability or risk of committing a Type I error is called α. The smaller the p-value, the lower the probability of committing Type I error. A problem in hypothesis testing is that, if we set a very small α (e.g., $p \leq 0.01$) in order to avoid a Type I error, we increase the probability of making a Type II error. This is the reason why in most researches, particularly on mental-cognitive disorders, α is conventionally set at 0.05, as a compromise between the two types of error.

16.3 Statistical Significance and Its Limitations

Statistical significance is the probability of a p-value to accurately reject the null hypothesis or to find a result at least as extreme as what was actually observed, if assumed that this hypothesis is true. However, statistical significance does not necessarily mean that the observed result is significant in practical, real-life terms. For example, in a clinical trial, a drug may show statistically significant but small or no practical significance or beneficial effect. On the contrary, an experimental drug may show no statistically significant but evident practical benefit. This is illustrated by Kirk [2] with a clinical trial using a new drug hypothesized to improve cognition in Alzheimer's disease. The researcher randomly assigns 12 Alzheimer patients to an experimental group and a placebo control group. Then, when analyzing their performance on intelligence tests, he runs a *t*-test and finds a $t(10) = 1.61$, $p = .14$, that is larger than .05, which indicates that the null hypothesis cannot be rejected, and this statistically not significant result is interpreted by him as not providing support for his hypothesis. However, in this research, the IQ of the experimental group was 13 points higher than that of the control group, with an estimated Cohen's *d* of .86, which represents a large effect with a 95% confidence interval from −.3 to 2.0, thus providing strong support for the researcher's hypothesis and requiring further studies to be replicated. Thus, a limitation of the *p*-value is that it is dependent on the sample size and does not indicate the size or the relevance of the observed effect. For instance, two studies with different sample sizes but identical in all other aspects may arrive to different conclusions, with the one with a larger sample size achieving statistically significant results, while the other one does not. Therefore, researchers are now recommended to always report *confidence intervals* and *effect sizes*, which convey what a *p*-value does not, namely, the magnitude and relative importance of an effect [3, 4]. On the other hand, Ioannidis [5] makes a case for not abandoning statistical significance, since it "is often the only piece of evidence processing that has a chance of being objectively assessed before experts, professional societies, and governmental agencies begin to review the data and make recommendations". He suggests that the statistical analysis and potential thresholds (*p*-values) should be specified in detail before conducting a research (and not afterwards), in order to avoid manipulation and hacking of the data for achieving positive ("significant") results. Since $p < 0.05$ is an easy to pass threshold, he has proposed lowering it to $p < 0.005$ for claiming statistical significance, besides using a large enough sample size [6].

16.4 Effect Size and Statistical Power

Effect size (ES) is a quantitative measure of the magnitude of the difference between the means of two treatment groups comprising an experimental group (that gets a new kind of intervention or therapy, e.g., a new rehabilitation technique for amnesia) and a control group (that gets a conventional therapy or no intervention at all). The ES may show if the therapy has a small, medium, or large effect. Usually one is interested not just in the difference between the means of the two groups (called *absolute* ES) but in the *standardized* ES that takes into account the variability of scores of every subject, particularly the Cohen's *d*, calculated by the formula:

$$d = \frac{\mu 1 - \mu 2}{\sigma}$$

where μ1 is the mean for one population, μ2 is the mean for the other population, and σ is the standard deviation for the population [7].

When we do not know the values of the population parameters, we use the equivalent statistics of the sample, namely, the means of each group (M1, M2) and the standard deviation of either group, when the variances of the two groups are homogeneous, as follows:

$$d = \frac{\text{M1} - \text{M2}}{s}$$

where M1 − M2 (the difference between the means of the groups) is divided by *s*, the standard deviation of either group (a negative sign in the result is disregarded). So, for two independent groups, the standardized ES indicates how many standard deviations the two means are separated from each other. ES can be classified as *small* ($d = 0.2$), *medium* ($d = 0.5$), and *large* ($d \geq 0.8$) [7]. Even if the ES is small, it may be important, for example, in a clinical trial with a new drug that saved the life of a small proportion of participants with a deadly disease [8, 9].

It has become more and more important to report research findings in terms of confidence intervals and ES, additionally to or instead of the statistical significance (*p*-value). This practice allows multiple ES of diverse studies (particularly the large ones) to be combined in a meta-analysis, taking into account the ES standard error, in order to verify if these studies produce a consistent effect. Differently from statistical significance (*p*-value), ES does not depend on sample size, although a smaller ES would require larger sample sizes to be detected.

Statistical power is the probability of avoiding Type II error by finding a statistically significant difference between interventions when such a difference actually exists. The probability of making a Type II error is represented by β, and consequently the power of a test is 1 − β. Statistical power depends on various factors, such as the aim of the research (e.g., testing a new drug that could save lives), study design (between-subjects versus within-subjects design), type of statistical test employed, α significance level, effect size, and sample size. Statistical power can be increased by using potent interventions with bigger effects, increasing sample size, and reducing measurement error [10].

ES and statistical power should be chosen before conducting a study, even though they can be calculated after the study has been concluded. When planning a study, ES may be chosen based on the literature data, consensus opinion of experts, or previous experience. For example, a clinical trial with an anti-hypertensive drug could aim to achieve, as the smallest treatment efficacy, a decrease of 5 mm in blood pressure, which could be taken as the predicted ES. As regards the statistical power, Cohen [7] and others [8] recommend 0.8 as a reasonable level of power [with this power, the probability of committing Type II error (β) is 1 − power = 1–0.8 = 0.2].

A power set at 0.8 (and consequently, $\beta = 0.2$) and α significance level at 0.05 will balance the risks of committing Type I and II errors. Accordingly, deciding beforehand the ES (*d*), the power, the α error probability, and the one- or two-tailed testing alternative are preconditions for calculating (with G*Power software, e.g., [11]) the minimal sample size needed to detect the smallest treatment difference or strength of association between an independent and a dependent variable.

16.5 One- or Two-Tailed Tests in Hypothesis Testing

A researcher may want to know if the mean score ($\bar{X}$) of an experimental group is greater than or less than the norm (μ), and not just different. When the researcher, based on previous knowledge or experience, hypothesizes that the sample mean will be "greater than", that is, in the right-hand side (upper tail) of the normal distribution or, on the contrary, "less than", in the left-hand side (lower tail) of the curve, the hypothesis testing is called *one-tailed* or *unidirectional*. When the researcher does not predict the direction of the outcome, the hypothesis testing is called *two-tailed* or *bidirectional*.

The one-tailed testing, with the region for rejecting *Ho* being in the right-hand side or in the left-hand side of the curve, requires smaller difference between the observed mean ($\bar{X}$) and the norm (μ) for attaining statistical significance. The two-tailed test, on the other hand, requires larger difference between $\bar{X}$ and μ for being statistically significant, since the probability $p \leq 0.05$ (or 5%) is divided and distributed in 0.025 on one tail and 0.025 on the other tail of the curve. Most psychological and educational researches are interested in larger differences in either direction (statistical significance of scores greater or lower than the norm) and adopt the more conservative two-tailed testing, which is less likely to commit Type I error.

Hypothesis on possible associations between variables may also be tested with one-tailed tests when the correlation is strongly hypothesized to be unidirectional, that is, positive or, on the contrary, negative, or with two-tailed tests, when we are willing to consider a higher correlation between variables in either direction in order to reject *Ho*, as preferred in most psychological researches.

16.6 Sample Size Calculation

Sample size needs to be calculated before the collection and analysis of data, so that enough number of subjects is enrolled in the study in order to rule out a meaningful difference between groups and answer the main research question, hypothesis, or purpose. In this regard, a common problem, particularly in clinical trials, is that about 10% of subjects drop out of the study for many reasons, and this percentage of subjects has to be additionally enrolled for performing the final data analyses with the minimum sample size planned.

Different study designs require different methods for sample size calculation. There are various formulas for calculating sample size, depending on the type of statistical analysis to be done (e.g., chi-squared, *t*-test; case-control or cohort studies; univariate, bivariate, or multivariate analyses, with qualitative or quantitative data). The type of statistical analysis in its turn determines other elements that will be needed for calculating sample size, such as standard deviation, alpha level, confidence interval, effect size, and power. If these elements are not available, the researcher may obtain them by looking for comparable published data or by performing a pilot study.

Sample size may be obtained by means of a formula or a software program or simply by using data of a similar study, particularly of descriptive studies published in indexed periodicals. As an example, for the investigation of the normal distribution of values of the Brazilian version of the Brief Repeatable Battery of Neuropsychological Tests (BRB-N; [12]), sample size was calculated with the computer program G*Power [11] by adopting effect size of 0.5, α error probability of 0.05, and power ($1 - \beta$ error probability) of 0.80 (for version A and B subgroups; two-tailed) and found that the minimal sample size would be 128 subjects, which divided 64 individuals for each subgroup. However, since most similar normalization studies had used samples of at least 150 individuals of the American, German, and Spanish population, we enrolled more than 200 subjects.

Sample size can be calculated with different formulas depending on whether it is a cross-sectional or longitudinal clinical interventional study. In clinical trials requiring *t*-test, analysis of variance or multivariate analysis, the formula for determining sample size is more complex, being recommended to consult a statistician, but there are various free software programs (including online calculators) that could be used:

http://www.psycho.uni-duesseldorf.de/aap/projects/gpower; *http://www.mc.vanderbilt.edu/prevmed/ps* [13]; and
http://hedwig.mgh.harvard.edu/sample_size/quan_measur/defs.html
(URL: http://hedwig.mgh.harvard.edu/sample_size/size.html).

16.7 The Problem of Small Sample

As we have seen, the larger the sample, the smaller the errors, the better the estimate of the population parameters and the more accurate the generalizations from the sample to the population, hence the relevance of getting a large sample. Small sample sizes increase the margin of errors and reduce the power of the study, that is, its ability to detect an effect or difference that in fact exists. In clinical trials, the use of small samples increases the risk of committing a large Type II error, with the serious consequence of failing to demonstrate a treatment difference that is really present. Unfortunately, most psychology and neuroscience researches use small samples sizes, and the consequences of this practice include overestimates of effect size and low reproducibility of results [14].

On the other hand, as opportunely put by Sturgis [15], it is crucial to distinguish between samples that are small because the population is hard to access and samples that are small because not enough effort has been put into the study. Studies on rare conditions (e.g., children with autism spectrum disorder) have to be conducted with small samples or single cases. Contrary to the hard "positivist" view considering as scientific research only those experiments with large samples and inferential statistical tests, small sample or single-case studies are true experiments that can demonstrate causal relations and have relevant practical implications. At the least, small sample studies may be considered as exploratory, as in pilot studies, whose data could be combined with those of similar studies in future meta-analysis.

Kazdin [16] has highlighted the enormous potential contribution of single-case studies, especially in the evaluation of intervention programs in everyday life at the level of the single case, which may be an individual person, an institution, or a business, each one considered as a unit, independently of the number of people involved. In such studies, he considers as the most fundamental design requirement the repeated observations of performance over time, with ongoing evaluation of the individual's performance on several occasions, as in the so-called ABAB design (Fig. 16.1).

ABAB design consists of an initial baseline phase (A phase), when behavior is repeatedly observed (evaluated) without any intervention until it appears to be stable. In Fig. 16.1, the baseline level of behavior (solid line) is assessed and projected (dashed line) to predict the level of behavior into the future, that is, into what will

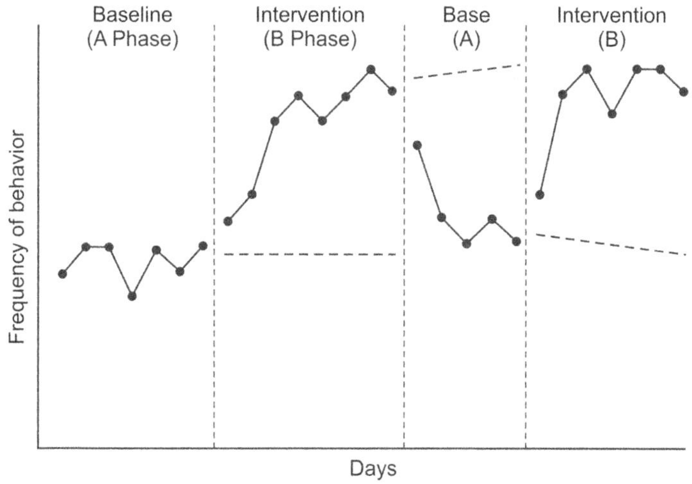

Fig. 16.1 Hypothetical data for an ABAB design. The solid lines in each phase reflect the actual data. The dashed lines indicate the level of performance projected or predicted from the previous phase. (From Kazdin AE, 2016. In: A. E. Kazdin, editor, Methodological issues & strategies in clinical research, fourth edition, American Psychological Association, with permission) [16]

be the following phase (B phase). If performance in this intervention (B) phase departs from the projected level of the baseline and then changes, this change could be due to the intervention itself or to some other influences operating at the onset of the intervention. To test this possibility, the intervention is withdrawn, and a second baseline condition is reintroduced. This second A phase (solid line) shows that the performance departs from a level near that of the final of the previous intervention and then returns to the level of the first baseline A phase, instead of following the dashed line, which would happen if there was some other influencing factor than the intervention. Then, when a second intervention (B phase) is reintroduced, performance departs from a level near that of the final of the previous baseline (second A phase) and then changes to a level similar to that of the final of the previous intervention, instead of following the third dashed line, thus strongly suggesting that the intervention was responsible for the observed changes. The withdrawal of a seemingly efficacious intervention could pose an ethical issue, but it is justified by the need to discard a possible false-positive result and by the posterior reintroduction and maintenance of the treatment. Otherwise, without this withdrawal, the continuation of a fake intervention would be ethically unacceptable.

As regards the issue of the generalizability of single-case studies findings, Kazdin [16] and Madden [17] remind us that there have not been concerns about the proper interventions and underpinnings of single-case research. Indeed, these interventions have wide generalizability and applicability of the findings. On the other hand, as stressed by Kazdin, generalizability of findings from between-groups research is hardly clear or automatic, firstly because experiments in psychology, education, and other areas rarely use random selection from the population; and secondly, the testing of the null hypothesis focuses just on means and measures of variability; so we do not know how many participants in fact responded and why, what makes it difficult to generalize the findings to the whole population of interest. Moreover, statistical significance does not always mean practical or clinical significance, in the same way that a statistically non-significant result could be practically or clinically meaningful.

Between-groups research remains, however, the best method for generalizing to the population of interest, to the extent that it is based on random selection of participants in a large enough sample and on control of influential variables or moderators. Moderators, as defined by Kazdin, are "those variables that may influence the direction or magnitude of change." For instance, in a clinical trial for depression, a moderator could be a family history of depression influencing (moderating) the effectiveness of the treatment, which could be more effective in individuals without such family history. Thus, the generalizability of the treatment efficacy would be valid for the subgroup of participants sharing that moderating characteristic, but not to the whole population of interest.

16.8 Conclusion

Analysis of the data regarding their generalization to the whole population or whether or not an independent variable (IV) does affect a dependent variable (DV) requires testing the *null hypothesis* (*Ho*) that there is no effect of an IV on a DV or correlation between variables in the population versus the *experimental hypothesis* (*H1*) that the IV does affect the DV or that there is correlation between variables. First we assume Ho is true, and only if Ho is rejected, can H1 be accepted. Here we can commit one of two types of errors: *Type I error*, rejecting Ho despite it is true (i.e., the intervention is in reality ineffective), and *Type II error*, rejecting H1 when it is true (i.e., the intervention is in fact effective). Hypothesis testing may be one-tailed, if we assume the sample mean is greater than or less than the norm (μ), or two-tailed, if we assume it is just different.

A limitation of the α significance level (p) for rejecting Ho is that it is dependent on the sample size and does not indicate the practical relevance of the observed effect. It is now recommended to use a lower p-value ($p \leq 0.005$), besides a large enough sample size, and to also report the *confidence interval* and *effect size* (ES) of the results. ES measures the difference between the means of two treatment groups taking into account the variability of scores of every participant subject, and it does not depend on sample size, but a large sample is required when ES is expected to be small.

Type II error can be avoided by establishing in the planning phase of the study its *statistical power*, based on the type of design, statistical test, p-value, effect size (d), and sample size. Usually, a power of 0.8, $p \leq 0.05$, and a large enough sample size will balance the risks of committing Type I and II errors. Smaller sample sizes reduce the power and can lead to errors, being justified in clinical trials only in studies of rare conditions, in which even single-case interventional studies (e.g., using Kazdin's ABAB design) can give great contribution. Sample size can be calculated (e.g., with the free G*Power software) taking into account the type of statistical test, p-value, effect size, and power. After finding the minimum sample size, it needs to be added by about 10% of subjects that commonly drop.

References

1. Seuc AH (1996) En defensa de la hipótesis nula: un comentario acerca de la significación estadística y la aceptación de la hipótesis nula. Bol Oficina Sanit Panam 120(3):218–224
2. Kirk RE (2009) Practical significance: a concept whose time has come. In: Gorard S (ed) Quantitative research in education. Sage, Thousand Oaks
3. Nuzzo R (2014) Statistical errors. Nature 506:150–152
4. Cumming G (2014) The new statistics: why and how. Psychol Sci 25(1):7–29
5. Ioannides JPA (2019) The importance of predefined rules and prespecified statistical analysis: do not abandon significance. JAMA 321(21):2067–2068. https://doi.org/10.1001/jama.2019.4582

6. Ioannides JPA (2018) The proposal to lower *P* value thresholds to .005. JAMA 319(14):1429–1430. https://doi.org/10.1001/jama.2018.1536
7. Cohen J (1988) Statistical power analyses for the behavioral sciences, 2nd edn. Erlbaum, Hillsdale
8. Clark-Carter D (1997) Doing quantitative psychological research: from design to report. Psychology Press Ltd, Hove
9. Rosnow RL, Rosenthal R (1989) Statistical procedures and the justification of knowledge in psychological science. Am Psychol 44(10):1276–1284
10. Sullivan GM, Feinn R (2012) Using effect size – or why the *P* value is not enough. J Grad Med Educ 4(3):279–282
11. Faul F, Erdfelder E, Lang A-G, Buchner A (2007) G*Power 3: a flexible statistical power analysis program for the social, behavioral, and biomedical sciences. Behav Res Methods 39:175–191
12. Damasceno A, Amaral JMSDS, Barreira AA, Becker J, Callegaro D, Campanholo KR, Damasceno LA, Diniz DS, Fragoso YD, Franco PS, Finkelsztejn A, Jorge FMH, Lana-Peixoto MA, Matta APDC, Mendonça ACR, Noal J, Paes RA, Papais-Alvarenga RM, Spedo CT, Damasceno BP (2018) Normative values of the brief repeatable battery of neuropsychological tests in a Brazilian population sample: discrete and regression-based norms. Arq Neuropsiquiatr 76(3):163–169
13. Dupont WD, Plummer WD (1990) Power and sample size calculations: a review and computer program. Control Clin Trials 11:116–128
14. Button KS, Ioannidis JPA, Mokrysz C, Nosek BA, Flint J, Robinson ESJ, Munafò MR (2013) Power failure: why small sample size undermines the reliability of neuroscience. Nat Rev Neurosci 14:365–376
15. Sturgis P (2006) Surveys and sampling. In: Breakwell GM, Hammond S, Fife-Schaw C, Smith JA (eds) Research methods in psychology, 3rd edn. Sage Publications, London
16. Kazdin AE (2016) Chapter 29: Single-case experimental research designs. In: Kazdin AE (ed) Methodological issues & strategies in clinical research, 4th edn. American Psychological Association, Washington, DC, pp. 459–483
17. Madden GJ (ed) (2013) APA handbook of behavior analysis, vol 1 & 2. American Psychological Association, Washington, DC

Chapter 17
Choosing a Statistical Test

17.1 Introduction

After the data have been collected and duly described, they are analyzed in terms of differences between groups or relationships between variables. Selection of a statistical test depends on the study design (independent groups versus repeated measures or matched samples), level of measurement (nominal or categorical, ordinal, interval, or ratio scales), and distribution of the data in the population. On the basis of these prerequisites, we can select a *parametric* (e.g., *t*-test) or a *non-parametric* test (e.g., Mann-Whitney U test).

Parametric tests make estimations of population parameters (means, standard deviations, proportions) based on inferences drawn from the sample data that has been collected. When the researcher draws samples and does experiments, his/her endeavor is always to study a population of interest, since it is usually impossible to collect data from all individuals of the whole population. This is also the reason for the existence of the science of statistics.

The use of parametric tests is based on the following assumptions: (1) the data (scores) are normally distributed in the parent population (as represented by a normal curve) and they have been randomly drawn; and (2) the level of measurement must be interval or ratio, continuous data. Some of these tests (ANOVA) require homogeneity of variances (i.e., data from multiple groups should have the same variance). Parametric tests are the most robust and accurate in detecting a significant treatment effect that truly exists, in this way avoiding Type II error. The validity and robustness of parametric tests (t-test, analysis of variance, correlation, regression) depend on the assumption that the population of data from which the samples are collected are normally distributed. This normality assumption of the gathered sample data may be evaluated visually by means of, for example, a histogram and more accurately by running a normality test as the Kolmogorov-Smirnov or preferably the most recommended Shapiro-Wilk test. Parametric tests can be used even when some of their assumptions are violated, for example, when the distribution of the

B. Damasceno, *Research on Cognition Disorders*,
https://doi.org/10.1007/978-3-030-57267-9_17

(continuous) data is skewed but the sample size is large (≥40). Nevertheless, when the data distribution is strongly skewed (showing a non-Gaussian, asymmetric curve), the use of parametric tests would lead to wrong conclusions. For example, if an experimental group has skewed data with a mean of 70 and median of 34, while a control group has a mean of 40 and median of 32, the use of a non-parametric test (e.g., the median test) would be the best option. An advantage of non-parametric tests is that they are not greatly affected by *outliers* (i.e., values much higher or much lower than the majority of the other values of the set of data), and outliers probably occurred in the data of these two groups, considering the huge difference between their means (70 versus 40).

Non-parametric tests are used when (1) the data are in nominal or ordinal scales; (2) the normality assumption is not satisfied, because the distribution of the sample is unknown or skewed toward one side (in this case being better measured by the median); and (3) the sample size is very small (<20). In these situations non-parametric tests are more efficient and powerful than the corresponding parametric ones. However, if all assumptions for a parametric test are satisfied and a non-parametric test is used instead, this can result in loss of information because the original data is converted in the order of size and only rank or signs are taken into account.

The choice of the appropriate statistical test depends on various factors, particularly the type of study design, level of measurement, and distribution of the data. As for the designs, they can be univariate, bivariate, and multivariate (or multivariable).

17.2 Univariate Analysis

Univariate analysis deals with a single variable taken from a group (e.g., age or IQ in a sample of the population), with descriptive or inferential purposes. The data is described in terms of frequency distribution (normal? skewed?), mean, median, mode, variance, standard deviation, and even using graphical methods (histograms). Inferences from the sample to the population may be done by means of appropriate statistical tests (χ^2 contingency test for nominal variable and one-sample *t*-test for interval, continuous variable).

17.3 Bivariate Analysis

Bivariate analysis investigates the relationship between two variables, for example, the possible influence of an independent on a dependent variable. It can also be descriptive, inferential, and even predictive (e.g., to predict the value of a dependent variable based on the known values of an independent variable by using a simple linear regression). In bivariate analysis, the choice of the statistical test depends on study design and type of data (Table 17.1).

Table 17.1 Summary guidelines for selecting appropriate parametric or their analogous nonparametric tests in bivariate analysis

Design and analysis type	Parametric tests	Nonparametric tests
Comparison of two independent groups	Independent groups *t*-test (for interval or ratio, continuous data)	Median test (for medians), or X^2, or Fisher's exact test (for nominal or ordinal data), or Mann-Whitney U test (for ordinal or interval non-normal data)
Comparison of two quantitative measurements taken from the same individuals (repeated measures) or from matched individuals (matched samples)	Paired *t*-test (for interval or ratio, continuous data)	Sign test or Wilcoxon signed-rank test
Comparison of means between three or more independent groups	One-factor independent groups analysis of variance (ANOVA)	Kruskal-Wallis test (for ordinal or interval non-normal data)
Comparison of three or more quantitative measurements taken from the same individuals (repeated measures) or from matched individuals (matched samples)	One-factor repeated measures analysis of variance (ANOVA)	Friedman χ^2 test
Estimation of degree of association or relationship between two quantitative variables	Pearson's correlation coefficient, simple linear regression	Spearman's rank correlation

In bivariate analysis, the most commonly used tests are the χ^2 (chi-squared) or Fisher's exact test for comparison of proportions (nominal data), the *t*-test for comparison of means (for interval, continuous data), and Pearson's correlation coefficient (r) for linear relationship between two continuous variables.

17.3.1 The Chi-Squared (χ^2) Test

The χ^2 test determines whether differences between observed sample values (proportions or percentages) and expected values are due to a true difference in the population or due to chance variation (sampling error). As illustration, we could test the null hypothesis that the proportion of subjects who got a disease is the same in the groups of vaccinated and nonvaccinated people (i.e., the vaccine gives no protection against the disease). The following two-way (2×2) contingency table (Table 17.2) shows the observed frequencies (*of*) and, in brackets, the expected frequencies (*ef*). The expected frequency (*ef*) for each cell, e.g., the cell for "vaccinated, free of disease," whose *ef* is 35, is obtained by multiplying the total for the row in which the cell occurs (59) by the total for the column in which that cell occurs (60) and then dividing the result by the overall total (100). In analysis of small samples with a 2×2 contingency table, when there are cells with less than five observations, Fisher's exact test is used instead of the χ^2.

Table 17.2 Contingency table for observed (*of*) and expected (*ef*) frequencies

Vaccination status	Free of disease	Diseased	Total
Vaccinated	41 (***35***)	18 (***24***)	59
Nonvaccinated	19 (***25***)	22 (***16***)	41
Total	60	40	100

Table 17.3 Chi-squared distribution

df	$\alpha = 0.05$	$\alpha = 0.01$
1	3.841	6.635
2	5.991	9.210
3	7.815	11.345
4	9.488	13.277
5	11.070	15.086

We calculate χ^2 with the formula $\chi^2 = \Sigma \frac{(of - ef)^2}{ef}$. Therefore,

$$\chi^2 = \frac{(41-35)^2}{35} + \frac{(19-25)^2}{25} + \frac{(18-24)^2}{24} + \frac{(22-16)^2}{16} = 1.03 + 1.44 + 1.50 + 2.25 = 6.22$$

Now, with this χ^2 equal to 6.22, we look for a cutoff point (critical value) that delimits the rejection region in the table for the chi-squared distribution (in part shown in Table 17.3).

In order to find the critical value in Table 17.3, first we have to determine the *degrees of freedom* (*df*) for χ^2. Degrees of freedom are items, observations, values, or scores that are free to vary or to be chosen between, as long as the sum of their frequencies in all categories (cells in the contingency (Table 17.2)) equals a fixed *n* (e.g., 100). One of the most clear explanations for the meaning of degrees of freedom is given by Patrick Runkel [1] in "What are degrees of freedom in Statistics?": "Suppose you have only 7 hats, and you want to wear a different hat every day of the week. On the first day, you can wear any of the 7 hats. On the second day, you can choose from the 6 remaining hats, on the third day you can choose from 5 hats, and so on. When day 6 rolls around, you still have a choice between 2 hats you haven't worn yet. But after you choose your hat for day 6, you have no choice for the hat that you wear on day 7. You *must* wear the one remaining hat. You had 7–1 = 6 days of "hat" freedom, in which the hat you wore could vary!". So, the larger the sample size, the higher the degrees of freedom.

Accordingly, for χ^2, degrees of freedom can be calculated as $df = (r - 1)(c - 1)$, where *r* is the number of rows and *c* is the number of columns in the contingency table; therefore, $df = (2 - 1)(2 - 1) = 1$. Now, for the level of significance of $\alpha = 0.05$ and the row of $df = 1$ in the table for the chi-squared distribution (Table 17.3), we find the cutoff value of 3.841. Since the χ^2 calculated was 6.22, larger than this critical value (thus falling in the rejection region), the null hypothesis of no protection of the vaccine may be rejected at this level of significance (0.05).

17.3.2 The t-Test

As mentioned before, the *t-test for two independent samples* requires that the data are continuous or possess at least interval scale of measurement and were randomly drawn from a population that is normally distributed. The null hypothesis, to be tested, is that the means of the two samples are equal (at $\alpha = 0.05$).

As illustration, suppose we have two groups of subjects: eight patients with medial temporal lobe epilepsy (group I) and ten normal controls (group II). Their scores on the delayed recall of a list of 15 words were as follows:

Group I: 7, 8, 10, 7, 11, 5, 6, 9.
Group II: 10, 13, 9, 12, 14, 13, 8, 12, 9, 11.
Group I: $n1 = 8$, mean score $\bar{x}1 = 7.8$.
Group II: $n2 = 10$, mean score $\bar{x}2 = 11.1$.
Degrees of freedom: calculated as $n1 + n2 - 2$ is equal to $8 + 10 - 2 = 16$.

First is calculated the pooled or "average" variance (sp^2) for the two samples:

$$sp^2 = \frac{\Sigma(x1 - \bar{x}1)^2 + \Sigma(x2 - \bar{x}2)^2}{n1 + n2 - 2}$$

where x1 is a raw score of group I and x2 a raw score of group II.

$$sp^2 = \frac{(7-7.8)^2 + (8-7.8)^2 + (10-7.8)^2 + \ldots\ldots + (10-11.1)^2 + (13-11.1)^2 + (9-11.1)^2 + \ldots\ldots}{8+10-2}$$

$$sp^2 = \frac{28.92 + 36.90}{8+10-2} = 4.41$$

Then t is calculated in order to verify the significance of the difference between the means of group I and group II:

$$t = \frac{\bar{x}1 - \bar{x}2}{\sqrt{sp^2(1/n1 + 1/n2)}} = \frac{7.8 - 11.1}{\sqrt{4.41(1/8 + 1/10)}} = -2.44$$

In conclusion, since the observed t (– 2.44) associated with 16 degrees of freedom and level of significance (α) of 0.05 is larger than the critical t (2.12) found in the table for t distribution (in part shown in Table 17.4), we can reject the null hypothesis and conclude that the mean scores of group I in the memory test is significantly lower than that of group II.

The *t-test for paired samples* evaluates the effect of a treatment based on measurements taken from the same individuals (or things) before and after the intervention ("repeated measures" design) or from matched individuals ("matched samples" design). The differences between each pair of measurements (in "repeated measures") or between individuals (in "matched samples") constitute a single sample of measurements, which is analyzed using a *one-sample t-test.*

Table 17.4 Table for t distribution

df	$\alpha = 0.05$	$\alpha = 0.01$
1	12.706	63.657
2	4.303	9.925
3	3.182	5.841
4	2.776	4.604
5	2.571	4.032
6	2.447	3.707
7	2.365	3.499
8	2.306	3.355
9	2.262	3.250
10	2.228	3.169
11	2.201	3.106
12	2.179	3.055
13	2.160	3.012
14	2.145	2.977
15	2.131	2.947
16	2.120	2.921

Table 17.5 Pre- and post-training data of a group of eight epilepsy patients submitted to memory rehabilitation

Patient number	Before training: ($x1$)	After training: ($x2$)	Differences: $x2 - x1 = d$	Squared differences: d^2
1	7	9	+ 2	4
2	8	8	0	0
3	10	12	+ 2	4
4	7	8	+ 1	1
5	11	12	+ 1	1
6	5	7	+ 2	4
7	6	8	+ 2	4
8	9	10	+ 1	1
Total	63	74	$\Sigma d = 11$	$\Sigma d^2 = 19$
Mean	7.87	9.25	1.37	

As illustration, suppose that our eight patients with medial temporal lobe epilepsy (evaluated at baseline visit) received regular memory training during 6 weeks and were thereafter reassessed to verify the effect of the intervention. Can it be concluded that the training significantly improved memory performance (at $\alpha = 0.05$), based on the results shown in Table 17.5? The null hypothesis states that the mean of the differences (between baseline and post-training evaluation) is equal to zero, that is, *Ho*: mean $D = 0$, where D is the true mean of the population of differences.

Thus, summarizing the data: sample size = n = 8; mean scores before training = $x1 = 7.87$; mean scores after training = $x2 = 9.25$; and degrees of freedom (*df*) for paired (repeated measures) samples = $n - 1 = 8–1 = 7$.

General procedure:

1. Find the differences of the values of the pairs of data and the mean of these differences:

$$\text{Mean of differences} = \frac{\Sigma d}{n} = \frac{11}{8} = 1.375$$

$$\text{Squared sum of differences} = \left(\Sigma d\right)^2 = 11^2 = 121$$

$$\text{Sum of squared differences}\left(\Sigma d^2\right) = 19$$

2. Calculate the variance (s2) of the differences:

$$s^2 = \frac{\Sigma d^2 - \frac{\left(\Sigma d\right)^2}{n}}{n-1} = \frac{19 - \frac{11^2}{8}}{8-1} = \frac{19 - 15.125}{7} = \frac{3.875}{7} = 0.553$$

3. Find the *t*-test value for paired samples, using the following formula (where *D* is the true population mean of differences, which is 0 under *Ho* hypothesis):

$$t = \frac{\text{Mean}\, d - D}{\sqrt{s^2 / n}} = \frac{1.375 - 0}{\sqrt{0.553/8}} = \frac{1.375}{0.262} = 5.248$$

4. Conclusion: since the calculated (observed) *t* value (5.248) is larger than that of the table for *t* distribution (2.365), with a significance level (α) of 0.05 and 7 degrees of freedom, the null hypothesis can be rejected, and, in practical terms, the training may have improved memory performance.

17.3.3 Correlation

Correlation is a test for measuring how variables are related, for example, people's height and weight. It provides information about the *direction* (positive or negative) and the *magnitude* (strength) of the relationship between variables (X and Y).

The first step is to put the data, measured at interval level, in a Cartesian two-dimensional *scatter plot* or *scatter diagram* formed by two axes: the horizontal (abscissa) axis where the values of X's (e.g., people's weight) are plotted and the vertical (ordinate) axis for the values of Y's (height). In the scatter diagram, each point represents the values of variables X and Y of each individual, and the distribution of points indicates the nature of the relationship between these variables. The arrangement of points on the diagram may follow a straight line (or nearly so) constituting a *linear* correlation. This line passes through the data points with the minimum distance between itself and all the points; hence, it can also be called the *best-fitting* line. The strength of a correlation between X and Y increases to the degree that the points in the scatter diagram concentrate around this imaginary straight line. A linear correlation can be *positive* (i.e., as X values get larger, so do Y values) or *negative* (as one variable gets larger, the other gets smaller). However, the arrangement of all points can also configure a *curvilinear* correlation; or the points may even be scattered in the form of a chaotic cloud, in this case indicating no (zero) correlation.

The second step is to determine the strength of the relationship between the variables. This is done most commonly using Pearson's product moment correlation coefficient (symbolized by r) or Spearman's rank order correlation coefficient (rs).

As prerequisites for the use of Pearson's r, (1) there must be a *linear* relationship between the two variables (X and Y) measured at *interval* or *continuous* level; (2) the data have been randomly sampled from the population; and (3) they are normally distributed. The coefficient r varies from −1 to +1. We use negative values, e.g., −1.00, −0.95, −0.50, and − 0.10, for indicating negative correlations, and positive values, e.g., +1.00, +0.95, +0.50, and + 0.10, for positive correlations. As regards the strength of the relationship between the variables, it becomes stronger as it approximates +1.00 or − 1.00 and weaker as it comes closer to 0.00 (absence of correlation). Two directionally opposite correlations as +1.00 and − 1.00, as well as +0.10 and − 0.10, have the same strength.

The third step is to calculate Pearson's r. This can be done by converting the data in z scores or simply working directly with the raw data by means of either of the following formulas:

$$r = \frac{N\Sigma XY - (\Sigma X)(\Sigma Y)}{\sqrt{\left[N\Sigma X^2 - (\Sigma X)^2\right]\left[N\Sigma Y^2 - (\Sigma Y)^2\right]}} \quad \text{or} \quad r = \frac{\Sigma XY - \frac{(\Sigma X)(\Sigma Y)}{N}}{\sqrt{\left[\Sigma X^2 - \frac{(\Sigma X)^2}{N}\right]\left[\Sigma Y^2 - \frac{(\Sigma Y)^2}{N}\right]}}$$

where r is Pearson's linear coefficient, N is the number of pairs of raw scores of X and Y, X is a raw score of variable X and Y is a raw score of variable Y.

As illustration, we could investigate a possible relationship between the memory scores of our eight temporal lobe epilepsy patients and their educational level. In Table 17.6, X is their memory scores and Y is their schooling years.

First, we calculate X^2, Y^2, XY, and the required sums (Σ). Then, we compute r by putting all the needed values, using the first formula:

$$r = \frac{8(431) - (63)(51)}{\sqrt{\left[8(525) - (63)^2\right]\left[8(357) - (51)^2\right]}} = \frac{3448 - 3213}{\sqrt{(4200 - 3969)(2856 - 2601)}} =$$

$$= \frac{235}{\sqrt{(231)(255)}} = \frac{235}{\sqrt{58905}} = \frac{235}{242.7} = +0.96$$

Table 17.6 Memory scores (X) and schooling years (Y) of eight epilepsy patients

Patients	X	X^2	Y	Y^2	XY
1	7	49	5	25	35
2	8	64	6	36	48
3	10	100	8	64	80
4	7	49	6	36	42
5	11	121	10	100	110
6	5	25	4	16	20
7	6	36	4	16	24
8	9	81	8	64	72
Total	$\Sigma X = 63$	$\Sigma X^2 = 525$	$\Sigma Y = 51$	$\Sigma Y^2 = 357$	$\Sigma XY = 431$

This coefficient ($r = + 0.96$) indicates a positive and high correlation between the patients' memory scores and their educational level. As an estimate of the true correlation in the population from which the samples were drawn, this observed coefficient is higher than the expected one at the level of significance (α) of 0.05 ($r = 0.7067$) and even of 0.01 ($r = 8343$), with 6 degrees of freedom. Here degrees of freedom are 2 less than the number of pairs in the sample (i.e., $df = n - 2 = 8 - 2 = 6$). So, the null hypothesis of no correlation can be rejected. Table 17.7 shows part of the table for Pearson's product moment correlation.

17.3.4 Simple Linear Regression

This is also a test for evaluating relationships between variables, but differently from correlation, here we have one dependent variable (DV), also called *criterion* variable, and one single independent variable (IV), also called *predictor* or *explanatory* variable. The regression analysis assumes a unidirectional functional dependence, so that the magnitude of the DV would be determined by the magnitude of the IV, but not on the contrary. The data are put as points scattered in a diagram in which the horizontal X-axis (abscissa) conventionally represents the predictor (IV or X variable) and the vertical Y-axis (ordinate), the criterion variable (DV or Y variable). Each point of the diagram represents a pair of X and Y values (e.g., X1–Y1, or X2–Y2, or X3–Y3, etc.). So, each point has an abscissa (e.g., X1) whose value is the perpendicular distance of the point from the vertical axis and an ordinate (e.g., Y1) whose value is its perpendicular distance from the horizontal axis. For example, in Fig. 17.1, for point A, X = 3 and Y = 2; for point B, X = 1 and Y = −2; and for point C, X = −2 and Y = −4.

A practical use of linear regression as a predictive model is to determine an unknown value of Y when a certain value of X is given. For this prediction, regression analysis requires the same prerequisites as those for correlation, namely, linear relationship between variables (which have to be highly correlated), interval, or continuous data that were randomly sampled and are normally distributed in the population.

Table 17.7 Pearson's product moment correlation

Df	α = 0.05	α = 0.01
1	.99692	.999877
2	.95000	.990000
3	.8783	.95873
4	.8114	.91720
5	.7545	.8745
6	.7067	.8343
7	.6664	.7977
8	.6319	.7646
9	.6021	.7348
10	.5760	.7079
11	.5529	.6835
12	.5324	.6614
13	.5139	.6411
14	.4973	.6226

As illustration, suppose we give a subject an injection of drug A and measure the changes of its plasma concentration (in mols/liter) as a function of the time (in minutes) after its administration (Table 17.8).

The regression line of these two variables can be calculated, since the scatter diagram shows a linear pattern (Fig. 17.2) and the correlation between these variables is very strong, with $r = 0.99$, which was found by means of the formula:

$$r = \frac{N\Sigma XY - (\Sigma X)(\Sigma Y)}{\sqrt{\left[N\Sigma X^2 - (\Sigma X)^2\right]\left[N\Sigma Y^2 - (\Sigma Y)^2\right]}}$$

The equation for finding the *regression line* (i.e., the *best-fitting* line) in order to predict values of a DV when there is just one IV (*X* variable) and one DV (*Y* variable) is

$$\text{DV} = a + (b \times \text{IV}) \text{ or } Y = a + (b \times X) \text{ or, for the population, } Y = \alpha + \beta X$$

in which *a* and *b* are called *linear coefficients*. The coefficient *a* (or α for the population), also called *intercept*, is the point in the vertical axis (i.e., the DV or *Y*-axis) crossed by the regression line, and it would be the value of the predicted DV (on the *Y*-axis) when the value of the IV (*X*-axis) is 0. The coefficient *b* (or *β* for the population) is the *slope* (also called *angular* or *regression* coefficient) of the line and represents changes in the DV for every change in the IV. The value of the slope indicates the direction and steepness of the line (going up from left to right, positive, or going down from left to right, negative). The larger the measure of the slope, the steeper the line.

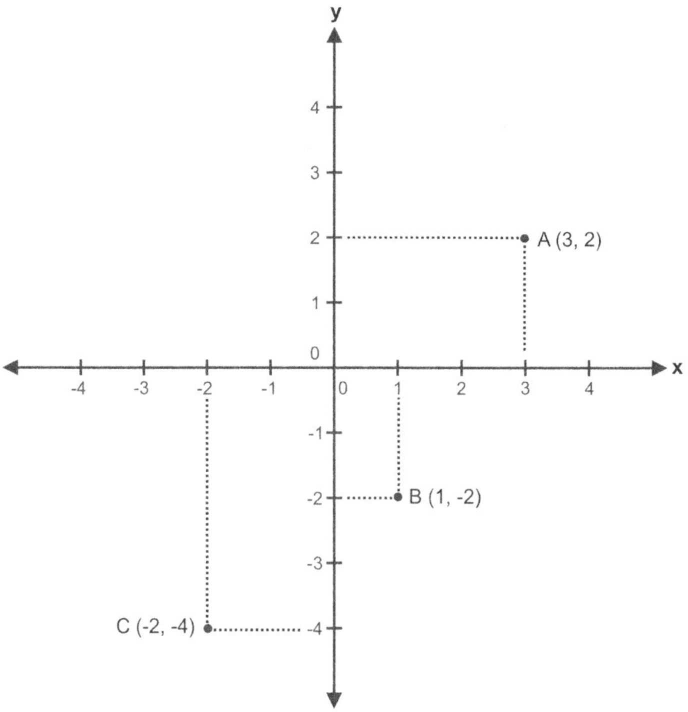

Fig. 17.1 Cartesian coordinate system

Table 17.8 Values of drug A plasma concentration (*Y*), in mols/liter, as a function of the time (*X*), in minutes, after its injection

X (time, min)	*Y* (s-drug A)	X^2	Y^2	*XY*
2	3	4	9	6
4	6	16	36	24
6	10	36	100	60
8	15	64	225	120
10	19	100	361	190
12	26	144	676	312
14	30	196	900	420
16	35	256	1225	560
18	38	324	1444	684
20	43	400	1849	860
$\Sigma X = 110$	$\Sigma Y = 225$	$\Sigma X^2 = 1540$	$\Sigma Y^2 = 3299.42$	$\Sigma XY = 1589.2$
Mean = 8.62	Mean = 17.65			

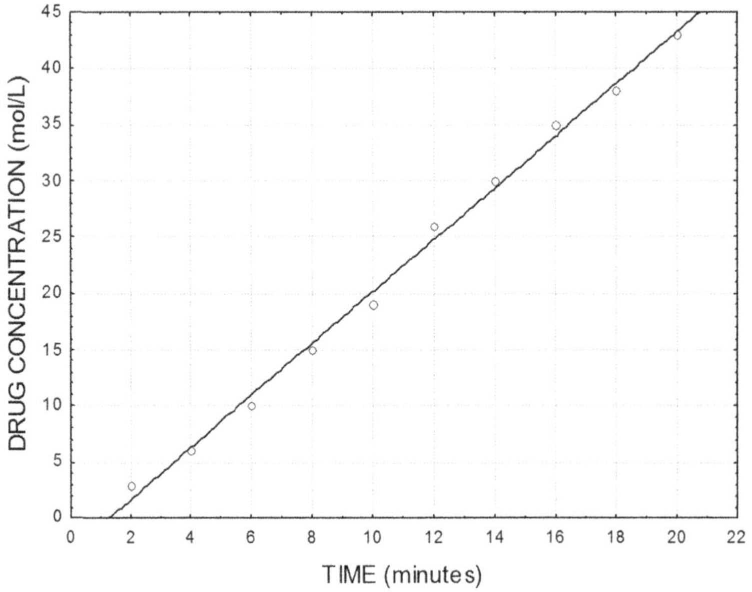

Fig. 17.2 Plasma concentration of the drug (in 10 mol/L) as a function of the time after its injection

In order to predict values of the DV by means of the formula DV = a + (b × IV), first we have to calculate the coefficient b as follows:

$$b = \frac{\left[n \times \text{total of}\left(\text{IV} \times \text{DV}\right)\right] - \left(\text{total for IV} \times \text{total for DV}\right)}{\left[n \times \text{total of}\left(\text{IV}^2\right)\right] - \left(\text{total for IV}\right)^2} = \frac{\left(n \times \Sigma XY\right) - \left(\Sigma X \times \Sigma Y\right)}{\left[n \times \Sigma\left(X^2\right)\right] - \left(\Sigma X\right)^2} =$$

$$= \frac{\left(8 \times 1589.2\right) - \left(69 \times 141.2\right)}{\left(8 \times 767\right) - \left(69\right)^2} = \frac{12713.6 - 9742.8}{6136 - 4761} = \frac{2970.8}{1375} = 2.16$$

After finding b (= 2.16), we determine the value of a with the formula:

$$a = \text{mean for DV} - \left(b \times \text{mean for IV}\right)$$

which is the same as

$$a = \text{mean for Y} - \left(b \times \text{mean for X}\right)$$

Therefore a = 17.65 − (2.16 × 8.62) = − 0.98

Now that we have the values of b (2.16) and a (− 0.98), we can calculate (predict) values of Y for any arbitrary values of X (provided that these arbitrary values are within the range of the observed X values), and, in this way, we can construct the regression line for the data. Conventionally, the predicted values of Y are indicated by $\hat{Y}$ (read "Y hat") and calculated with the formula:

$$\hat{Y} = a + (b \times \mathrm{X})$$

For example, if $X = 2$, then $\hat{Y} = -0.98 + (2.16 \times 2) = 3.34$. For $X = 15$, $\hat{Y} = -0.98 + (2.16 \times 15) = 31.42$; and for $X = 9$, $\hat{Y} = -0.98 + (2.16 \times 9) = 18.46$; and so on.

Zar [2] cautions that "it is an unsafe procedure to extrapolate from regression equations, that is, to predict $\hat{Y}$ values for X values outside the observed range of X... For values of X above and below this range, the function may not be the same (i.e., a and/or b may be different); indeed, the relationship may not even be linear in such ranges... If there is good reason to believe that the described function holds for X values outside the range of those observed, then we may cautiously extrapolate. Otherwise, beware."

17.4 Correlation, Regression, Plausibility, and Causality

Another danger to be avoided when two variables are correlated is to assume that one is causing the variance of the other. Obviously, there are some criteria that may strengthen the suspicion of a causal association between variables or events, such as (1) the strength of the association (the larger the correlation ratio, the higher the probability that one variable or event is causing the other); (2) consistency (the more often the association appears under diverse circumstances, the more likely it is to be causal); (3) temporal relationship (exposure to the putative causal factor precedes the onset of the other); and (4) specificity of the association (the extent to which the occurrence of one variable predicts the occurrence of another) [3]. Either case, the relationship between the variables or events should be plausible, that is, consistent and explicable according to the existing scientific knowledge. The problem here is that the relationship between one variable (IV) and the other (DV) may be mediated by their joint relationship with a third confounding variable. A way to eliminate confounding (if this was not previously done with randomization and matching) and come near to a causal relationship is by using a multivariable analysis. However, "statistics alone cannot prove that a relationship between a risk factor and an outcome is causal" [4]. The best procedure to identify a causal association is by experimentally manipulating the IV and looking for effects on the DV. If such effects consistently occur, we can conclude there is a causal relation between the two variables.

17.5 Multivariable Analysis

Mental and cognitive disorders typically have diverse causes and potential confounders. For this reason, psychology research usually deals with multiple variables, thus requiring a *multivariable analysis* in order to determine the unique (independent) influence or contribution of different factors to a single outcome. For example, cognitive impairment in neurological conditions (e.g., epilepsy, multiple sclerosis, Alzheimer's disease) may be caused by various factors (isolated or combined), such as the brain dysfunction itself, anxiety, depression, fatigue, sleep disturbance, and side effect of drugs. In such situations, there can be multiple independent and dependent variables. To find out which of these factors is the primary or predominant contributor to the patient's cognitive impairment, it is necessary to submit them (1) to a detailed qualitative analysis if we are dealing with a single case or (2) to a statistical multivariable analysis in the case of a group study, in order to simultaneously assess the independent contribution of each of these factors or *confounders*. As defined by Katz [4], "confounding occurs when the apparent association between a risk factor and an outcome is affected by the relationship of a third variable to the risk factor and the outcome; and the third variable is called a confounder". For example, fatigue (especially cognitive fatigue) can impair cognitive performance, but a third factor, sleep disturbance, can independently cause fatigue and cognitive impairment. In reality, what we have is an *interaction* between risk (or causal) factors in such a way that the effect or impact of a risk factor on outcome is modified (increased or decreased) by the effect of another factor. Multivariable analysis can eliminate confounding when this has not been already done by means of randomization and matching in the design phase of the study.

The choice of a multivariable test depends mainly on the nature of the outcome variable (interval, continuous; ordinal; or nominal, categorical) and the hypothesized relationship between variables. The most used tests in clinical research are the *multi-way analysis of variance* (*ANOVA*), the *multiple linear regression* (for interval, continuous data), the *multiple logistic regression* (for dichotomous variables, e.g., male or female, dead or alive), and the *proportional hazards analysis* (for determining the relationship between several risk factors, considered simultaneously, and time to a clinical event or death).

17.5.1 Analysis of Variance (ANOVA)

ANOVA is commonly used in cognitive-behavioral researches for determining differences between the means of three or more independent groups. Its assumptions are that the samples are randomly and independently selected, the groups have the same variance (homogeneity of variances or homoscedasticity), and the data are continuous or have at least an interval scale of measurement as well as normal distribution in the population. ANOVA evaluates whether or not there is significant difference between the true means of the populations from which the groups were extracted. Decision-making is done by means of *F statistic*, which is obtained by dividing the *variance among groups* (distance between the means of the various groups) by the *variance within groups* (distance between the raw scores and the means of each group), that is,

$$F = \frac{\text{Variance among groups}}{\text{Variance within groups}}$$

Thus, the larger the differences between the sample means (the numerator in the formula) while variance within groups remains unchanged, the larger the *F* statistic and safer the decision to reject the null hypothesis (*Ho*) of "equal means." If the observed *F* is higher than the cutoff point found in the ANOVA table (partly shown in Table 17.9), then *Ho* is rejected.

In Table 17.9, we have in the columns the numerator degrees of freedom (*dfnumerator* = number of groups or samples minus 1) and in the rows the denominator degrees of freedom (*dfdenominator* = total number of measurements in all groups minus the number of groups). For example, if we have four groups (A, B, C, D) with ten measurements or participants in each group, *dfnumerator* = 4–1 = 3, and *dfdenominator* = 40–4 = 36. The cutoff *F* in the table is found in the cell where the numerator *df* intercepts the denominator *df*.

A limitation of ANOVA is that it only informs us that there is a global difference between groups, but not where (between which groups) the differences are. This problem could be solved by using *t*-tests for multiple separate comparisons between the various groups (e.g., A × B, A × C, A × D, B × C, B × D, C × D) and for each dependent variable, but this would generate too many comparisons and, for this reason, increase the probability of finding at least one significant *t*-value (≤ 0.05) just by chance (when *Ho* is really true), thus leading to a Type I error. This limitation of using multiple *t*-tests is commonly overcome by means of *Bonferroni adjustments*, whose most simplified version is to divide the original α-level (e.g., 0.05) by the number of times the *t*-test is repeated, for example, $0.05 \div 4 = 0.0125$, which would turn out to be the new criteria for considering as significant the result of any of the repeated tests (0.0125, and not 0.05). On the other hand, Bonferroni adjustment has its own limitations: (1) even though it reduces the risks of Type I error, it increases the chances of a Type II error; and (2) it does not take into account the simultaneous interrelationships between variables, which are best tackled with appropriate multivariable analysis [5].

Thus, after ANOVA has detected significant differences between groups (means), the best way for localizing the differences between particular pairs of groups or means is by using post hoc analysis for multiple comparisons taking into account the significant *F* found. This is done most commonly with the Tukey test, but other post hoc tests as Newman-Keuls, Scheffé, Dunnett, and Duncan can also be used. With the Tukey test, a difference between two means is considered statistically significant if it is equal or larger than Tukey's HSD ("honestly significant difference"). (For calculation of Tukey's HSD, see Clark-Carter, 1997).

Table 17.9 ANOVA table with probabilities of the F-distribution for α = 0.05 according to degrees of freedom (df) of the numerator (df1) and denominator (df2)

	df1								
df2	1	2	3	4	5	6	7	8	9
1	161.45	199.50	215.71	224.58	230.16	233.99	236.77	238.88	240.54
2	18.51	19.00	19.16	19.25	19.30	19.33	19.35	19.37	19.38
3	10.13	9.55	9.28	9.12	9.01	8.94	8.89	8.85	8.81
4	7.71	6.94	6.59	6.39	6.26	6.16	6.09	6.04	6.00
5	6.61	5.79	5.41	5.19	5.05	4.95	4.88	4.82	4.77
6	5.99	5.14	4.76	4.53	4.39	4.28	4.21	4.15	4.10
7	5.59	4.74	4.35	4.12	3.97	3.87	3.79	3.73	3.68
8	5.32	4.46	4.07	3.84	3.69	3.58	3.50	3.44	3.39
9	5.12	4.26	3.86	3.63	3.48	3.37	3.29	3.23	3.18
10	4.96	4.10	3.71	3.48	3.33	3.22	3.14	3.07	3.02
11	4.84	3.98	3.59	3.36	3.20	3.09	3.01	2.95	2.90
12	4.75	3.89	3.49	3.26	3.11	3.00	2.91	2.85	2.80
13	4.67	3.81	3.41	3.18	3.03	2.92	2.83	2.77	2.71
14	4.60	3.74	3.34	3.11	2.96	2.85	2.76	2.70	2.65
15	4.54	3.68	3.29	3.06	2.90	2.79	2.71	2.64	2.59
16	4.49	3.63	3.24	3.01	2.85	2.74	2.66	2.59	2.54
17	4.45	3.59	3.20	2.96	2.81	2.70	2.61	2.55	2.49
18	4.41	3.55	3.16	2.93	2.77	2.66	2.58	2.51	2.46
19	4.38	3.52	3.13	2.90	2.74	2.63	2.54	2.48	2.42
20	4.35	3.49	3.10	2.87	2.71	2.60	2.51	2.45	2.39

17.5.2 Multiple Regression

Multiple regression is an extension of the simple linear regression, with the same prerequisites (linear relationship between variables that are normally distributed and interval or continuous data that were randomly sampled). It is used when we have one dependent variable (DV or criterion) and more than one independent variable (IVs or predictors). Multiple regression can simultaneously verify the independent contribution of various predictors (IVs) to the outcome (DV) and may in this way disclose confounders. In psychological studies, there are usually several IVs that have to be taken into account and controlled. For example, a patient's performance on a test of verbal learning and delayed recall of word list (DV) may be influenced by his age, education, and attention level (IVs). Besides, there are overlaps among these IVs and, consequently, in the variance they explain in the DV. In this situation, a multiple regression is needed for investigating the relation between a DV and a single IV adjusted for the effects of one or more other IVs. Lewis [6] suggests that predictors and potential confounders should be chosen beforehand, in the planning phase of a clinical research, giving preference to include variables that (1) "from previous work are most likely to be associated with outcome," (2) "are the most clinically relevant," (3) "are reliably and accurately measured," (4) "distinguish between patients," (5) "have the least missing data," and (6) "do not measure the same underlying effect as another included variable."

In multiple linear regression, the predicted value of the DV ($\hat{Y}$) is calculated with a formula that is an extension of that for the simple linear regression, $\hat{Y} = a + b1X1 + b2X2 + b3X3 + bnXn$ or, for the general population,

$$\hat{Y} = \alpha + \beta 1X1 + \beta 2X2 + \beta 3X3 + \ldots + \beta nXn,$$

where $X1$ to Xn is the number of relevant IVs and $b1$ (or $\beta 1$), $b2$ ($\beta 2$), $b3$ ($\beta 3$), and bn (βn) are the partial regression coefficients. According to the formula above, $\hat{Y}$ is linearly dependent upon the simultaneous influence of $X1$, $X2$, $X3$, and Xn. The intercept α is the value of Y when $X1$, $X2$, X ... Xn are zero. β (beta-weight) is used when both the criterion and the predictor variables are converted to z-scores (standardized) and indicates how much Y increases (in standard deviations) when the predictor variable (e.g., $X1$) increases by one standard deviation while the other predictor variables are held constant. $\beta 1$, for example, measures the extent to which Y is related to $X1$ after removing the effect of $X2$, $X3$ ... Xn on both Y and $X1$.

There are various types of multiple regression, depending on how the IVs are chosen and put in the model, if all at once, as with *standard multiple regression*, or one at a time, as with *stepwise regression*. The complex calculations involved in multiple regression are nowadays done by means of computer software programs, if needed after consultation with a biostatistician.

Another issue is the sample size needed for multiple regression. Some authors [5, 7] recommend a sample size in excess of 100 for the results to be reliable, while others [4, 8] suggest at least 10–20 per independent variable. A more precise sample size calculation should be done by means of power analysis, taking into account the number of predictors (including potential confounders), effect size, standard deviation, alpha (α, usually set at 0.05, two-tailed), and beta (β, usually 0.20). On the basis of this information, the sample size can be calculated by means of free computer programs, such as:

http://www.psycho.uni-duesseldorf.de/aap/projects/gpower
http://www.power-analysis.com/specifications.htm
http://hedwig.mgh.harvard.edu/sample_size/quan_measur/defs.html
http://home.clara.net/sisa/sampship.htm

17.6 Conclusion

Selection of a statistical test depends on study design, level of measurement, and distribution of the data in the population. Parametric tests (e.g., *t*-test, ANOVA) for estimating population parameters require that the data are interval, discrete, or continuous, normally distributed in the parent population, and randomly drawn from it. These tests are the most robust and accurate for detecting a significant treatment effect that truly exists, thus avoiding Type II error. Non-parametric tests (e.g., chi-squared χ^2, median and sign tests, Mann-Whitney) are used for nominal or ordinal data that do not satisfy the normality assumption and when the sample size is very small (<20 observations). If the data satisfy the assumptions for a parametric test, the use of a non-parametric one results in loss of information.

Bivariate analysis most commonly uses the χ^2 or Fisher's exact test, *t*-test, ANOVA, and Pearson's correlation coefficient (*r*). The χ^2 is for countable nominal data, determining whether or not the frequency of a certain observation in a sample differs significantly from its expected frequency. Fisher's exact test is used when a 2x2 contingency table has cells with less than five observations. The *t*-test compares means of two independent groups ("independent groups *t*-test") or of two repeated measures taken from the same or matched individuals ("paired *t*-test"). Non-parametric tests equivalent to the independent groups *t*-test are the χ^2, Mann-Whitney U, and median test and to the paired *t*-test, the sign test and Wilcoxon signed-rank test. Comparison of means of three or more independent groups is done with the one-factor independent groups ANOVA or the non-parametric equivalent Kruskal-Wallis test. Comparison of three or more repeated measures taken from the same or matched individuals is done with one-factor repeated measures ANOVA or with its non-parametric equivalent Friedman χ^2 test. Degree of association between two variables is made with Pearson's correlation coefficient or, when there is one dependent variable (DV) and one single independent predictor variable (IV), with simple linear regression, and in case of ordinal data, with their equivalent non-parametric Spearman's rank correlation. The finding of correlation between variables, however strong it may be, does not prove there is a causal relationship between them, unless an experimental manipulation of the IV has shown a consistent effect on the DV (outcome).

Multivariable analysis determines the independent contribution of different factors or IV (confounders) to a single outcome (DV), with tests chosen on the basis of the nature of the outcome variable (if interval, continuous; ordinal; or nominal) and on the hypothesized relationship between variables. The most used are the multi-way ANOVA, multiple linear regression, multiple logistic regression, and proportional hazards analysis.

References

1. Runkel P (2016) What are degrees of freedom in Statistics? Available from: https://www.qualitydigest.com/inside/statistics-column/042116-what-are-degrees-freedom-statistics.html; freely available in http://blog.minitab.com/blog/statistics-and-quality-data-analysis
2. Zar JH (1984) Biostatistical analysis, 2nd edn. Prentice-Hall, Inc, Englewood Cliffs
3. Mausner J, Bahn A (1974) Epidemiology: an introductory text. W. B. Saunders Company, Philadelphia
4. Katz MH (2006) Multivariable analysis: a practical guide for clinicians, 2nd edn. Cambridge University Press, Cambridge

5. Breakwell GM, Hammond S, Fife-Schaw C, Smith JA (2006) Research methods in psychology, 3rd edn. SAGE Publications, London, pp 36–37
6. Lewis S (2007) Regression analysis. Pract Neurol 7:259–264
7. Kerlinger FN, Pedhazur EJ (1973) Multiple regression in behavioral research. Holt, New York
8. Feinstein AR (1996) Multivariable analysis: an introduction. Yale University Press, New Haven

Part V
Methodological Issues in Research on Selected Conditions

Chapter 18
Cognitive Research on Early Multiple Sclerosis

18.1 Introduction

Multiple sclerosis (MS) is a chronic inflammatory, autoimmune, demyelinating, and progressive disease of the central nervous system (CNS), affecting more frequently Caucasian women (about twice as men) in the ages 20 through 40 years. MS is characterized by lesions (plaques) widespread in the brain, spinal cord, and optic nerve and disseminated in time, presenting a relapsing-remitting course in the majority of patients. There is involvement of white matter (WM), even the normal-appearing WM, as well as of gray matter (GM), particularly in the cerebral cortex, thalamus, basal ganglia, hippocampus, and cerebellum [1–10]. Besides inflammatory demyelination, there is axonal transection and neuronal loss, even in the early course of the disease, contributing to progressive brain atrophy as well as physical and cognitive disability. The most common initial clinical manifestation is sensory-motor (>50% of cases). Rarely the first symptoms are cognitive-behavioral, which may present as aphasia [11], agnosia [12], memory deficits [13, 14], epileptic seizure, confusional psychosis, or dementia.

The disease usually presents two main clinical courses [15, 16]: (1) *relapsing-remitting* MS (RRMS), the most common, characterized by episodes of acute exacerbation of symptoms (relapses) and partial or full recovery, with stable course between the relapses. and (2) *progressive* MS, with steadily increasing objectively documented neurological disability independent of relapses, occurring after an initial relapsing course, with or without acute exacerbations during the progressive course – the *secondary-progressive* MS (SPMS) or showing a continuous progressive accumulation of disability from onset, which persists after at least 1 year, the *primary progressive* MS (PPMS).

Cognitive deficits in MS patients have a highly negative impact on their work and social activities, independent of the degree of physical disability [17], hence the need of an early diagnosis of the disease as well as identification and analysis of these deficits for their treatment to be more effective.

B. Damasceno, *Research on Cognition Disorders*,
https://doi.org/10.1007/978-3-030-57267-9_18

18.2 The Problem of Early MS Diagnosis

MS diagnosis is based on the demonstration of dissemination of lesions in space and time in the CNS, and it can be established as long as there is no better explanation for the clinical presentation, what requires the exclusion of alternative diagnosis by means of history, physical neurological examination, and imaging and laboratory tests. Since the 2010 revised McDonald criteria [18], the disease can be diagnosed very early, already in the first attack by means of a single baseline brain MRI demonstrating the simultaneous presence of asymptomatic gadolinium-enhancing and nonenhancing MS typical lesions. The 2017 revision of McDonald criteria [16] additionally established that "in patients with a typical clinically isolated syndrome and clinical or MRI demonstration of dissemination in space, the presence of CSF-specific oligoclonal bands allows a diagnosis of MS; symptomatic lesions can be used to demonstrate dissemination in space or time in patients with supratentorial, infratentorial, or spinal cord syndrome; and cortical lesions can be used to demonstrate dissemination in space" [16]. According to these criteria, "attack," "exacerbation," "relapse," and (when it is the first episode) "clinically isolated syndrome" (CIS) are synonyms defined as "patient-reported symptoms or objectively observed signs typical of a focal or multifocal acute or subacute inflammatory demyelinating event in the CNS, with duration of at least 24 hours, in the absence of fever or infection."

A problem for the early diagnosis of MS is that most neurologists consider as "attack" only sensory-motor symptoms, such as paresthesia, sensory loss, paresis, ataxia, visual deficit, urinary urgency and/or incontinence. Cognitive-behavioral disturbances are considered as atypical for MS, being often undervalued for the diagnosis and prognosis of the disease. Another problem refers to the detection of cognition disorders in early MS, since there are controversies regarding (1) the definition of "cognitive deficit" or "cognitive impairment" and (2) what tools are necessary and appropriate to assess cognitive dysfunction in early MS [19].

18.3 Cognitive Impairment

Cognitive impairment affects up to 65% of all MS patients, even early in the disease course manifested as a clinically isolated syndrome, with greater dysfunction in the secondary-progressive phase [19–21]. MS impairs various cognitive domains, mainly attention, executive function, efficiency of information processing, and episodic memory but sparing basic language abilities [22–25]. Even social cognition may be impaired in MS patients, as manifested in tests of theory of mind and facial emotion recognition, with negative impact in their social interaction with other people and quality of life [26]. Reduction of processing speed is the most common cognitive deficit in MS patients and may secondarily cause impairment in timed tests of executive functions, working memory, and abstract reasoning.

"Cognitive impairment" has been defined with the "all or none," "impaired," or "intact" approach, based on existence or absence of any cognitive abnormality or on the "categorical" approach, by classifying the number of failed subtests that measures different cognitive functions, for example, 0–2 tests failed, no impairment; 3–5, mild impairment; and > 5, moderate impairment (as did Amato et al. [21]). Sumowsky et al. [24] reminded us that the low scores in some of the subtests may be due to impairment of information processing speed or memory function alone, thus leading to different estimates of the prevalence of cognitive dysfunction in the disease. These authors [24] suggest future studies "should better characterize groups as impaired in isolated or combined deficits (e.g., memory impaired but speed intact; speed and memory impaired), and also utilize purer measures of each cognitive domain (e.g., latent variables or composite domain scores)." In this regard, similar to what was proposed by Jak et al. [27] and Bondi et al. [28] for defining cognitive impairment in early Alzheimer's disease, here also an appropriately designed qualitative and actuarial neuropsychological battery could contribute to a safer diagnosis of cognitive impairment in one or more of the domains most affected by MS, namely, cognitive processing speed and episodic memory. Reliability could be increased by requiring impaired scores in two subtests for each domain, for instance, for memory, Selective Reminding Test (SRT delayed recall with inclusion of a recognition task), California Verbal Learning Test (CVLT), or Rey Auditory Verbal Learning Test (RAVLT), and for information processing speed, Symbol Digit Modalities Test (SDMT) and Paced Auditory Serial Addition Test (PASAT). In addition, sensitivity could also be increased by defining cognitive impairment as –1SD and not −1.5SD (or –2SD) below normal, as typically defined in most studies. With this lower threshold (–1SD), we could also detect the cognitive decline complained by patients with high premorbid cognition but who now keep performing within the average range of −1.5SD. Since detection of cognitive decline is relevant for establishing disease prognosis as well as for choice or change of disease modifying drugs, all new MS cases should undergo a short baseline cognitive evaluation (e.g., with the Brief Repeatable Battery of Neuropsychological Tests, BRB-N).

18.4 Cognitive Impairment and MS Neuropathology

Cognitive dysfunction may manifest itself as a disease relapse without accompanying sensory-motor symptoms, thus being the only indicator of disease activity, which can be confirmed by neuropsychological tests (e.g., Symbol Digit Modalities Test) and MRI markers [29]. Besides, even subclinical MRI disease activity (asymptomatic gadolinium-enhancing lesions) along with high burden of cortical lesions and callosal atrophy contributes to cognitive dysfunction manifested as low performance in neuropsychological tests [30].

Deficit of processing speed and higher-order cognitive functions could be explained by a disconnection mechanism due to lesions in strategic WM tracts (corpus callosum, superior and inferior longitudinal fasciculus, cingulum, fornices, and tracts connecting prefrontal cortical regions) and to a lesser degree by diffuse abnormalities in the normal-appearing WM of the same tracts, as shown in MRI diffusion tensor imaging (DTI) studies [31–34]. These myelinated WM tracts are essential for the rapid transfer, association, and simultaneous syntheses of multiple information required by working memory and complex attention tasks, as in the Symbol Digit Modalities Test (SDMT) and Paced Auditory Serial Addition Task (PASAT) [1, 35]. Resting-state fMRI studies have also found dysfunction within and between large-scale neuronal networks in relapsing-remitting MS patients, with decreased functional connectivity in regions of the salience (SN), executive control (ECN), working memory (WMN), default mode (DMN), sensory-motor, and visual networks, and this dysfunction has been correlated to disability and T2 lesion volumes [36]. However, it has been shown that WM overall lesion burden does not fully explain the severity of cognitive impairment in MS. GM demyelination and atrophy (by neurite transection and reduced synapse and glial densities; [37, 38]) also contribute to cognitive impairment, reducing processing speed, and particularly visuospatial and verbal, semantic, and episodic memories, mainly when affecting the neocortex, hippocampus, and thalamus [2, 39–42]. On the other hand, besides the contribution of WM and GM pathology, the patient's cerebral and cognitive reserve may also explain the variable severity of the resultant cognitive syndrome in different subjects [43].

Most authors agree that GM atrophy, particularly neocortical, is the main contributor to real impairment of cognitive performance not explained by reduced processing speed seen in timed tasks as SDMT and PASAT. These were the tasks employed by the few studies that found a minor role of GM damage in the cognitive impairment, besides the limitations of the MRI techniques used for detecting GM lesions/atrophy, namely, double inversion recovery (DIR) [44] and diffusion tensor imaging (DTI) [45]. DIR misses the majority of GM lesions observed by microscopy, in particular the most frequent cortical lesion type in MS, namely, the subpial cortical or type III lesions [4, 46]; and the diffusion tensor imaging (DTI) model assumes that there is a single predominant orientation of fibers traveling within the voxel, and this constitutes its major limitation as regards neocortical and subcortical GM structures with voxels containing complex fiber architecture [47].

18.5 Influence of Depression, Fatigue, Sleep Disturbance, Comorbidities, and Side Effect of Drugs on Cognitive Dysfunction

Cognitive function in MS patients is also affected by other factors than the lesions, such as depression, anxiety, fatigue, sleep disturbance, comorbidities, and side effect of drugs (e.g., benzodiazepines, baclofen, antidepressants). MS-related visual and sensory-motor symptoms including pain may also influence performance on neuropsychological tasks, confounding the interpretation of test results.

Depression is present in up to 60% of MS patients and may manifest itself as depressive or asthenoemotional symptoms, anxiety, and even as major depression, with suicide risk in over a quarter of patients, particularly in cases with social isolation and alcohol abuse [23, 48–50]. Asthenoemotional or neurasthenic syndrome is more frequent than major depression, being characterized, in variable degree, by increased mental fatigability, concentration difficulties with secondary forgetfulness, anxiety, insecurity, emotional lability, low tolerance, and increased irritability (sometimes with fits of rage). Depressive or asthenoemotional symptoms affect cognitive performance, especially if they are accompanied by fatigue, insomnia, and lack of motivation, above all in tasks requiring high-level sustained attention, processing speed, executive functioning, working memory, and episodic memory learning [51]. Etiologically, depression has been related both to (1) MS immune-inflammatory pathology itself and impaired functional connectivity, mainly in the circuits interconnecting inferior medial prefrontal and limbic structures (thalamus, hippocampus, amygdala, hypothalamus, and even basal ganglia) and in the ascending monoaminergic brainstem pathways [52–56] and to (2) psychosocial factors such as uncertainty, helplessness, inadequate coping strategies, loss of recreational opportunities, social isolation, high levels of stress, and fatigue [57].

Fatigue affects 60–90% of MS patients, with 40% of them experiencing it as their most disabling symptom [58, 59]. Fatigue is a syndrome constituted by asthenia (tiredness at rest), increased fatigability, and pathological exhaustibility with exercise and stress. Fatigue is felt by the patient as being extremely tired or exhausted, even after rest or sleep, a subjective sensation of lack of all energies for physical and/or mental work, distinct from sadness or weakness, causing detrimental effects on life quality, social and occupational functioning, with 67% of patients experiencing it on a daily basis [60]. *Cognitive fatigue* is a subjective feeling of decreased ability to engage in intense, prolonged, and continuous mental (cognitive) activity, and it can be objectively measured as a decrement in task performance [61, 62]. Etiologically, fatigue can be primary or secondary [59, 63]. *Primary fatigue* is caused by (1) regional (rather than global) MS pathology (demyelination, axonal damage) in WM and GM of strategic brain regions, mainly in prefrontal, temporal, and thalamic regions, with loss of cortical-subcortical connectivity [63, 64]; (2) cytokines released by the immune-mediated inflammatory process [65]; and (3) neuroendocrine dysfunction related to lesions in the hypothalamus and autonomic pathways [66]. *Secondary fatigue* may be a consequence of depression, cognitive impairment, sleep disturbance, medication side effect, reduced activity due to impaired physical and mental strength, and comorbidities (e.g., chronic urinary infection) [63].

Sleep complaints are common in up to 67% of MS patients, manifested as insomnia, obstructive sleep apnea, restless leg syndrome, periodic limb movement, narcolepsy-cataplexy syndrome, and REM sleep behavior disorder [59, 67]. Insomnia in its turn may be due to nocturia, bladder incontinence, leg spasms, pain, discomfort, medication side effects, depression, anxiety, or bad sleep hygiene [68]. In this study by Stanton et al. [68], the most common cause of middle or terminal insomnia was nocturia (72%) and pain or discomfort (22%), while anxiety and racing mind were the main cause of initial insomnia (28%). In fatigue studies that took into account disease severity as well as depression and sleep as covariants, sleep disturbance was the greatest contributor to fatigue [69, 70]. The pathophysiological mechanism of sleep disorder in MS is multifactorial, involving lesions in the brainstem-hypothalamic circuits that regulate circadian sleep-wake cycle, melatonin dysregulation, and decreased functional connectivity between the thalamus and frontal regions [71–73].

Evaluation of depression and fatigue in MS patients is a challenging task, because they are subjective overlapping syndromes, with fatigue being a key component of the diagnosis of depression according to the DSM-5 criteria [74]. Even more challenging is the complex relationship between depression, fatigue, sleep disturbance, and cognitive impairment (Fig. 18.1). Asthenoemotional syndrome or depression causes cognitive deficits, which impair social-occupational functioning, leading to reactive depression. Additionally, depression is often accompanied by fatigue and insomnia, which also cause cognitive deficits, reduced work capacity, unemployment, bad life quality, and a chronic state of preoccupations that cause more insomnia and fatigue, and so on, in a vicious circle.

The assessment and differential diagnosis of these disturbances require a detailed history taking as well as a qualitative and phenomenological analysis of the symptoms, in order to establish which of them is the primary or predominant and, for this reason, in need to be first tackled with pharmacological or non-pharmacological therapy. The phenomenological analysis may be based on a standardized instrument or, in clinical practice, on a detective-like interview looking for a detailed description of the symptoms by the patient regarding how he/she subjectively experiences them.

Some of the most used scales for depression and fatigue have limitations. For instance, the Montgomery-Åsberg Depression Rating Scale (MADRS) [75] and the Beck Depression Inventory (BDI) [76] are considered to have low construct validity for depression and fatigue [34]. For this reason, a shorter (seven items) version of the BDI, the BDI-Fast Screen (BDI-FS), was elaborated and validated, prioritizing thought content (e.g., negative self-evaluation, feelings of worthlessness, or

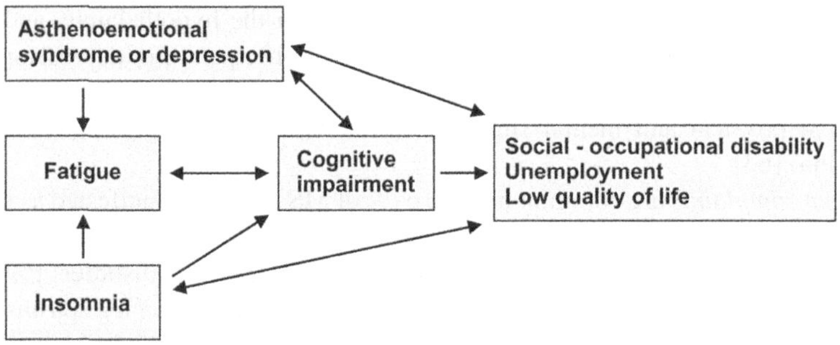

Fig. 18.1 Interactions between depression and asthenoemotional syndrome, fatigue, sleep disturbance, social-occupational disability, and cognitive impairment

inappropriate guilt) and mood (e.g., dysphoria, anhedonia) and excluding items in which depression is confounded with fatigue and cognitive impairment [77, 78]. As regards the assessment of fatigue, one of the most used instruments, the Fatigue Severity Scale (FSS) [79] measures only physical fatigue, leaving aside the cognitive and the psychosocial fatigue, which are undertaken by the Modified Fatigue Impact Scale (MFIS) [80, 81] and by the Fatigue Scale for Motor and Cognitive Functions, with better phenomenological description and severity grading (FSMC) [82].

18.6 Cognitive Assessment

Assessment of cognition in MS patients has not been in the focus of the neurologist's clinical practice or even in clinical trials with disease modifying drugs, in spite of the negative impact of cognitive dysfunction in the patient's social-occupational activities and general mental health. Investigation of sustainability and long-term performance of various outcome measures, including NEDA ("no evidence of disease activity") status, has suggested that the incorporation of cognitive tests into combined clinical and cognitive composite measures can more accurately predict disease outcome in the following years [83]. Clinical trials commonly use the Expanded Disability Status Scale (EDSS) [84], which is biased toward the sensory-motor function, offering a rough estimate of cognitive function, besides its problems with standardization and poor inter-rater reliability. The introduction of the MS Functional Composite (MSFC) [85] has offered several advantages since it is standardized, reproducible, and more sensitive to changes in neurological status; and it has a test for information processing speed and working memory (Paced Auditory Serial Addition Test), but it leaves aside other frequently impaired cognitive domains, as episodic memory.

Several often used screening instruments, such as the Mini-Mental State Examination (MMSE) [86], the Clock Drawing Test (CDT) [87], and the MS Neuropsychological Screening Questionnaire (MSNQ) [88], have limited power to diagnose MS typical cognitive dysfunctions. The widely most used, the MMSE, requires good hand and visual functions, which are frequently compromised by paresis, ataxia, as well as visual disturbances related to optic neuritis (reduced visual acuity) and/or cerebellar-brainstem lesions (nystagmus, saccadic dysmetria, internuclear ophthalmoplegia). Alternative short screening tests more suitable for MS patients with such sensory-motor difficulties are, for instance, the Short Orientation-Memory-Concentration test (SOMC) [89] and the Cognitive Abilities Screening Instrument – Short version (CASI-S) [90–92], which contain the MMSE items most predictive of cognitive dysfunction, namely, register, recall, and orientation [93].

On the other hand, the use of comprehensive psychometric batteries by trained neuropsychologists is not feasible outside specialist centers, besides these batteries being time-consuming and not designed to detect MS-specific cognitive dysfunctions.

For this reason, brief neuropsychological batteries have been developed, which cover the cognitive domains most often compromised in the disease (Table 18.1). The most widely used are the Brief Repeatable Battery of Neuropsychological Tests (BRB-N) [20, 94], with the Brazilian version by Damasceno et al. [95]; the Minimal Assessment of Cognitive Function in Multiple Sclerosis (MACFIMS) [22]; and, more recently, the Brief International Cognitive Assessment for Multiple Sclerosis (BICAMS) [96, 97], with the Brazilian version by Spedo et al. [98].

The BRB-N comprises the following tests:

1. *Selective Reminding Test* (SRT) [99] for verbal learning of a list of 12 unrelated words presented in up to 6 consecutive trials, for the subject to recall as many words as possible; after each trial, the examiner repeats only the words the subject could not recall; and after 20 min, the subject tries to recall the list again (delayed recall). SRT has versions A and B, with different lists of 12 words.
2. *10/36 Spatial Recall Test* (SPART) [100] for visual-spatial learning by reproducing immediately, in three trials, the pattern of 10 checkers on a 6×6 checkerboard viewed for 10 s; and then, after 20 min, in the delayed recall, the subject tries to replicate the pattern again.
3. *Symbol Digit Modalities Test* (SDMT) [101] for sustained selective attention and information processing speed; and the subject has to associate, as quickly as possible, nine different symbols with nine single digits (1–9) during 90 s.
4. *Paced Auditory Serial Addition Test* (PASAT) [102] for information processing speed, sustained attention, and working memory, in which the subject listens to an audio recording of 61 digits presented every 3 s, adds each new digit to the one immediately prior to it, and provides each sum orally as quickly as possible.

Table 18.1 Most used short neuropsychological batteries and their subtests for assessing MS cognitive dysfunction: Brief Repeatable Battery of Neuropsychological Tests (BRB-N), Minimal Assessment of Cognitive Function in Multiple Sclerosis (MACFIMS), and Brief International Cognitive Assessment for Multiple Sclerosis (BICAMS)

Cognitive domain	BRB-N	MACFIMS	BICAMS
Visual-spatial perception		JLO	
Verbal memory	SRT	CVLT-II	CVLT-II T1-5
Visual-spatial memory	SPART	BVMT-R	BVMT-R T1-3
Information processing speed and sustained attention	SDMT, PASAT	SDMT, PASAT	SDMT
Verbal fluency	WLG (semantic)	COWAT (phonologic)	
Executive function		D-KEFS	

Abbreviations: *SRT* Selective Reminding Test, *SPART* 10/36 Spatial Recall Test, *SDMT* Symbol Digit Modalities Test, *PASAT* Paced Auditory Serial Addition Test, *WLG* Word List Generation, *JLO* Judgment of Line Orientation, *CVLT-II California Verbal Learning Test* second edition, *BVMT-R* Brief Visuospatial Memory Test-Revised, *COWAT* Controlled Oral Word Association Test, *D-KEFS* Sorting Test from the Delis-Kaplan Executive Function System

5. *Word List Generation* (WLG) for semantic verbal fluency, the subject spontaneously produces names of a given category (vegetables and fruits in version A; animals in version B).

The MACFIMS includes the following tests:

1. *Controlled Oral Word Association Test* (COWAT) [103]: the subject generates as many words as possible in successive 1-min trials, beginning with each of three designated letters.
2. *Judgment of Line Orientation* (JLO) [103]: the subject has to identify the angle defined by two stimulus lines from among those defined by a visual array of lines covering 180 degrees.
3. *California Verbal Learning Test* second edition (CVLT-II) [104]: the examiner reads 16 words, and the subject has to repeat as many words as possible, in 5 learning trials; and after 25 min, the subject has to spontaneously recall all the words again and then to recognize them in a yes or no forced-choice recognition task.
4. *Brief Visuospatial Memory Test-Revised* (BVMT-R) [105]: the examiner shows to the subject a matrix of six visual designs, which the subject is asked to reproduce using paper and pencil, and taking as much time as needed; and there were three free-recall trials followed by 25-min delayed recall and yes or no recognition trials.
5. *Paced Auditory Serial Addition Test* (PASAT) [101]: Rao's adaptation was employed in the MACFIMS [105].
6. *Symbol Digit Modalities Test* (SDMT) [100]: Rao's adaptation was employed [106].
7. *Sorting Test* from the *Delis-Kaplan Executive Function System* (D-KEFS) [107]: the examiner presents to the subject six cards each depicting a single word, with the varied cards allowing conceptual sorting according to at least eight different principles (e.g., card shape, color, or semantic association among words) and with a time limit of 4 min for each of two card sets.

BRB-N and MACFIMS have comparable sensitivity to cognitive impairment in MS [108]. MACFIMS requires double as much time to be applied (90 min), but it has stronger psychometric properties, its BVMT-R test appears to be more sensitive than the 10/36 SPART, and its auditory verbal learning test (CVLT-II) has the advantage of including a delayed recognition task, which may allow distinguishing between a problem of accessing the learned words (due to attentional deficit, depression, anxiety, or frontal dysfunction) and an impairment of consolidation (due to an entorhinal-hippocampal dysfunction). On the other hand, while the 10/36 SPART is a task of visual-spatial location recall in which the subject needs just to put the checkers in the correct place, the BVMT-R requires the individual to retrieve six unique designs as well as to draw them accurately in the correct locations on the page and for this reason can be influenced by visual deficit and hand paresis, ataxia, or apraxia (potential confounders). Both BRB-N and MACFIMS may be influenced by demographic factors (age, gender, education) and by MS sensory-motor symptoms, besides the PASAT subtest showing significant practice effect [109]. The BICAMS is a shorter battery that assesses the cognitive functions most frequently affected in MS patients, taking 15 min to be applied without need of any special equipment and comprising three tests:

Symbol Digit Modalities Test (SDMT), for information processing speed, consists of nine single digits paired with nine abstract symbols, and the subject has to say, as quickly as possible, the number that corresponds with each symbol. This test is considered the best predictor of MS patient's cognitive impairment in both the BRB-N and MACFIMS [108].

California Verbal Learning Test (CVLT-II T1-5) [104], for verbal memory (immediate recall), comprises a list of 16 words which are read to the subject 5 times in the same order; after each reading of the list, the subject has to recall as many words as possible in any order.

Brief Visuospatial Memory Test-Revised (BVMT-R T1-3), for visual memory (immediate recall), requires the subject to inspect a 2×3 stimulus array of abstract geometric figures presented for 10 s, consisting in three learning trials. After each trial, the array is removed, and the subject is required to draw the array from memory, with the correct shapes in the correct positions.

BICAMS was recommended by a consensus of MS specialists with the aim "not to be either a cognitive screen or full neuropsychological assessment, but rather a brief monitoring instrument" that could "assist therapeutic decision-making" concerning both adjustment at work and home and start or shift in disease modifying drug (DMD) treatment, particularly as regards its effect on cognitive impairment [110]. It was also constructed with the aim of maximizing widespread international use, being suitable for research and everyday clinical practice in small centers, and it can be administered by neurologists or healthcare workers without neuropsychological training [97, 110, 111].

Thus, it is challenging to study complex mental functions in a disease that is also complex and ever changing, presenting cognitive dysfunction even in its early phase in ¼ of patients [21]. The use of comprehensive time-consuming neuropsychological batteries is not viable in most MS practitioner's clinics and small centers, besides many of them having subtests which are non-informative as regards MS typical cognitive dysfunctions. The introduction of shorter batteries as BRB-N and MACFIMS has been a long waited advance for the assessment of MS cognitive status, which can now be better followed-up and monitored with the BICAMS. A remaining problem in many studies of MS cognitive impairment is the lack of control tasks (counterproofs) to verify the influence of confounding variables on the tests proposed (e.g., the lack of subtests for attention or perception as control tasks for verbal or visual learning tests as CVLT, RAVLT, or BVMT-R) or without analyzing the possible influence of these variables by means of appropriate statistical tests. In Amato et al.'s study [21], for instance, 22 (44%) of 50 MS patients had depression as classified by the Hamilton Rating Scale, but the influence of this variable on cognitive performance was not statistically analyzed. Another limitation of most studies is that the evaluation of episodic memory (e.g., word list learning and delayed recall) is restricted to the processes of encoding and free-recall, leaving untested the recognition, and for this reason being unable to conclude about the memory mechanism affected.

18.7 Conclusion

Multiple sclerosis (MS) is an autoimmune, inflammatory, and degenerative disease of the central nervous system (CNS) with lesions disseminated in time (relapses) and space of both white (WM) and gray matter (GM). Most patients present a relapsing-remitting course (RRMS) followed by a secondary-progressive phase (SPMS) and increasing damage to cognition networks, impairing mainly (in up to 65% of cases) information processing speed (IPS), attention, executive function, and episodic memory, with negative impact on social-occupational activities. Clinical onset with cognitive symptoms is rare, thus posing difficulties for the early diagnosis of the disease. Reduction of IPS is mostly explained by lesions in WM tracts crucial for rapid transfer and simultaneous syntheses of multiple information, as occurred in timed tests (e.g., PASAT and SDMT), but neocortical, hippocampal, and thalamic GM atrophy may be the main contributors to real cognitive impairment. Cognitive dysfunction is also due to depression, fatigue, sleep disturbance, drug side effects, and comorbidities, which influence each other in a vicious circle. MS frequently causes depression and fatigue, which overlap with each other and should be differentiated with scales focusing only on depression (e.g., BDI-FS) or on fatigue [e.g., FSMC].

Assessment of cognition has been neglected in MS clinical practice and drug trials. The often used instruments (EDSS, MSFC, MMSE) and even classical psychometric batteries leave aside MS typical cognitive dysfunctions, besides requiring good visual and hand function, often compromised. For these reasons, they have been replaced by more suitable and shorter batteries (BRB-N, MACFIMS, and BICAMS) especially designed for evaluating the cognitive functions most affected by the disease. As compared to BRB-N, MACFIMS has stronger psychometric properties and adds assessment of executive function and delayed recognition of word lists, making possible to differentiate a prefrontal from an entorhinal-hippocampal dysfunction, but its visual-spatial recall subtest (BVMT-R) requires good visual and manual function for retrieving and drawing six unique designs, while that of BRB-N needs just to put the checkers in the correct place. Both BRB-N and MACFIMS tasks may be influenced by age, gender, education, and MS sensory-motor symptoms, besides their PASAT subtest showing significant practice effect. BICAMS is the shortest, includes three subtests (SDMT, CVLT-II, and BVMT-R), and is easier to be administered by neurologists and healthcare workers. A remaining problem in MS cognitive research is the lack of control tasks (counterproofs) or appropriate multivariable statistical analysis for verifying the influence of confounding variables (e.g., depression, deficit of attention, and perception) on performance in these batteries (e.g., in CVLT-II and BVMT-R learning tasks).

References

1. Sanfilipo MP, Benedict RH, Weinstock-Guttman B, Bakshi R (2006) Gray and white matter brain atrophy and neuropsychological impairment in multiple sclerosis. Neurology 66:685–692
2. Houtchens MK, Benedict RH, Killiany R et al (2007) Thalamic atrophy and cognition in multiple sclerosis. Neurology 69:1213–1223
3. Sicotte NL, Kern KC, Giesser BS et al (2008) Regional hippocampal atrophy in multiple sclerosis. Brain 131(4):1134–1141
4. Geurts JJG, Barkhof F (2008) Grey matter pathology in multiple sclerosis. Lancet Neurol 7(9):841–851
5. Batista S, Zivadinov R, Hoogs M, Bergsland M, Heininen-Brown M, Dwyer MG et al (2012) Basal ganglia, thalamus and neocortical atrophy predicting slowed cognitive processing in multiple sclerosis. J Neurol 259:139–146
6. Filippi M, Rocca MA, Horsfield MA, Hametner S, Geurts JJG, Comi G, Lassmann H (2013) Imaging cortical damage and dysfunction in multiple sclerosis. JAMA Neurol 70(5):556–564
7. Minagar A, Barnett MH, Benedict RHB, Pelletier D, Pirko I, Sahraian MA, Frohman E, Zivadinov R (2013) The thalamus and multiple sclerosis: modern views on pathologic, imaging, and clinical aspects. Neurology 80(2):210–219
8. Damasceno A, Damasceno BP, Cendes F (2014) The clinical impact of cerebellar grey matter pathology in multiple sclerosis. PLoS One 9(5):e96193. https://doi.org/10.1371/journal.pone.0096193.eCollection
9. Rocca MA, Barkhof F, De Luca J, Frisén J, Geurts JJG, Hulst HE, Sastre-Garriga J, Filippi M, for the MAGNIMS Study Group (2018) The hippocampus in multiple sclerosis. Lancet Neurol 17:918–926
10. Azevedo CJ, Cen SY, Khadka S, Liu S, Kornak J, Shi Y, Zheng L, Hauser SL, Pelletier D (2018) Thalamic atrophy in multiple sclerosis: a magnetic resonance imaging marker of neurodegeneration throughout disease. Ann Neurol 83(2):223–234. https://doi.org/10.1002/ana.25150
11. Achiron A, Ziv I, Djaldetti R, Goldberg H, Kuritzky A, Melamed E (1992) Aphasia in multiple sclerosis: clinical and radiologic correlations. Neurology 42:2195–2197
12. Okuda B, Tanaka H, Tachibana H, Iwamoto Y, Takeda M, Kawabata K, Sugita M (1996) Visual form agnosia in multiple sclerosis. Acta Neurol Scand 94:38–44
13. Pelosi L, Geesken JM, Holly M, Hayward M, Blumhardt LD (1997) Working memory impairment in early multiple sclerosis: evidence from an event-related potential study of patients with clinically isolated myelopathy. Brain 120:2039–2058
14. Coebergh JAF, Roosendall SD, Polman CH, Geurts JJ, van Woerkom TCAM (2010) Acute severe memory impairment as a presenting symptom of multiple sclerosis: a clinical case study with 3D double inversion recovery MR imaging. Mult Scler 16(12):1521–1524
15. Lublin FD, Reingold SC, Cohen JA, Cutter GR, Sørensen PS, Thompson AJ, Wolinsky JS et al (2014) Defining the clinical course of multiple sclerosis: the 2013 revisions. Neurology 83(3):278–286
16. Thompson AJ, Banwell BL, Barkhof F, Carrol WM, Coetzee T, Comi G et al (2018) Diagnosis of multiple sclerosis: 2017 revisions of the McDonald criteria. Lancet Neurol 17:162–173
17. Amato MP, Portaccio E, Goretti B, Zipoli V, Hakiki B, Giannini M et al (2010) Cognitive impairment in early stages of multiple sclerosis. Neurol Sci 31(Suppl 2):211–214
18. Polman CH, Reingold SC, Banwell B, Clanet M, Cohen JA, Filippi M et al (2011) Diagnostic criteria for multiple sclerosis: 2010 revisions to the McDonald criteria. Ann Neurol 69:292–302
19. Achiron A, Barak Y (2003) Cognitive impairment in probable multiple sclerosis. J Neurol Neurosurg Psychiatry 74:443–446
20. Rao SM, Leo GJ, Bernardin L, Unverzagt F (1991) Cognitive dysfunction in multiple sclerosis: I. frequency, patterns, and prediction. Neurology 41(5):685–689

21. Amato MP, Ponziani G, Siracusa G, Sorbi S (2001) Cognitive dysfunction in early-onset multiple sclerosis: a reappraisal after 10 years. Arch Neurol 58(10):1602–1606
22. Benedict RHB, Cookfair D, Gavett R, Gunther M (2006) Validity of the minimal assessment of cognitive function in multiple sclerosis (MACFIMS). J Int Neuropsychol Soc 12(4):549–558
23. Chiaravalotti ND, De Luca J (2008) Cognitive impairment in multiple sclerosis. Lancet Neurol 7(12):1139–1151
24. Sumowsky JF, Benedict R, Enzinger C, Filippi M, Geurts JJ, Hamalainen P et al (2018) Cognition in multiple sclerosis: state of the field and priorities for the future. Neurology 90:278–288
25. Paul F (2016) Pathology and MRI: exploring cognitive impairment in MS. Acta Neurol Scand 134(Suppl. 200):24–33. https://doi.org/10.1111/ane.12649
26. Cotter J, Firth J, Enzinger C, Kontopantelis E, Yung AR, Elliot R, Drake RJ (2016) Social cognition in multiple sclerosis: a systematic review and meta-analysis. Neurology 87:1727–1736
27. Jak AJ, Bondi MW, Delano-Wood L, Wierenga C, Corey-Bloom J, Salmon DP, Delis DC (2009) Quantification of five neuropsychological approaches to defining mild cognitive impairment. Am J Geriatr Psychiatry 17:368–375
28. Bondi MW, Edmonds EC, Jak AJ, Clark LR, Delano-Wood L et al (2014) Neuropsychological criteria for mild cognitive impairment improves diagnostic precision, biomarker associations, and prediction of progression. J Alzheimers Dis 42:275–289
29. Benedict RH, Morrow S, Rodgers J, Hojnacki D, Bucello MA, Zivadinov R, Weinstock-Guttman B (2014) Characterizing cognitive function during relapse in multiple sclerosis. Mult Scler 20:1745–1752
30. Damasceno A, Damasceno BP, Cendes F (2015) Subclinical MRI disease activity influences cognitive performance in MS patients. Mult Scler Relat Disord 4(2):137–143
31. Dineen RA, Vilisaar J, Hlinka J et al (2009) Disconnection as a mechanism for cognitive dysfunction in multiple sclerosis. Brain 132:239–249
32. Roosendaal SD, Geurts JJG, Vrenken H, Hulst HE, Cover KS, Castelijns JA, Pouwels PJ, Barkhof F (2009) Regional DTI differences in multiple sclerosis patients. NeuroImage 44(4):1397–1403
33. Mesaros S, Rocca MA, Kacar K et al (2012) Diffusion tensor MRI tractography and cognitive impairment in multiple sclerosis. Neurology 78(13):969–975
34. Rocca MA, Amato MP, De Stefano N et al (2015) Clinical and imaging assessment of cognitive dysfunction in multiple sclerosis. Lancet Neurol 14:302–317
35. Lockwood AH, Linn RT, Szymanski H, Coad ML, Wack DS (2004) Mapping the neural systems that mediate the paced auditory serial addition task (PASAT). J Int Neuropsychol Soc 10:26–34
36. Rocca MA, Valsasina P, Martinelli V, Misci P, Falini A, Comi G et al (2012) Large-scale neuronal network dysfunction in relapsing-remitting multiple sclerosis. Neurology 79:1449–1457
37. Wegner C, Esiri MM, Chance SA et al (2006) Neocortical neuronal, synaptic, and glial loss in multiple sclerosis. Neurology 67:960–967
38. Dutta R, Chang A, Doud MK, Kidd GJ, Ribaudo MV, Young EA, Fox RJ, Staugaitis SM, Trapp BD (2011) Demyelination causes synaptic alterations in hippocampi from multiple sclerosis patients. Ann Neurol 69(3):445–454
39. Roosendaal SD, Geurts JJG, Vrenken H, Hulst HE, Cover KS, Castelijns JA, Pouwels PJ, Barkhof F (2009) Regional DTI differences in multiple sclerosis patients. NeuroImage 44(4):1397–1403
40. Calabrese M, Agosta F, Rinaldi F et al (2009) Cortical lesions and atrophy associated with cognitive impairment in relapsing-remitting multiple sclerosis. Arch Neurol 66:1144–1150
41. Nelson F, Datta S, Garcia N et al (2011) Intracortical lesions by 3T magnetic resonance imaging and correlation with cognitive impairment in multiple sclerosis. Mult Scler 17(9):1122–1129

42. Preziosa P, Rocca MA, Pagani E, Stromillo ML, Enzinger C, Gallo A, Hulst HE et al (2016) Structural MRI correlates of cognitive impairment in patients with multiple sclerosis: a multicenter study. Hum Brain Mapp 37(4):1627–1644
43. Sumowsky JF, Rocca MA, Leavitt VM et al (2014) Brain reserve and cognitive reserve protect against cognitive decline over 4.5 years in MS. Neurology 82:1776–1783
44. Papadopoulou A, Muller-Lenke N, Naegelin Y et al (2013) Contribution of cortical and white matter lesions to cognitive impairment in multiple sclerosis. Mult Scler 19:1290–1296
45. Llufriu S, Martinez-Heras E, Fortea J, Blanco Y et al (2014) Cognitive functions in multiple sclerosis: impact of gray matter integrity. Mult Scler 20(4):424–432
46. Seewann A, Kooi E-J, Roosendaal SD, Pouwels PJW, Wattjes MP, van der Valk P et al (2012) Postmortem verification of MS cortical lesion detection with 3D DIR. Neurology 78:302–308
47. Lanyon LJ (2012) Chapter 7: Diffusion tensor imaging: structural connectivity insights, limitations and future directions. In: Bright P (ed) Neuroimaging – methods. InTechOpen, pp 137–162, ISBN 978-953-51-0097-3
48. Minden SL, Schiffer RB (1991) Depression and mood disorders in multiple sclerosis. Neuropsychiatry 4:62–77
49. Feinstein A (2011) Multiple sclerosis and depression. Mult Scler J 17(11):1276–1281
50. Boeschoten RE, Braamse AMJ, Beekman ATF, Cuijpers P, van Oppen P, Dekker J, Uitdehaag BMJ (2017) Prevalence of depression and anxiety in multiple sclerosis: a systematic review and meta-analysis. J Neurol Sci 372:331–341
51. Arnett PA, Barwick FH, Beeney JE (2008) Depression in multiple sclerosis: review and theoretical proposal. J Int Neuropsypchol Soc 14:691–724
52. Feinstein A, Roy P, Lobaugh N, Feinstein K, O'Connor P, Black S (2004) Structural brain abnormalities in multiple sclerosis patients with major depression. Neurology 62(4):586–590
53. Sabatini U, Pozzilli C, Pantano P, Koudriavtseva T, Padovani A, Millefiorini E, Di Biasi C, Gualdi GF, Lenzi M (1996) Involvement of the limbic system in multiple sclerosis patients with depressive disorders. Biol Psychiatry 39(11):970–975
54. Bakshi R, Czarnecki D, Shaikh ZA et al (2000) Brain MRI lesions and atrophy are related to depression in multiple sclerosis. Neuroreport 11:1153–1158
55. Colasanti A, Guo Q, Giannetti P, Wall MB, Newbould RD, Bishop C et al (2016) Hippocampal neuroinflammation, functional connectivity and depressive symptoms in multiple sclerosis. Biol Psychiatry 80:62–72
56. Geest Q, Boeschoten RE, Keijzer MJ, Steenwijk MD, Pouwels PJW, Twisk JWR, Smit JH, Uitdehaag BMJ, Geurts JJG, Oppen P, Hulst HE (2019) Fronto-limbic disconnection in patients with multiple sclerosis and depression. Mult Scler J 25(5):715–726
57. Feinstein A (2007) The clinical neuropsychiatry of multiple sclerosis. Cambridge University Press, New York
58. Fisk JD, Pontefract A, Ritvo PG, Archibald CJ, Murray TJ (1994) The impact of fatigue on patients with multiple sclerosis. Can J Neurol Sci 21(1):9–14
59. Strober LB (2015) Fatigue in multiple sclerosis: a look at the role of poor sleep. Front Neurol 6:21. https://doi.org/10.3389/fneur.2015.00021
60. Krupp LB, Alvarez LA, LaRocca NG, Scheinberg LC (1988) Fatigue in multiple sclerosis. Arch Neurol 45(4):435–437
61. Schwid SR, Tyler CM, Scheid EA, Weinstein A, Goodman AD, McDermott MP (2003) Cognitive fatigue during a test requiring sustained attention: a pilot study. Mult Scler 9:503–508. https://doi.org/10.1191/1352458503ms946oa
62. Gergelyfi M, Jacob B, Olivier E, Zénon A (2015) Dissociation between mental fatigue and motivational state during prolonged mental activity. Front Behav Neurosci 9:176. https://doi.org/10.3389/fnbeh.2015.00176
63. Patejdl R, Penner IK, Noack TK, Zettl UK (2016) Multiple sclerosis and fatigue: a review of the contribution of inflammation and immune-mediated neurodegeneration. Autoimmun Rev 15(3):210–220

64. Rocca MA, Parisi L, Pagani E, Copetti M, Rodegher M, Colombo B, Comi G, Falini A, Filippi M (2014) Regional but not global brain damage contributes to fatigue in multiple sclerosis. Radiology 273:511–520
65. Morris G, Berk M, Valder K, Maes M (2015) Central pathways causing fatigue in neuroinflammatory and autoimmune illnesses. BMC Med:13–28. https://doi.org/10.1186/s12916-014-0259-2
66. Huitinga I, Erkut ZA, van Beurden D, Swaab DF (2004) Impaired hypothalamus-pituitary-adrenal axis activity and more severe multiple sclerosis with hypothalamic lesions. Ann Neurol 55(1):37–45
67. Fleming WE, Pollak CP (2005) Sleep disorders in multiple sclerosis. Semin Neurol 25:64–68
68. Stanton BR, Barnes F, Silver E (2006) Sleep and fatigue in multiple sclerosis. Mult Scler 12(4):481–486
69. Strober LB, Arnett PA (2005) An examination of four models predicting fatigue in multiple sclerosis. Arch Clin Neuropsychol 20(5):631–646
70. Ghajarzadeh M, Sahraian MA, Fateh R, Daneshmand A (2012) Fatigue, depression and sleep disturbances in Iranian patients with multiple sclerosis. Acta Med Iran 50(4):244–249
71. Brass SD, Duquette P, Proulx-Therrien J, Auerbach S (2010) Sleep disorders in patients with multiple sclerosis. Sleep Med Rev 14(2):121–129
72. Melamud L, Golan D, Luboshitzky R, Lavi I, Miller A (2012) Melatonin dysregulation, sleep disturbances and fatigue in multiple sclerosis. J Neurol Sci 314(1–2):37–40
73. van Geest Q, Westerik B, van der Werf YD, Geurts JJ, Hulst HE (2017) The role of sleep on cognition and functional connectivity in patients with multiple sclerosis. J Neurol 264(1):72–80
74. American Psychiatric Association (2013) Diagnostic and statistical manual of mental disorders, 5th edn. Author, Washington, DC
75. Montgomery SA, Åsberg M (1979) A new depression scale designed to be sensitive to chance. Br J Psychiatry 134:382–389
76. Beck AT, Ward CH, Mendelson M, Mock J, Erbaugh J (1961) An inventory for measuring depression. Arch Gen Psychiatry 4:561–571
77. Beck AT, Steer RA, Brown GK (2000) BDI-fast screen for medical patients: manual. Psychological Corporation, San Antonio
78. Benedict RH, Fishman I, McClellan MM, Bakshi R (2003) Validity of the beck depression inventory-fast screen in multiple sclerosis. Mult Scler 9:393–396
79. Krupp LB, LaRocca NG, Muir-Nash J, Steinberg AD (1989) The fatigue severity scale. Application to patients with multiple sclerosis and systemic lupus erythematosus. Arch Neurol 46(10):1121–1123
80. Fisk JD, Pontefract A, Ritvo PG, Archibald CJ, Murray TJ (1994) The impact of fatigue on patients with multiple sclerosis. Can J Neurol Sci 21(1):9–14
81. Téllez N, Rio J, Tintoré M, Nos C, Galán I, Montalban X (2005) Does the modified fatigue impact scale offer a more comprehensive assessment of fatigue in MS? Mult Scler 11(2):198–202
82. Penner IK, Raselli C, Stöcklin M, Opwis K, Kappos L, Calabrese P (2009) The Fatigue Scale for Motor and Cognitive Functions (FSMC): validation of a new instrument to assess multiple sclerosis-related fatigue. Mult Scler 15(12):1509–1517
83. Damasceno A, Pimentel-Silva LR, Damasceno BP, Cendes F (submitted) Long-term performance of outcome measures in multiple sclerosis. Eur J Neurol
84. Kurtzke JF (1983) Rating neurologic impairment in multiple sclerosis: an expanded disability status scale (EDSS). Neurology 13(11):1444–1452
85. Cutter GR, Baier ML, Rudick RA, Cookfair DL, Fischer JS, Petkau J et al (1999) Development of a multiple sclerosis functional composite as a clinical trial outcome measure. Brain 122:871–882
86. Folstein MF, Folstein SE, McHugh PR (1975) "Mini-mental state". A practical method for grading the cognitive state of patients for the clinician. J Psychiatr Res 12(3):189–198

87. Barak Y, Lavie M, Achiron A (2002) Screening for early cognitive impairment in multiple sclerosis patients using the clock drawing test. J Clin Neurosci 9(6):629–632
88. Benedict RH, Munschauer F, Linn R, Miller C, Murphy E, Foley F, Jacobs L (2003) Screening for multiple sclerosis cognitive impairment using a self-administered 15-item questionnaire. Mult Scler 9(1):95–101
89. Katzman R, Brown T, Fuld P, Peck A, Schechter R, Schimmel H (1983) Validation of a short orientation-memory-concentration test of cognitive impairment. Am J Psychiatry 140(6):734–739
90. Teng EL, Hasegawa K, Homma A, Imai Y, Larson E, Borenstein AR, Sugimoto K, Yamaguchi T, Sasaki H, Chiu D (1994) The Cognitive Abilities Screening Instrument (CASI): a practical test for cross-cultural epidemiological studies of dementia. Int Psychogeriatrics 6:45–58
91. Teng EL, Larson EB, Lin KN, Graves AB, Liu HC (1998) Screening for dementia: the Cognitive Abilities Screening Instrument – Short Version (CASI-Short). Presentation at the annual convention of the American Psychological Association San Francisco
92. Damasceno A, Delicio AM, Mazo DFC, Zullo JFD, Scherer P, Ng RTY, Damasceno BP (2005) Validation of the Brazilian version of mini-test CASI-S. Arq Neuropsiquiatr 63(2-B):416–421
93. Magaziner J, Bassett SS, Hebel JR (1987) Predicting performance on the mini-mental state examination. Use of age- and education-specific equations. J Am Geriatr Soc 35(11):996–1000
94. Boringa JB, Lazeron RH, Reuling IE, Ader HJ, Pfennings L, Lindeboom J, de Sonneville LM, Kalkers NF (2001) The brief repeatable battery of neuropsychological tests: normative values allow application in multiple sclerosis clinical practice. Mult Scler 7(4):263–267
95. Damasceno A, Amaral JMSDS, Barreira AA, Becker J, Callegaro D, Campanholo KR, Damasceno LA, Diniz DS, Fragoso YD, Franco PS, Finkelsztejn A, Jorge FMH, Lana-Peixoto MA, Matta APDC, Mendonça ACR, Noal J, Paes RA, Papais-Alvarenga RM, Spedo CT, Damasceno BP (2018) Normative values of the brief repeatable battery of neuropsychological tests in a Brazilian population sample: discrete and regression-based norms. Arq Neuropsiquiatr 76(3):163–169
96. Langdon DW, Amato MP, Boringa J, Brochet B, Foley F, Fredrikson S, Hämäläinen P, Hartung H-P, Krupp L, Penner IK, Reder AT, Benedict RHB (2012) Recommendations for a Brief International Cognitive Assessment for Multiple Sclerosis (BICAMS). Mult Scler 18(6):891–898
97. Benedict RHB, Amato MP, Boringa J, Brochet B, Foley F, Fredrikson S, Hamalainen P, Hartung H, Krupp L, Penner I, Reder AT, Langdon D (2012) Brief International Cognitive Assessment for MS (BICAMS): international standards for validation. BMC Neurol 12:55. http://www.biomedcentral.com/1471-2377/12/55
98. Spedo CT, Frndak SE, Marques VD, Foss MP, Pereira DA, Carvalho LF, Guerreiro CT, Conde RM, Fusco T, Pereira AJ, Gaino SB, Garcia RB, Benedict RHB, Barreira AA (2015) Cross-cultural adaptation, reliability, and validity of the BICAMS in Brazil. Clin Neuropsychol 29(6):836–846. https://doi.org/10.1080/13854046.2015.1093173
99. Buschke H, Fuld PA (1974) Evaluating storage, retention, and retrieval in disordered memory and learning. Neurology 24(11):1019–1025
100. Rao SM (1990) Cognitive function study group, NMSS. A manual for the brief repeatable battery of neuropsychological tests in multiple sclerosis. New York, National Multiple Sclerosis Society
101. Smith A (1982) Symbol digit modalities test (SDMT). Manual (revised). Los Angeles, Western Psychological Services
102. Gronwall DM (1977) Paced auditory serial-addition task: a measure of recovery from concussion. Percept Mot Skills 44(2):367–373
103. Benton AL (1994) Neuropsychological assessment. Annu Rev Psychol 45:1–23
104. Delis DC, Kramer JH (2000) California verbal learning test: CVLT-II; Adult version; Manual
105. Benedict RH (1997) Brief visuospatial memory test-revised: professional manual. Psychological Assessment Resources, Inc, Odessa

106. Rao SM (1991) A manual for the brief repeatable battery of neuropsychological tests in multiple sclerosis. New York, National Multiple Sclerosis Society
107. Delis DC, Kaplan E, Kramer JH (2001) Delis-Kaplan Executive Function System (D-KEFS). Psychological Corporation, San Antonio
108. Strober L, Englert J, Munschauer F, Weinstock-Guttman B, Rao S, Benedict RH (2009) Sensitivity of conventional memory tests in multiple sclerosis: comparing the Rao brief repeatable neuropsychological battery and the minimal assessment of cognitive function in MS. Mult Scler 15(9):1077–1084
109. Bever CT, Grattan L, Panitch HS, Johnson KP (1995) The brief repeatable battery of neuropsychological tests for multiple sclerosis: a preliminary serial study. Mult Scler 1:165–169
110. Langdon DW, Amato MP, Boringa J, Brochet B, Foley F, Fredrikson S, Hämäläinen P, Hartung H-P, Krupp L, Penner IK, Reder AT, Benedict RHB (2012) Recommendations for a Brief International Cognitive Assessment for Multiple Sclerosis (BICAMS). Mult Scler 18(6):891–898
111. Langdon DW, Amato M, Boringa J et al (2011) The Brief International Cognitive Assessment for Multiple Sclerosis (BICAMS): first consensus steps towards a brief universal cognitive assessment for MS. Neurology 76:A479

Chapter 19
Temporal Lobe Epilepsy

19.1 Introduction

Epilepsy is a chronic syndrome characterized by recurrent seizures with different clinical manifestations associated with occasional or intermittent paroxysmal discharges of brain neurons. Temporal lobe epilepsy (TLE) is the most common (approximately 40% of adult epilepsy), usually associated with temporal-limbic lesions, memory decline, and drug resistance, but presenting good outcome after resection of the epileptogenic focus. The seizures often arise from medial temporal structures (hippocampus, amygdala, parahippocampal gyrus), but the neuronal discharges may originate in other brain regions (e.g., occipital) then spreading to the medial temporal lobe. This is the so-called medial temporal lobe epilepsy (MTLE), which may present itself as (1) a simple partial seizure (SPS), with rising epigastric sensation, fear, "déjà vu" or "jamais vu" experience, paleness, sudoresis, and sometimes olfactory or gustative sensations, or (2) complex partial seizure (CPS), with motionless staring gaze, absence, and automatisms (oro-alimentary, vocal or gestural), with duration from 2 to 10 min, presenting postictal confusion, somnolence, disorientation, and impairment of attention, memory, and language. MTLE patients usually have previous history of febrile seizures in infancy, status epilepticus, and cases of epilepsy in the family [1, 2].

MTLE patients may present interictal disturbances of memory and reasoning as well as depressive or asthenoemotional symptoms, and rarely psychotic disorder, which may be due to the underlying brain lesion or subclinical epileptogenic activity, side effect of antiepileptic drugs (AED), especially phenobarbital, phenytoin, primidon, and topiramate, or to a combination of all these factors. AEDs, particularly topiramate, may further worsen the epilepsy-related memory impairment of these patients [3].

B. Damasceno, *Research on Cognition Disorders*,
https://doi.org/10.1007/978-3-030-57267-9_19

19.2 Neurophysiological and Neuroimaging Investigation

Neurophysiological investigation of MTLE includes electroencephalography (EEG) with or without video telemetry (for behavioral-electroencephalographic correlation). Interictal EEG may be normal or show non-epileptiform (slow waves) and/or epileptiform discharges (acute waves), unilateral or bilateral, synchronous or asynchronous, in the anterior temporal regions. Functional neuroimaging may also contribute to the diagnosis of the epileptogenic focus. Positron emission tomography (PET) is the most used in the interictal period and may reveal a focal hypometabolic region concordant with seizure onset, while single-photon emission computed tomography (SPECT) may show delimited area of hyperperfusion in the temporal region during a seizure, corresponding to the epileptogenic focus, thus contributing to the neurosurgical decision [4].

Structural MRI may be normal or show decrease of hippocampal volume (atrophy) in T1 and increase of signal in T2 acquisitions, correlated to hippocampal sclerosis (HS) [1, 5]. In MTLE patients with HS, there is progressive diffuse gray matter atrophy further extending to other extrahippocampal structures of the medial temporal region (entorhinal and perirhinal cortices, parahippocampal gyrus) and even to the entire lateral temporal lobe, unilateral or bilaterally, often asymmetric, involving as well as the insula, frontal, and occipital lobes ipsilateral to the epileptogenic zone, and bilateral thalamus, even in patients that have been seizure free for two or more years [6, 7]. Extrahippocampal gray matter atrophy involving entorhinal, perirhinal cortices, and more distant limbic and frontal structures as the cingulate and orbitofrontal cortex contribute to further worsening of general and particularly of verbal memory in patients with left MTLE [8].

In functional MRI studies, both right and left MTLE patients with HS have widespread abnormal large-scale network connectivity, particularly affecting the hippocampus, contralateral mesial temporal structures, the default mode network [9–14], and the connectivity between the basal ganglia-thalamus circuitry and the cortex, particularly in left TLE, as well as in frontal, and parietal/occipital lobe epilepsy [15].

Histopathology in chronic MTLE patients with HS shows progressive neuronal loss and astrocytic proliferation (gliosis) in hippocampal fields CA1, CA3, and CA4, with relative preservation of CA2 (ILAE classification type I, "classical HS"), with further extension to the adjacent dentate gyrus, parahippocampal gyrus, and amygdala ("mesial temporal sclerosis" or "HS plus") [16]. There may additionally be subtle cortical temporal dysplasias (type IIIa) and even dual pathology (cavernoma, dysembryoplastic neuroepithelial tumor, or ganglioglioma) accompanying the HS [17].

19.3 Neuropsychological Assessment

Neuropsychological investigation should include not only cognition but also emotion, personality, and quality of life, which usually deteriorate in the chronic course of epilepsy. First step is an initial interview, which may contribute to establish empathy and rapport with the patient, to avoid future "noise" in the testing as well as to get some idea on his/her intellectual level, discourse, personality, previous skills, attitudes, and worries, which can influence test performance and make difficult the interpretation of its results. For example, an average score on a test of mental arithmetic would represent a marked decline from the premorbid level in a patient who was a qualified accountant, while a score below the normative mean does not necessarily represent an acquired deficit in an individual who previously had modest abilities [18]. Second step is the proper neuropsychological examination by means of a basic battery of tests, which in most epilepsy center includes an estimate of premorbid cognitive competence and intelligence with the Wechsler Adult Intelligence Scale-Revised (WAIS-R); assessment of attention with WAIS-R digit span; visual-spatial perception with Rey Complex Figure [19].; language (Boston Naming, FAS Verbal Fluency, Token Test) [20–22]; memory (Wechsler Memory Scale-Revised or Rey Auditory Verbal Learning) [23, 24], executive function, and mental flexibility (Stroop, Wisconsin Card Sorting, Trail Making) [21, 25, 26].

Neuropsychological assessment of patients with MTLE, particularly in those with drug-resistant seizures, may reveal a mild-to-moderate episodic (verbal and nonverbal) memory deficit as well as scores of language and intellectual functions below the mean of the healthy population [27]. The memory impairment is usually correlated to the hippocampal atrophy detected by MRI volumetry and cell counting of this region [1, 28, 29].

Traditionally, the aim and challenge of the preoperative neuropsychological evaluation have been to establish the side and local of the temporal lobe dysfunction, blindly to the results of other laboratory investigations. As reminded by Baxendale and Thompson [30], lateralization and localization of lesions and seizure foci are now better performed by new neuroimaging techniques, but a comprehensive, qualitative, and quantitative assessment remains essential for establishing a baseline neuropsychological profile, which (1) contributes to the postoperative prognosis when correlated to the data of other presurgical investigations (EEG, MRI, PET, SPECT), (2) helps the patient to make an informed decision, and (3) forms the basis of a tailor-made preemptive rehabilitation program implemented prior to the surgery in order to minimize the postsurgical cognitive morbidity. Besides this, a careful comprehensive neuropsychological evaluation can diagnose a deficit of attention or receptive language and thus help to disclose potential confounds in the fMRI procedure and guide the interpretation of its results [30]. With the evaluation of potential confounders as handedness and language dominance by means of a standardized questionnaire and language fMRI tasks, fMRI can even predict memory decline after temporal lobe resection [31, 32]. Moreover, such a comprehensive neuropsychological battery could also assess the confounding effect of cognitive fatigue in a lengthy testing paradigm in the fMRI scanner.

As regards the localization diagnosis, when the neuropsychological, video-EEG-telemetry, and neuroimaging (MRI, PET, SPECT) data, independently gathered, are convergent, that is, show the same brain local of the dysfunction, then a safer surgical decision may be taken, and good postsurgical results can be predicted, resulting in elimination or reduction of the seizures in 58% to 64% of the cases. In this regard, as suggested by Milner [33] and Jones-Gotman [34], the choice of the neuropsychological tests would take into account the functional difference between the two temporal lobes (the so-called material-specific memory model, MSMM), with the left one (dominant) mediating memory for verbal material (names, list of words or numbers) and the right one, memory for nonverbal material (faces, locals, abstract designs). Thus, based on the MSMM, in order to detect a double dissociation in the functions of the temporal lobes, (1) the test material would be polarized as much as possible as for its verbal versus nonverbal (visual, spatial) characteristics (e.g., employing a list of abstract words versus a series of abstract figures); (2) the tests should consist in learning tasks, by presenting the material repeated times; and (3) the verbal and nonverbal tests should be equivalent as for the type of memory activity required (encoding, recall, or recognition), so that recall (or recognition) of one test could be compared with recall (or recognition) of the other test [34]. According to Jones-Gotman (1996), two of the most used tests (Wechsler Memory Scale and Rey Complex Figure) are not well polarized into the verbal versus nonverbal nature of their material nor are they matched as concerns the kind of memory activity involved (encoding, recall, recognition), so they are not suitable for comparisons between the hemispheres.

Other studies [35–37], including ours [38–40], have confirmed the material-specific memory model as concerns the relation between deficit of verbal memory and epileptogenic focus or lesion in the left temporal lobe, but not between nonverbal (visual, spatial) memory deficit and epileptogenic focus or lesion in the right temporal lobe, probably due to the verbalizability of the material employed in the visual tests and because visual-spatial memory has a more diffuse and bilateral brain representation. Moreover, the MMSM was constructed on the basis of temporal lobectomy case studies and has not been sufficiently validated in unoperated cases.

Indeed, more recent studies have challenged the strong version of the MSMM with its implicit assumption of verbal and nonverbal memories as unitary, internally homogeneous, and fully lateralized functions, without taking into account their different subtypes (heterogeneities) (e.g., for visual memory, subtypes could be maze learning, navigation, scene recognition, abstract designs, object location, or spatial position) nor considering task specificities (e.g., for verbal memory: learning of unrelated arbitrary versus semantically related paired associates, consisting in learning of syllables, digits, or words in pairs so that one member of the pair evokes recall of the other) [30, 41, 42]. Moreover, there is evidence of impairment of nonverbal (visual, spatial) memory in cases with left hippocampal sclerosis and left anterior temporal lobe resection [43] and of verbal memory after right temporal lobe resection [44]. Besides, left temporal lobe presents a lateral-medial specialization for verbal memory, with the anterior portion of the inferior temporal gyrus processing semantically related paired associates, the perirhinal region mediating arbitrary paired associates, and the hippocampus protecting (consolidating) newly learned information from the effects of interference [45, 46]. Additionally, neuroimaging studies have indicated a dynamic interaction between the left and right medial temporal regions, depending on the specific tasks used [41, 47].

In conclusion, impairment of memory and other cognitive functions in MTLE patients results from an interaction between various factors, such as the epileptogenic focus and associated network disruptions, the underlying brain lesion, and side effect of AEDs, besides other influential variables, such as an earlier age at seizure onset, longer duration of epilepsy, and higher seizure frequency. The interplay is even more complex if we consider the interfunctional relationships of memory with attention, perception, language, intellectual-executive function, and mood state, all of which are involved in the execution of neuropsychological tasks, and should be evaluated and taken into account; otherwise the finding of low memory scores cannot safely be attributed to a specific or primary memory disturbance.

19.4 Conclusion

Medial temporal lobe epilepsy (MTLE) is caused by paroxysmal neuronal discharges arising mainly from the hippocampus, amygdala, and parahippocampal gyrus. It evolves with atrophy of medial and neighboring lateral temporal lobe as well as widespread abnormal connectivity in large-scale networks, impairing memory and intellectual functions. MTLE is usually drug resistant but responds to surgical resection of the epileptogenic focus (EF) with reduction or elimination of seizures in the majority of cases. Thus, the challenge of the surgery is to completely remove the EF with minimum or no neurological side effects, what is achieved when the electroencephalography, neuroimaging, and neuropsychological investigation converge, showing the same brain local of the lesion or EF. For this endeavor, the choice of neuropsychological tests should take into account the functional difference between the two temporal lobes, with the left one (dominant) mediating verbal, and the right one, the nonverbal memory (according to the so-called material specific memory model, MSMM), using polarized learning tests (verbal versus nonverbal, e.g,. list of abstract words versus series of abstract figures) and evaluating the same memory process (encoding, recall, or recognition). The strong version of the MSMM assuming that verbal and nonverbal memories are homogeneous and fully lateralized have been challenged, particularly as regards the relation between visual-spatial memory and right temporal lesion, probably because nonverbal memory has a more widespread and bilateral representation. In fact, there are cases of temporal sclerosis or resection in the left side impairing nonverbal memory and in the right side affecting verbal memory. In spite of this, if a well- designed neuropsychological battery finds, for example, high scores of verbal contrasting with low scores of visual-spatial memory in a right-handed individual is highly indicative of a right temporal lobe dysfunction.

In summary, impairment of memory and other cognitive functions in MTLE result from interaction of various factors such as the EF and associated network disruptions, the underlying brain lesion, side effect of antiepileptic drugs, and higher seizure frequency. Additionally, disorders of attention, perception, and mood (anxiety, depression) can affect performance in memory tasks secondarily leading to low scores.

References

1. Engel J, Willimson PD, Wieser HG (1997) Mesial temporal lobe epilepsy. In: Engel J, Pendley TA (eds) Epilepsy: a comprehensive textbook. Lippincott-Raven Pyblishers, Philadelphia, pp 2417–2426
2. Cendes F, Andermann F, Dubeau F et al (1993) Early childhood prolonged febrile convulsions, atrophy and sclerosis of mesial structures, and temporal lobe epilepsy: an MRI volumetric study. Neurology 43:1083–1087
3. Loring DW, Williamson DJ, Meador KJ, Wiegand F, Hulihan J (2011) Topiramate dose effects on cognition: a randomized double-blind study. Neurology 76:131–137
4. Cendes F, Theodore WH, Brinkmann BH et al (2016) Neuroimaging of epilepsy. Handb Clin Neurol 136:985–1014
5. Cendes F, Andermann F, Gloor P et al (1993) Atrophy of mesial structures in patients with temporal lobe epilepsy: cause or consequence of repeated seizures? Ann Neurol 34:795–801
6. Cendes F, Kobayashi E (2000) Temporal lobe epilepsy. In: Guerreiro CAM, Guerreiro MM, Cendes F, Lopes-Cendes I (eds) Epilepsia. Lemos Editorial, São Paulo, pp 201–213. (in Portuguese)
7. Alvim MK, Coan AC, Campos BM, Yasuda CL, Oliveira MC, Morita ME, Cendes F (2016) Progression of gray matter atrophy in seizure-free patients with temporal lobe epilepsy. Epilepsia 57(4):621–629
8. Bonilha L, Alessio A, Rorden C, Baylis G, Damasceno BP, Min LL, Cendes F (2007) Extrahippocampal gray matter atrophy and memory impairment in patients with medial temporal lobe epilepsy. Hum Brain Mapp 28(12):1376–1390
9. Pereira FR, Alessio A, Sercheli MS, Pedro T, Bilevicius E, Rondina JM, Ozelo HF, Castellano G, Covolan RJ, Damasceno BP, Cendes F (2010) Asymmetrical hippocampal connectivity in mesial temporal lobe epilepsy: evidence from resting state fMRI. BMC Neurosci 11:66
10. Pittau F, Grova C, Moeller F, Dubeau F, Gotman J (2012) Patterns of altered functional connectivity in mesial temporal lobe epilepsy. Epilepsia 53:1013–1023
11. Voets NL, Beckmann CF, Cole DM, Hong S, Bernasconi A, Bernasconi N (2012) Structural substrates for resting network disruption in temporal lobe epilepsy. Brain 135:2350–2357
12. Yasuda CL, Chen Z, Beltramini GC, Coan AC, Morita ME, Kubota B, Bergo F, Beaulieu C, Cendes F, Gross DW (2015) Aberrant topological patterns of brain structural network in temporal lobe epilepsy. Epilepsia 56(12):1992–2002. https://doi.org/10.1111/epi.13225
13. Vaughan DN, Rayner G, Tailby C, Jackson GD (2016) MRI-negative temporal lobe epilepsy: a network disorder of neocortical connectivity. Neurology 87:1934–1942
14. Campos BM, Coan AC, Yasuda CL, Casseb RF, Cendes F (2016) Large-scale brain networks are distinctly affected in right and left mesial temporal lobe epilepsy. Hum Brain Mapp 37:3137–3152
15. Výtvarová E, Mareček R, Fousek J, Strýcek O, Rector I (2017) Large-scale cortico-subcortical functional networks in focal epilepsies: the role of the basal ganglia. Neuroimage Clin 14:28–36
16. Thom M (2014) Review: hippocampal sclerosis in epilepsy: a neuropathological review. Neuropathol Appl Neurobiol 40:520–543
17. Malmgren K, Thom M (2012) Hippocampal sclerosis: origins and imaging. Epilepsia 53(Suppl.4):19–33. https://doi.org/10.1111/j.1528-1167.2012.03610.x)
18. Crawford JR, Garthwaite PH (2002) Investigation of the single case in neuropsychology: confidence limits on the abnormality of test scores and test score differences. Neuropsychologia 40(8):1196–1208
19. Osterrieth PA (1944) Le test de copie d'une figure complexe. Arch Psychol 30:206–356
20. Kaplan EF, Goodglass H, Weintraub S (1983) The Boston naming test, 2nd edn. Lea & Febiger, Philadelphia
21. Lezak MD (1995) Neuropsychological assessment, 3rd edn. Oxford University Press, New York

22. De Renzi E, Vignolo LA (1962) The token test: a sensitive test to detect disturbances in aphasics. Brain 85:665–678
23. Wechsler D (1987) Wechsler memory scale-revised manual. The Psychological Corporation, San Antonio
24. Rey A (1964) L'examen clinique en psychologie. Presses Universitaires de France, Paris
25. Stroop JR (1935) Studies of interference in serial verbal reactions. J Exp Psychol 18:643–662
26. Heaton RK, Chelune GJ, Talley JL et al (1993) Wisconsin card sorting test. Manual. Psychological Assessment Resources, Odessa
27. Hermann BP, Seidenberg M, Schoenfeld J, Davies K (1997) Neuropsychological characteristics of the syndrome of mesial temporal lobe epilepsy. Arch Neurol 54:369–376
28. Sass KJ, Lencz T, Westerveld M, Novelly RA, Spencer DD, Kim JH (1991) The neural substrate of memory impairment demonstrated by the intracarotid amobarbital procedure. Arch Neurol 48:48–52
29. Jones-Gotman M, Brulot M, McMackin D, Cendes F et al (1993) Word and design list learning deficits related to side of hippocampal atrophy as assessed by volumetric MRI measurements. Epilepsia 34(Suppl. 6):71
30. Baxendale S, Thompson P (2010) Beyond localization: the role of traditional neuropsychological tests in an age of imaging. Epilepsia 51(11):2225–2230. https://doi.org/10.1111/j.1528-1167.2010.02710.x
31. Sidhu MK, Stretton J, Winston GP, Symms M, Thompson PJ, Koepp MJ, Duncan JS (2015) Memory fMRI predicts verbal memory decline after anterior temporal lobe resection. Neurology 84:1512–1519
32. Cendes F (2015) Can fMRI predict memory decline after temporal lobe resection? Nat Rev Neurol 11:372–374
33. Milner B (1972) Disorders of learning and memory after temporal lobe lesions in man. Clin Neurosurg 19:421–446
34. Jones-Gotman M (1996) Psychological evaluation for epilepsy surgery. In: Shorvon S, Dreifuss F, Fish D, Thomas D (eds) The treatment of epilepsy. Blackwell Science, Oxford, pp 621–630
35. Hermann BP, Seidenberg M, Schoenfeld J, Davies K (1997) Neuropsychological characteristics of the syndrome of mesial temporal lobe epilepsy. Arch Neurol 54:369–376
36. Baxendale SA, Thompson PJ, van Paesschen W (1998) A test of spatial memory and its clinical utility in the pre-surgical investigation of temporal lobe epilepspy patients. Neuropsychologia 36:591–602
37. Jones-Gotman M, Harnadek MCS, Kubu CS (2000) Neuropsychological assessment for temporal lobe epilepsy surgery. Can J Neurol Sci 27(Suppl 1):S39–S43
38. Leone AA, Damasceno BP, Cendes F, Guerreiro CAM (2001) Memory deficits in patients with temporal lobe epilepsy. J Int Neuropsychol Soc 7:429
39. Alessio A, Damasceno BP, Camargo CHP, Kobayashi E, Guerreiro CAM, Cendes F (2004) Differences in memory performance and other clinical characteristics in patients with mesial temporal lobe epilepsy with and without hippocampal atrophy. Epilepsy Behav 5:22–27
40. Alessio A, Pereira FR, Sercheli MS, Rondina JM, Ozelo HB, Bilevicius E, Pedro T, Covolan RJ, Damasceno BP, Cendes F (2013) Brain plasticity for verbal and visual memories in patients with mesial temporal lobe epilepspy and hippocampal sclerosis: a fMRI study. Hum Brain Mapp 34(1):186–199
41. Saling MM (2009) Verbal memory in mesial temporal lobe epilepsy: beyond material specificity. Brain 132(Pt 3):570–582
42. Willment KC, Golby A (2013) Hemispheric lateralization interrupted: material-specific memory deficits in temporal lobe epilepsy. Front Hum Neurosci 7:546. https://doi.org/10.3389/fnhum.2013.00546
43. Glikmann-Johnston Y, Saling MM, Chen J, Cooper KA, Beare RJ, Reutens DC (2008) Structural and functional correlates of unilateral mesial temporal lobe spatial memory impairment. Brain 131(Pt 11):3006–3018. https://doi.org/10.1093/brain/awn213

44. Gleissner U, Helmstaedter C, Schramm J, Elger CE (2002) Memory outcome after selective amygdalo-hippocampectomy: a study in 140 patients with temporal lobe epilepsy. Epilepsia 43:87–95
45. Weintrob DL, Saling MM, Berkovic SF, Berlangieri SU, Reutens DC (2002) Verbal memory in left temporal lobe epilepsy: evidence for task-related localization. Ann Neurol 51(4):442–447
46. Lillywhite LM, Saling MM, Briellmann RS, Weintrob DL, Pell GS, Jackson GD (2007) Differential contributions of the hippocampus and rhinal cortices to verbal memory in epilepsy. Epilepsy Behav 10(4):553–559
47. Kennepohl S, Sziklas V, Garver KE, Wagner DD, Jones-Gotman M (2007) Memory and the medial temporal lobe: hemispheric specialization reconsidered. NeuroImage 36:969–978

Chapter 20
Mild Cognitive Impairment and Early Dementia

20.1 Introduction

Aging is often accompanied by cognitive complaints distributed in a continuum ranging from sporadic and isolated failures of memory in normal subjects until full-blown dementia, whose main cause, in up to 70% of cases, is Alzheimer's disease (AD), with a prevalence estimated in 40 million patients worldwide. Isolated and mild memory complaints are common and have been described as "benign senescent forgetfulness," "age associated memory impairment," and lastly as "mild cognitive impairment." However, the mental disorders of aging are not restricted to memory but usually affect other cognitive functions (attention, executive functions, language, and visual-spatial abilities) as well as noncognitive domains manifesting as apathy, increased psychic fatigability and irritability, anxiety, affective lability, sadness, easy cry, and clear depression. Indeed, depression is more common in the elderly, usually manifested as atypical, with predominant somatic and cognitive complaints.

The diagnosis of AD is a challenge. On the one hand, up to 30% of patients with clinically typical AD dementia have normal biomarkers and no AD neuropathology, and more than 20% of typical cases older than 80 years have instead "limbic-predominant age-related TDP-43 encephalopathy" (LATE) or other conditions. On the other hand, up to 40% of cognitively normal elderly have positive AD biomarkers and neuropathological changes, besides about 20% of these normal elderly never developing dementia, even in their 90s, as shown by community-based long-term follow-up studies. All these findings and facts make a case against research criteria and frameworks based exclusively on biological biomarkers without taking into account clinical symptoms or functional impairment, which are the main characteristics of any disease. It is here that the neuropsychological evaluation plays a central role in characterizing the cognitive and behavioral changes typical of AD as well as in staging and following the disease.

B. Damasceno, *Research on Cognition Disorders*,
https://doi.org/10.1007/978-3-030-57267-9_20

20.2 Dementia

Dementia is a syndrome that may have different causes (brain diseases), and its diagnostic criteria have advanced by no more requiring obligatory memory impairment (amnesia) and by including changes of behavior and personality.

According to NIA-AA core clinical criteria [1], *dementia syndrome* is diagnosed when there is (1) cognitive and behavioral symptoms that are not explained by delirium or major psychiatric disorder, interfere with the ability to function at work or at usual daily activities, and represent decline from previous levels of functioning; (2) cognitive impairment detected by history taking (from the patient or knowledgeable informant) as well as by objective cognitive assessment ("bedside mental status examination or neuropsychological testing"); (3) cognitive or behavioral changes involving at least two of the following domains: (a) memory; (b) reasoning, executive functions and judgment; (c) visuospatial abilities; (d) language; and (e) personality and behavior.

The requirement of obligatory memory impairment in former diagnostic criteria (ICD-10, DSM-III, NINCDS-ADRDA) was probably due to the higher prevalence of AD as a cause of dementia, even though it was known that this disease may have non-amnestic presentations, such as the syndromes of posterior cortical atrophy, logopenic primary progressive aphasia, or behavioral frontal variant. Amnesia as initial symptom is even less frequent in vascular and frontotemporal dementia.

According to NIA-AA criteria, "significant interference in the ability to function at work or in usual daily activities" remains decisive for differentiating dementia from mild cognitive impairment. These criteria emphasize that this differentiation is a "clinical judgment made by a skilled clinician on the basis of the individual circumstances of the patient and the description of daily affairs of the patient obtained from the patient *and* from a knowledgeable informant." Thus, it is up to the clinician to make this judgment, which may sometimes be very difficult. For instance, what is a significant interference? Would be judged as dementia a college teacher's difficulties with episodic and semantic memory or a company CEO's failures with high-level complex executive tasks, which are in themselves mild from the point of view of normative scores, but at the same time severe enough to make these professionals inappropriate for keeping their jobs? Here is an area where a comprehensive neuropsychological assessment and detailed functional evaluation could help the clinician to make a more accurate and safe decision. Or in a reverse situation, would be judged as dementia the cognitive difficulties of an illiterate peasant presenting evident logopenic aphasic symptoms, episodic memory impairment, disorientation on official time, and inability to plan and execute complex activities, but not severe enough for impeding him to function well at his ordinary work and to maintain independence in his usual daily activities?

NIA-AA core clinical criteria for *probable AD dementia* further requires (1) presence of dementia, (2) with insidious onset and clear-cut worsening of cognitive symptoms, (3) initial and predominant deficits (evident on history and examination) in one of the following categories: (a) amnestic presentation (but with evidence of cognitive dysfunction in at least one other cognitive domain), or (b) non-amnestic presentation, which could be manifested in language (predominant word-finding difficulties) or visuospatial abilities or executive function (requiring deficits in other cognitive domains different from that of each of these presentations); and (4) this diagnosis of probable AD dementia should not be applied when there is evidence of concomitant cerebrovascular disease or prominent features of Lewy body dementia, behavioral variant frontotemporal dementia, semantic or nonfluent/agrammatic variant of primary progressive aphasia, or another neurological or decompensated non-neurological medical condition, or use of medication with evident cognitive side effects (polypharmacy dementia).

According to these criteria, the certainty of the diagnosis of probable AD is increased when there is (1) cognitive decline based on progressive deficits documented by subsequent evaluations, or (2) evidence of a causative genetic mutation (in APP, PSEN1, or PSEN2 genes), or (3) evidence of AD pathophysiological process, i.e., presence of biomarkers of brain amyloid-beta (Aβ) protein deposition (low CSF Aβ1-42 and positive PET amyloid imaging) and biomarkers of downstream neuronal degeneration or injury (elevated CSF tau, both total tau and phosphorylated tau; decreased FDG uptake on PET in temporoparietal cortex; disproportionate atrophy on MRI in medial, basal and lateral temporal lobe, and medial parietal cortex). The use of a fixed cut-off tau/Aβ42 ratio for CSF diagnosis of AD (e.g., >0.52) has its limitations and caveats, which have been highlighted by Lehmann et al. [2], for instance, (1) not taking into account p-tau (highly specific for AD); (2) using fixed ratios requires having similar values for Aβ42 and tau in the different laboratories, what is challenging; and (3) deciding for presence or absence (yes/no answer) of AD based only on CSF biomarkers, without considering a multimodal (even clinical) probabilistic approach to establish the diagnosis of AD.

20.3 Mild Cognitive Impairment and Prodromal Alzheimer's Disease

The term "mild cognitive impairment" (MCI) refers to a disorder of cognition that, differently from dementia, preserves the ability to carry out common activities of daily life (e.g., household chores), even though presenting some difficulties with more complex instrumental tasks. It has a prevalence of 3–19%, particularly above 65 years age, and about 35% of the cases convert to AD dementia within a 3-year follow-up, with an annual conversion rate of 5–10%, while that of normal controls is 1–2% per year [3]. A smaller proportion (11%) of MCI patients do improve to the extent that the underlying cause is resolved, e.g., cardiorespiratory disease, metabolic or endocrine dysfunction, depression, or severe psychosocial stress [4]. The more the cognitive domains affected, the higher the risk of MCI conversion to AD, particularly when there is deficit of both episodic memory delayed recall and executive functions associated with psychological and behavioral disturbances. The main challenge is to accurately diagnose the underlying etiology in every individual patient, especially because, in most cases, MCI is AD in an early prodromal phase, when new drugs could have their highest efficacy. This challenge has pressed the development of more accurate clinical criteria, with inclusion of biomarkers of the disease [5, 6]. Clinical diagnostic criteria for MCI have undergone revisions since the first one proposed by investigators of the Mayo Clinic, which required unique or predominant subjective and objective impairment of memory, with preserved independence in daily life activities [7, 8]. Besides the *single-domain amnesic MCI* (aMCI), other non-memory types of cognitive impairment were afterward taken into account: *multi-domain MCI*, affecting executive functions, visuospatial skills, and language, with or without memory dysfunction, and *single-domain non-memory MCI*, restricted, for example, to language or executive control [9–11]. Multi-domain MCI (mdMCI) can have varied etiology (degenerative, vascular, toxic-metabolic, traumatic, psychiatric), and it is more prevalent than aMCI [12].

Amnestic multi-domain MCI usually converts to AD, while the nonamnestic one most probably evolves to a non-Alzheimer dementia as the Lewy body dementia [13], Parkinson's disease [14], vascular cognitive impairment [15], as well as frontotemporal dementia, particularly in patients presenting prominent psychiatric and related behavioral symptoms in the absence of important cognitive impairment (so-called mild behavioral impairment, MBI) [16]. The introduction of the amnestic multi-domain MCI subtype represents an advance for improving sensitivity and specificity of AD diagnosis, considering the heterogeneous initial presentations of the disease. Neuropathological changes most often start in the medial temporal lobe (entorhinal cortex and hippocampus), giving amnesia as first and predominant symptom, and then spreading to temporal and parietal neocortex (including posterior cingulate and precuneus) as well as to dorsolateral and ventral-medial prefrontal regions, in this way additionally impairing other non-memory functions (language, visuospatial skills, executive functions, emotion regulation, behavior, and personality). Even when the disease starts with a non-memory disturbance (aphasia, apraxia, dysexecutive syndrome), it presents afterward amnestic symptoms, which may be detected even early by means of a comprehensive neuropsychological evaluation.

International working groups have further developed clinical criteria for improving the diagnostic and prognostic accuracy in cases of MCI suspect of being due to AD [5, 6]. The National Institute on Aging and Alzheimer's Association criteria for diagnosis of MCI due to AD (NIA-AA; [5]) comprise two levels of recommendations: the *Core Clínical Criteria*, to be used in all clinical settings without the need of highly specialized tests or procedures, and the *Clinical Research Criteria*.

I. *Criteria for the clinical and cognitive syndrome* comprise: (1) presence of concern about a change in cognition relatively to a previous level of functioning, as informed by the patient, a knowledgeable informant, or a skilled clinician; (2) objective evidence of impairment in one or more cognitive domains (memory, executive function, attention, language, visuospatial skills); (3) preservation of independence in functional abilities, although having mild problems performing complex instrumental tasks (e.g., paying bills, shopping, preparing special meals); (4) absence of dementia, that is, the cognitive impairment is sufficiently mild that it does not interfere in the ability to function at work or in usual daily activities; (5) the individual's scores on cognitive tests are typically 1 or 1.5 standard deviations below the mean of his/her age and education matched peers; and (6) etiology of the MCI clinical and cognitive syndrome consistent with AD according to a detailed and skilled clinical evaluation, results of neuroimaging, laboratory tests, and neuropsychological assessment, which ruled out other etiologies, or history consistent with familial AD, that is, the presence of one or more first-degree relatives having the disease or autosomal genetic mutations for AD (APP, PSEN1, and PSEN2 genes), or patient with one or two ε4 alleles in the apolipoprotein E gene, which gives increased risk for AD.

II. *Clinical Research Criteria* for MCI is intended to be used only in research settings and incorporates additionally the use of following AD biomarkers: reduced levels of Aβ1-42 and elevated levels of total tau (T-tau) and phosphorylated tau (P-tau) in the cerebrospinal fluid (CSF); amyloid deposition in the brain as assessed by positron emission tomography (amyloid-PET); medial temporal lobe atrophy on structural MRI; or a reduced glucose metabolism in temporoparietal regions on fluorodeoxyglucose PET (FDG-PET).

These biomarkers have also been more recently recommended by the International Working Group (IWG-2) criteria for diagnosis of AD and even for the prodromal phase of the disease [6]. With the IWG-2 criteria, the diagnosis of the *typical amnestic form of AD* is more simplified, requiring the presence of (1) episodic memory decline over more than 6 months as the first and most important clinical symptom, with objective evidence of low free-recall that is not normalized by cuing, which is highly correlated with hippocampal dysfunction and (2) the presence of one of the following biomarkers supporting the underlying AD pathology: decreased Aβ1-42 together with increased T-tau or P-tau in CSF, increased tracer retention on amyloid-PET, or AD autosomal dominant mutation present (in PS1, PS2, or APP genes).

These biomarkers are also required by IWG-2 criteria for diagnosis of *atypical AD* manifested as one of the following specific clinical phenotypes whose symptoms have early, progressive, and predominant presentation: (1) the *posterior cortical atrophy variant*, with the occipitotemporal subtype (impairment of visual identification of objects, faces, or symbols) and the more common biparietal subtype (visuospatial dysfunction, eye-hand dyscoordination, limb apraxia, neglect, or Balint syndrome); (2) the *logopenic variant* (progressive aphasia characterized by predominant difficulties with retrieval of single word and repetition of sentences but sparing semantic, syntactic and motor speech abilities); (3) the *behavioral frontal variant*, with apathy, executive dysfunction, disinhibited and stereotyped behaviors; and (4) *Down's syndrome variant* of AD characterized by early executive dysfunction and predominant behavioral changes [6]. IWG-2 criteria also define *mixed AD*, characterized by clinical and biomarker evidence for both AD and vascular or Lewy body disease.

20.4 Controversies Surrounding Biomarkers in the Early Stages of Alzheimer's Dementia

A first controversy regards the differentiation between biomarkers of AD diagnosis and biomarkers of AD progression. According to the IWG-2 criteria (differently from that of NIA-AA), downstream topographical biomarkers such as hippocampal atrophy on MRI and temporoparietal hypometabolism on FDG-PET are considered to lack pathological specificity for AD as they may be found in other diseases. Even hippocampal atrophy, considered to be a robust MRI predictor of conversion from prodromal AD to the dementia stage [17], can be found in other conditions such as old age, limbic encephalitis, Lewy body, and frontotemporal dementia, and it may not be present in early-onset nonamnestic (atypical) variants of AD. On the other hand, these topographical markers may show longitudinal changes typical of AD and, in this way, can monitor and measure disease course [6]. Repeated volumetric MRI can measure the rate of hippocampal atrophy over time, which is two to four times faster in AD than in normal aging [18]. In the same way, repeated FDG-PET can also show changes in the map of regional hypometabolism, which are linked to the clinical symptoms and deficits of the disease, thus serving as a sensitive biomarker of its stage and progression.

Another controversy is about the role of fibrillar Aβ deposits in AD. Focal extracellular accumulation of insoluble fibrillar Aβ (neuritic or senile plaques) and intracellular neurofibrillary tangles (NFTs) composed of hyperphosphorylated tau protein are considered the pathological hallmarks of the disease. The *amyloid hypothesis* assumes that Aβ accumulation initiates a cascade of pathological events causing synapse loss, formation of Aβ plaques and tau tangles, neuron loss, and subsequently dementia. Putative main supports for this hypothesis have been cases of early-onset AD (EOAD) caused by mutations of the amyloid precursor protein (APP) gene, mapped to chromosome 21, or cases of Down syndrome with triple copy of APP (trisomy 21). The sequential cleavage of APP (a transmembrane protein) by the β- and γ-secretases produces smaller peptides, Aβ peptides, among which the most neurotoxic are those constituted by 42 and 43 amino acids (Aβ42 and Aβ43). Thus, in cases of APP gene mutations or Down's syndrome, there would be abnormal processing of APP, overproduction, aggregation, and deposition of Aβ, subsequently driving hyperphosphorylation of tau protein, formation of intracellular tau aggregates (neurofibrillary tangles), and damage of synapses and neurons.

This invariant temporal sequence of pathological events has also been questioned [19, 20]. Some studies show that intraneuronal tau aggregates and MRI measures of brain atrophy (neurodegeneration) can appear decades before the deposition of Aβ plaques [21]. The amyloid hypothesis invariant temporal sequence has been supported by cases of early onset AD (EOAD), but these cases constitute only 5% of all AD cases [22]. The majority of AD cases have late onset (LOAD), associated with other genetic risk factors, particularly the *apolipoprotein E ε4 genotype* (APOE4; [23]), and the *triggering receptor expressed on myeloid cells 2 gene* (TREM2 gene; [24, 25]. APOE *ε4* genotype is the strongest genetic risk factor for LOAD, while the ε2 allele is protective [23]. APOE4 is a 299 glycoprotein expressed in the human brain predominantly by astrocytes and microglia and has high affinity for binding to (and sequestering) the soluble Aβ oligomer, besides enhancing the proteolytic degradation of Aβ within microglia cell and the ability of astrocytes to clear diffuse Aβ deposits [26–28]. TREM2 is a cell surface receptor (transmembrane glycoprotein) specifically expressed by microglia. Guerreiro R et al. (2013) and Jonsson T et al. (2013) identified a rare mutation (R47H) in the TREM2 gene, associated with increased risk (odds ratio > 3) for AD. This mutation leads to TREM2 deficiency, in this way impairing two main microglial functions necessary for containing (encapsulating) the inflammatory processes of fibrillar Aβ plaques, namely, phagocytosis (for clearance of amyloid proteins) and suppression of cytokine production and secretion [29–31]. R47H mutation results in reduced TREM2 binding affinity to Aβ42 oligomers as well as in decreased number of microglia around Aβ plaques, thus leading to greater diffusion and toxicity of Aβ oligomers [32, 33]. Interestingly, although APOE4 and TREM2 genotypes are not directly related to the APP gene, they contribute to increased AD risk at least in part by reducing brain clearance of Aβ, thus showing that microglia (neuroinflammation) is directly involved in the pathogenesis of the disease.

Another issue concerns whether or not Aβ accumulation is *necessary* or *sufficient* to produce the clinical symptoms of MCI and dementia [34]. Extracellular deposits of Aβ occur in normal aging, though they are more prevalent in AD. In quantitative histopathological studies, the number of insoluble Aβ plaques does not correlate with the degree of cognitive decline or dementia severity [35], while tau pathology does it [36]. There is a weak correlation between plaque load and cognitive scores, even though, as a general rule, the higher the number of plaques, the more severe the cognitive decline [37]. On the other hand, many patients presenting clinically typical AD dementia do not show enough AD pathological changes on PET imaging or autopsy. For these reasons, the amyloid hypothesis has shifted toward defining soluble Aβ oligomers as the toxic agent that impairs synaptic plasticity and consequently cognitive behavioral functions [38]. Indeed, there has been increasing evidence supporting this role of Aβ oligomers. Soluble oligomers of Aβ42 extracted from human AD brain and injected into healthy mouse hippocampus inhibit long-term potentiation, enhance long-term synaptic depression, induce progressive spine loss via downregulation of NMDA receptors and subsequently removal of AMPA receptors, thus decreasing synapse number and dendritic spine density, and impairing memory and learning [39–41].

In AD, intraneuronal accumulation of Aβ oligomers precedes its extracellular deposition, impairing the intracellular transport of brain-derived neurotrophic factor (BDNF), recycling endosomes, and mitochondria, causing mitochondrial dysfunction as well as damage of synapses and dendritic spines, independently of tau [42, 43]. On the other hand, it is well-known that Aβ oligomers induce tau hyperphosphorylation [41], by which tau protein undergoes intraneuronal posttranslational modifications, loses its affinity to the microtubules, and then aggregates into oligomers and NFTs, leading to disintegration of microtubules, in this way impairing intracellular transport of neurotrophic factors and organelles. Besides, there is growing evidence that Aβ oligomers may act synergistically with oligomeric forms of tau and soluble α-synuclein to promote synaptic dysfunction in AD [44, 45]. Moreover, soluble toxic aggregates (oligomers) of Aβ, tau, and α-synuclein can seed and propagate transynaptically by prion-like mechanisms (via endosomes and exosomes), spreading the disease in different regions of the brain, and consequently impairing the large-scale neurofunctional networks of cognition [46–48]. Additionally, Aβ oligomers seeds can act as a template for the aggregation of other proteins (PrP^c, TDP-43) generating overlapping phenotypes with other different neurodegenerative disorders [49].

All these findings suggest that aggregation of both Aβ and tau, especially as oligomers, is necessary and sufficient to produce AD dementia to the extent they cause widespread synaptic dysfunction and destruction. The rare cases of "tangle-only" or "plaque-only" dementia are probably associated with other brain pathologies [50]. Mutations in the gene of the microtubule-associated protein tau (MAPT gene) lead to tau aggregation (NFTs and neurodegeneration) and cause familial frontotemporal dementia (FTDP-17) but not AD.

Alzheimer's disease results from a complex interplay between genetic, environmental, and age-associated comorbid factors. In the majority of late-onset AD cases, with increasing age predominates the pathological contribution of other concomitant brain conditions, such as cerebrovascular diseases (CVDs), sequelae of former traumatic brain injuries or chronic exposure to neurotoxic agents, dyslipidemia, diabetes, hippocampal sclerosis, and α-synuclein deposition as Lewy bodies (abundant in more than 50% of AD cases; [51]). As summarized by Nelson et al. [52], "together, neurodegenerative diseases, CVD, and other aging-associated brain diseases weaken the apparent association between AD pathology and antemortem cognitive impairment."

Indeed, CVDs are the most prevalent concomitant pathologies in the brains of aged individuals, detectable in 75–90% of persons older than 90 years [52]. CVDs may be hypertensive, inflammatory, amyloidogenic, embolic, large- and small-vessel ischemic disease, and even microinfarcts (with diameter of 0.2–0.5 mm). Microinfarcts (MIs) are common in patients with AD (43%) and even in nondemented older individuals (24%) [53]. There is increasing evidence that MIs play a relevant additive, synergistic, and independent role in AD pathogenesis and cognitive impairment, even in those cases without atherosclerosis or cerebral amyloid angiopathy (the most important risk factor for MIs in AD). A probable mechanism by which MIs cause cognitive impairment could be that they are widespread and accompanied by diffuse hypoperfusion, hypoxia, oxidative stress, and inflammation, particularly in the watershed areas of the tertiary association cortex (in frontal and temporoparietal regions), and hence could damage large-scale neurofunctional networks and explain many of AD's cognitive and behavioral disorders [54–56]. MIs are more numerous in the watershed areas of middle and posterior cerebral arteries, i.e., parieto-occipital and parietotemporal cortical borderzones, which become early affected by Aβ accumulation, MIs, and afterward tau pathology, what could explain the high frequency of some of the earliest neocortical symptoms in the course of AD, e.g., word-finding difficulties. In this regard, Adamczuk et al.'s fMRI study of the associative-semantic system in cognitively intact older adults is quite illustrative. They examined whether amyloid load (as determined by ^{18}Flutemetamol PET) affects fMRI response during associative-semantic (confrontation naming) versus visuospatial processing, and they found that higher activity in the left posterior middle temporal gyrus correlated positively with increased amyloid load [57]. Higher amyloid load was correlated with slower confrontation naming. Interestingly, these cortical borderzones are among the regions that afterward become hypometabolic and/or atrophied in patients with MCI or AD [56, 58].

20.5 Preclinical AD and the Case Against an Exclusively Biological Definition of the Disease

Preclinical AD is defined as an asymptomatic or presymptomatic phase of the disease with evidence of typical pathophysiological processes or proven autosomal dominant mutation. One of the main reasons for introducing this diagnostic category has been the need to treat the disease as earlier as possible, since anti-Aβ clinical trials for AD in mild to moderate phase dementia failed to demonstrate clinical benefit, in spite of evidence that the trial resulted in decreased Aβ burden according to biomarker or autopsy evidence [34]. The intention is to treat AD early pathological processes (e.g., by lowering Aβ burden and/or decreasing neurofibrillary tangle formation) in order to prevent subsequent neurodegeneration as well as to delay the conversion to full-blown MCI or dementia.

NIA-AA proposed research criteria for preclinical AD [34] classifying it in three stages: *stage 1* characterized by asymptomatic amyloidosis, with high PET amyloid tracer retention or low CSF Aβ1-42 but negative markers of neuronal injury (tau, FDG, structural MRI); *stage 2*, asymptomatic amyloidosis plus evidence of one or more of following markers of neurodegeneration: elevated CSF T-tau/P-tau; neuronal dysfunction on FDG-PET or functional MRI (i.e., hypometabolism in posterior cingulate, precuneus, and/or temporoparietal cortices); cortical thinning (in lateral and medial parietal, posterior cingulate, and lateral temporal cortices) and/or hippocampal atrophy on structural MRI; and *stage 3*, amyloidosis plus markers of neurodegeneration plus subtle cognitive decline relatively to a baseline level of cognition, with poorer performance on more challenging tests but still performing within normal range on standard cognitive measures.

Afterward, the IWG-2014 [6] and IWG-2016 [59] proposed more simplified research criteria for diagnosis of AD in its *preclinical* asymptomatic phase, without considering stages of the disease and requiring the presence of at least one biomarker of AD pathology, which may be decreased Aβ1-42 together with increased T-tau or P-tau in CSF or increased retention on fibrillar amyloid PET; or the presence of AD autosomal dominant mutation (in PS1, PS2, APP, or other genes). The IWG-2016 defines preclinical AD in a cognitively unimpaired (CU) individual with abnormal Aβ and normal tau (A+T–) as "at risk for AD, asymptomatic Aβ+" and in a CU individual with normal Aβ and abnormal tau (Aβ–T+) as "at risk for AD, asymptomatic T+."

More recently, the NIA-AA has proposed a research framework intended for observational and interventional research, and not as guidelines for diagnostic criteria to be used in routine clinical care [60]. In this framework, AD is defined *biologically* as a continuum comprising (1) *Alzheimer's pathologic change* (not yet AD), with Aβ (*A*) positivity but without tau (*T*) or neurodegeneration (*N*) biomarkers [*A*+*T*–(*N*)–]; (2) *Alzheimer's disease*, with [*A*+*T*+(*N*)–] or [*A*+*T*+(*N*)+]; and (3) *Alzheimer's and concomitant suspected non Alzheimer's pathologic change* [*A*+*T*–(*N*)+]. As in the IWG-2016 criteria for preclinical AD, the diagnosis of the disease is based on its underlying pathologic processes (documented by in vivo biomarkers or postmortem examination), not on clinical symptoms or signs, which are regarded as neither sensitive nor specific for AD neuropathologic change, since, as it is argued, even a multi-domain amnestic dementia can be produced by other diseases besides AD. In fact, among patients with clinically typical AD dementia, 10–30% have normal PIB-PET or CSF Aβ42 and no AD neuropathology [50], and more than 20% (up to 50%) of cases older than 80 years have "limbic-predominant age-related TDP-43 encephalopathy" (LATE) as the underlying cause, according to large community-based autopsy series [61].

This framework as well as the IWG-2016 pose some problems. The first one is to settle the diagnosis of a disease without taking into account symptoms, signs, and functional impairment. The concept of disease is quite complex, comprising biological, medical, cultural, and anthropological aspects. The reduction of AD diagnosis to just a biological construct carries the risk of diagnosing the disease in people who will never develop mental-cognitive-behavioral dysfunctions or dementia. As cautioned by Khachaturian et al. [62] in an Editorial of Alzheimer's & Dementia, "just about every cognitively normal person >65 years has a few plaques and tangles in the brain," hence the need for "linking a semiquantitative evaluation of plaques and tangles to the probability that they may account for the cognitive impairment" or for making "accurate predictions of meaningful cognitive impairment in an individual with a positive biomarker."

The use of biomarkers alone to diagnose AD in an asymptomatic individual is problematic, since up to 40% of cognitively normal elderly have abnormal Aβ-biomarkers and AD neuropathologic changes [63]. Besides this, we know from clinical practice and prospective cohort studies that not all elderly become demented, even in their 90s. For instance, the Betula Project followed-up under 15 years a cohort of 1954 healthy adults aged 35–85 at baseline, all living in northeast Sweden (registered in Umeå city). The longitudinal trajectories of their episodic memory were assessed by means of validated tasks and not only global screening tests [64, 65]. After 15 years, 18% were classified as maintainers, 13% as decliners, and 68% as average performers. Thus, almost 20% (one fifth) maintained their high-level memory performance observed at baseline, and even increased it a little, probably due to practice effect (see the highest curve in Fig. 20.1).

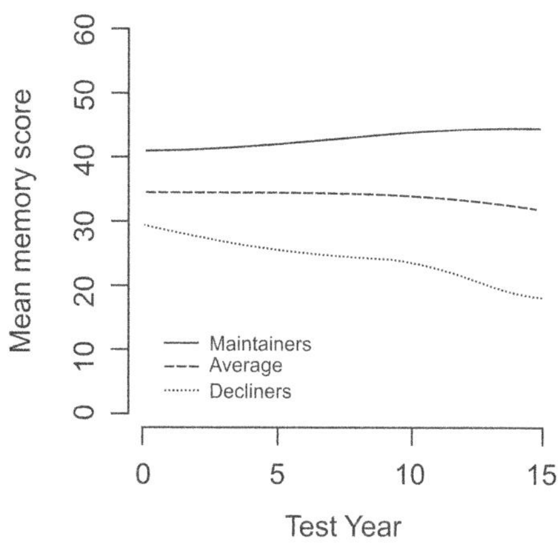

Fig. 20.1 Average test scores for 1558 participants (maintainers, average performers, and decliners) after 15 years follow-up in the Betula Project. (From Josefsson et al., 2012, JAGS, with permission of John Wiley & Sons, Inc.)

Participants with highest performance had similar or better results of memory and cognitive tests than those of younger adults, and they tended to have higher educational level (had got good grades on school exams), had been more physically active, were women, had been living with someone, and were carriers of the met allele of the catechol-O-methyltransferase (COMT) gene, which is involved in the degradation of dopamine. Former studies by researchers of the Betula Project had shown that carriers of the Met/Met genotype (with low COMT activity) performed better on episodic and semantic memory than carriers of the Val allele (with higher enzyme activity) [66]. On the other hand, decliners tended to be less educated, not active in the labor force, and had higher prevalence of apolipoprotein E ε4 allele, which is a risk factor for AD [23]. Thus, the exclusion of clinical (mental, cognitive, behavioral) symptoms and signs is not enough justified, since they are the main characteristics of any disease, even of diseases without measurable neuropathological changes, as a disabling anxiety neurosis. A better approach in preclinical or prodromal AD, particularly at the individual level, would be a combination of biological (CSF, imaging) and neuropsychological biomarkers put in an algorithm that could give a prediction of the disease in the form of a probability statement (as proposed by Khacharturian et al. [62]). In this algorithm, each putative biomarker could get a weight based on evidence derived from longitudinal studies of large enough population-based samples. Besides this, a temporal parameter could be added to the algorithm in order to detect dynamic changes in isolated or combined biomarkers, since a phenomenon is best understood if we know and take into account its temporal, historical dimension. These temporal parameters could be, for instance, annual tax of atrophy in AD relevant structures (e.g., hippocampal volume reduction, cortical thinning in lateral and medial parietal, posterior cingulate, and lateral temporal cortices); metabolic changes in posterior cingulate, precuneus, and/or temporoparietal cortices on FDG-PET or functional MRI; CSF T-tau/P-tau ratio; and qualitative and quantitative changes on standardized and validated neuropsychological tests, particularly in those assessing memory, language, visuospatial, and executive domains. This approach could be applied to investigations of both individuals and groups.

Recent studies have provided evidence for the relevance of including cognitive evaluation in the diagnosis of AD, even in its preclinical phase. Wolk et al. [67] followed-up 232 amnestic MCI patients from 2009 to 2014 and found the highest probability (hazard ratio) of AD when a positive Aβ PET scan, plus reduced hippocampal volume on high-resolution MRI, and poor cognitive status (MMSE plus immediate and delayed Logical Memory-II) were combined, giving an 8.45 times greater risk of progressing to probable AD (more than 90% converted to AD). Papp et al. [68] and Schindler et al. [69] could identify early decline of free and cued memory (by means of the Free and Cued Selective Reminding Test, FCSRT) in normal older adults, which was associated with high CSF tau/Aβ42 ratio or elevated β-amyloid burden on PiB PET imaging. In another study of preclinical AD by Landau et al. [70], 142 cognitively normal older adults, all considered amyloid negative at baseline, were followed-up with 18F-florbetapir PET scans and standardized tests for memory and executive functions during an average of 3.9 years. A greater Aβ accumulation was associated with greater composite score declines in the memory domain, even though not in the executive function domain. This study highlights the value of including cognitive (particularly memory) testing in preclinical AD, even when Aβ accumulation is still within the Aβ-negative range.

Cognitive decline has also been associated with changes in brain networks in AD patients, particularly in the default mode network [71–73]. In order to predict cognitive decline in preclinical AD, a recent study by Buckley et al. [74] submitted 237 clinically normal elderly (aged 63–90 years) to Aβ imaging with PiB PET and resting-state functional connectivity MRI (rs-fMRI). Baseline connectivity in four cognitive networks (default mode, salience, dorsal attention, and frontoparietal control) was used to predict longitudinal changes in the Preclinical Alzheimer Cognitive Composite (PACC), which comprises WMS Logical Memory IIa delayed recall, Mini-Mental State Examination (MMSE), WAIS-R Digit Symbol Substitution Test, and the Free and Cued Selective Reminding Test (FCSRT). Baseline connectivity in the default, salience, and control networks predicted longitudinal PACC decline after a median follow-up of 3 years, particularly in those individuals with combined higher Aβ burden and lower connectivity in the default mode network (DMN), which supports episodic memory. In such individuals, this combination could represent synaptic dysfunction by accumulation of Aβ oligomers in the DMN and other areas of high intrinsic connectivity [74, 75].

On the other hand, fMRI studies of preclinical AD subjects have shown initially increased activity correlated with higher amyloid burden in brain regions that later on become hypometabolic or atrophic as the disease progresses to its early clinical stages. This has been found in two critical hubs of cognition network, namely, the hippocampal formation for episodic memory [34] and the left posterior middle temporal gyrus for lexical-semantic retrieval [57]. This initial hyperactivity phase has been interpreted as due to deposition of soluble Aβ oligomers in synapses and neurons (before plaque formation), disrupting balance of synaptic excitation and inhibition, and consequently leading to dysfunction of local and large-scale networks [76].

In the study by Adamczuk et al. [57], 56 cognitively normal subjects (52–74 years age) underwent neurolinguistic assessment, 18F-flutemetamol PET, and a functional MRI paradigm using confrontation naming versus a visuoperceptual task as control condition. Activity in the left posterior middle temporal gyrus was higher with higher amyloid levels, which were correlated with slower confrontation naming.

Besides cognitive decline, psychological and behavioral symptoms also occur in preclinical AD, such as loneliness, apathy, and "subthreshold" anxious-depressive symptoms (defined as scoring ≤ 10 on the 30-item Geriatric Depression Scale, thus not fulfilling the criteria for major depression). These psychological and behavioral symptoms have been associated with higher amyloid-β burden and neurodegeneration as measured by PiB PET, MRI hippocampal volumetry, and cerebral 18F-fluorodeoxygucose (FDG) metabolism [77–79]. In preclinical AD, defined by amyloid positivity, early affective changes (such as increased emotional reactivity, anxiety, irritability) are associated with increased connectivity in regions of the salience network (right anterior insula and superior temporal sulcus), in contrast to the decreased connectivity observed in the default mode network [80–82].

In summary, the exclusion of clinical symptoms and signs from the diagnosis of preclinical AD is not scientifically justified, and we should be cautious in undertaking long-term interventional drug trials (as proposed by the NIA-AA Research Framework) based only on biological biomarkers, even when targeting tau pathology (more closely related to cognitive deficits) instead of anti-Aβ treatments, which have as yet failed despite being successful in removing or reducing brain deposits of β-amyloid. There is enough evidence that the inclusion of neuropsychological markers could help to make a better selection of patients for such trials and to come to a safer decision regarding the real efficacy of the drugs. And besides, the common occurrence of undesirable side effects should be taken into account, particularly considering the long-term treatment (years), and that many of these people, with or without the drug, would never develop Alzheimer's dementia, in spite of having positive biomarkers.

20.6 Preclinical and Prodromal AD: Neuropsychological Issues

Neuropsychology is in a unique and privileged position for (1) doing a qualitative and phenomenological analysis of the patient's symptoms by means of a comprehensive and deepened evaluation, searching for dissociations which could contribute to disclose the impaired basic mechanisms (mental operations) and, in this way, to diagnose the local or regional distribution of the brain dysfunction or lesion, and (2) for yielding a baseline of psychological, behavioral, and cognitive disturbances for future comparisons, be it in clinical trials or simply for following-up the evolution of the syndrome and for coming to a safer differential diagnosis of the suspect disease.

As regards AD, the neuropsychological evaluation can identify its earliest and subtle cognitive and behavioral changes, and so contribute to a more accurate diagnosis of the disease in its initial phase characterized by heterogeneous pathological and neuropsychological presentations [20, 83]. These heterogeneous initial manifestations have been classified firstly by Petersen [9] and Winblad [84] in different MCI subtypes, based on the following conventional criteria: (1) single domain amnesic MCI, affecting only or predominantly declarative memory (episodic, semantic, or prospective); (2) single domain non-amnesic (impairing language or visuospatial or executive function); (3) multi-domain amnesic; or (4) multi-domain non-amnesic MCI. More recently, other authors [85–87], based on actuarial neuropsychological approach and cluster analysis, have found three MCI subtypes: amnesic (isolated memory impairment), dysnomic (affecting mainly naming but also declarative memory), and dysexecutive/mixed (with significant deficit in executive function, attention, naming, and memory). As recognized by these authors, a limitation was the lack of assessment of visuospatial functions, usually affected early in prodromal AD.

Thus, a thorough qualitative and actuarial evaluation may disclose patterns or profiles of dysfunction in cognition (including high-level discursive social interaction and problem-solving) as well as in mood and behavior, which could characterize typical or atypical AD. To attain this goal, at least four cognitive domains commonly affected by the disease should be assessed, namely, the executive/attentional, language, episodic memory, and visuospatial [15, 88]. Several authors have given evidence that detailed actuarial neuropsychological data strongly correlate with neuroimaging and CSF biomarkers and contribute to the differential diagnosis between AD, in its different initial presentations, and other dementing disorders, such as the frontotemporal lobe degeneration, vascular cognitive impairment, and Lewy body disease [89–91]. In this regard, Edmonds et al. [87] found that the MCI subtypes had different (although partly overlapping) MRI patterns of cortical thinning (atrophy), which was seen primarily in bilateral medial and lateral temporal lobe regions in the amnesic MCI, or mainly in lateral (predominantly left) and medial temporal lobe as well as in frontal lobe regions in the dysnomic MCI, or was widespread bilaterally in frontal, temporal, parietal, and cingulate cortices in the dysexecutive/mixed MCI. For these authors, the patterns of cortical thinning observed across the three MCI subtypes suggest a progression of the disease, from a mild (amnesic) to a possible intermediate (dysnomic) and then to a severe (dysexecutive/mixed) stage, corresponding to the neuropathological Braak stages I-II (transentorhinal) through III-IV (hippocampal-limbic) and V-VI (necortical).

20.7 Limitations of Conventional Criteria for MCI and Prodromal AD

Unfortunately, most studies of preclinical and prodromal AD have trusted in a single cognitive test (e.g., Mini-Mental State Examination or delayed recall of a story) plus evaluation of common daily life functions (usually by means of CDR global scores).

This approach has resulted in inaccurate diagnoses, since impaired performance on a single neuropsychological test is common in neurologically normal adults [88, 92, 93]. The ADNI criteria for MCI, for instance, requires: (1) subjective memory complaints reported by the patient, his/her companion, or clinician; (2) objective memory deficit defined as scoring below an education-adjusted cut-off score on delayed recall of Story A of the WMS-R Logical Memory Test; (3) global CDR score of 0.5; and (4) sufficiently preserved performance on activities of daily life (i.e., absence of dementia).

These criteria have some limitations. First, story recall may be less sensitive to early MCI than tests of learning, delayed recall, and recognition of list of unrelated words, as measured, for instance, with the Rey Auditory Verbal Learning Test (RAVLT) or the Free and Cued Selective Reminding Test (FCSRT), whose failure is highly suggestive of temporolimbic (hippocampal) amnesia [68]. In story recall, on the contrary, words are semantically and coherently interconnected in a narrative, for this reason being more easily recalled, provided that neocortical regions (prefrontal, lateral temporal, and inferior parietal) are relatively preserved, as occur in the early phases of AD. A second limitation is the use of the global CDR score, heavily based on memory score, since memory is considered the primary category, and all others (Orientation, Judgment and Problem-solving, Community Affairs, Home and Hobbies, and Personal Care) are secondary. So, if we have a case with memory score of 0.5 and three secondary categories scoring 0 on one side of memory (e.g., Orientation = 0, Home and Hobbies = 0, and Personal Care = 0) while two secondary categories are scored 1 on the other side (e.g., Judgment and Problem-Solving = 1, and Community Affairs = 1), in this case, the global CDR score is equal to that of memory (= 0.5). In such a case, the use of the global CDR score would undervalue relevant information regarding instrumental activities of daily life (IADL) given in the scale by the items Judgment and Problem-Solving and Community Affairs, in this way failing to detect significant cognitive and functional changes in prodromal (MCI phase) AD, which could be indicative of further progression of the disease. This has been shown by Chang et al. [94] in a study of 283 MCI individuals, divided in two subgroups (intact IADL and impaired IADL) according to their scores on the three CDR categories assessing IADL (Judgment & Problem Solving, Community Affairs, and Home & Hobbies). They found that the IADL impaired MCI subgroup had worse episodic memory (on RAVLT delayed recall and recognition) and executive functions (on Trail Making Test Part B and Digit Symbol Test) as well as more widespread gray matter loss in frontal and parietal regions and higher percentage of subjects progressing to AD. For these reasons, researchers have looked for other alternatives to the global CDR score, including the CDR Scale Sum of Boxes scores (CDR-SOB) for its having increased range of values that make possible to detect smaller changes within and between dementia stages (i.e., through global CDR scores 0, 0.5, 1.0, 2.0, and 3.0), thus allowing to differentiate between MCI and very early AD. In this regard, O'Bryant et al. [95] studied 1577 participants (110 controls, 202 with MCI, and 1265 with probable AD) and found following optimal ranges of CDR-SOB corresponding to the global CDR scores: 0.5–4.0 for a global CDR score of 0.5; 4.5–9.0 for a global score of 1.0; 9.5–15.5 for a global score of 2.0; and 16.0–18.0 for a global score of 3.0. A third limitation of the CDR scale pointed out by Chang et al. [94] is the possibility of biases in the informant's report on IADL items, hence the need of an objective assessment of such abilities, for example, by means of subject-performed tasks that have better discriminative and predictive power.

In comparison with the ADNI criteria, the actuarial neuropsychological approach for MCI developed by Jak et al. [96] and Bondi et al. [97] represents an advance, since (1) it balances sensitivity (defining impairment below −1SD as opposed to −1.5 or −2 SDs of the ADNI and Petersen's and Winblad's criteria) and reliability (requiring two impaired scores within a domain as opposed to a single impaired score); (2) it uses two subtests for each of the main cognitive domains: memory (RAVLT delayed recall and delayed recognition), language [Boston Naming Test (30-items) and Category Fluency (animals)], and speed/executive function (Trail Making Test A and B); and (3) it includes scores of instrumental activities of daily living (Functional Assessment Questionnaire, FAQ). By this approach, MCI is diagnosed if any one of the following three criteria are met: (1) impaired score (defined as >1 SD below the age-corrected normative mean) on both subtests within at least one cognitive domain; (2) one impaired score (>1 SD below age-corrected normative mean) in each of the three cognitive domains; or (3) score on the FAQ = 9 indicating dependence in three or more daily activities. As recognized by these authors, a limitation is the lack of assessment of visuospatial functions, which could increase the reliability of their criteria.

These criteria have reduced the false-positive diagnostic errors. For instance, in a study by Bondi et al. [97], MCI was identified in less than 50% (401 subjects) of those 846 subjects that had been diagnosed as having MCI according to the ADNI criteria. Furthermore, in the ADNI sample of participants that had been classified as MCI, Edmonds et al. [86] found one-third (34%) of individuals which performed within normal limits in an extensive actuarial neuropsychological testing, besides showing low rate of progression to dementia as well as strong relationships between cognition and AD biomarkers.

Thus, a comprehensive, qualitative, and actuarial investigation may contribute to an accurate diagnosis of AD to the extent that it can (1) identify the earliest and subtle neuropsychological changes that occur in the preclinical and prodromal phase of the disease; (2) relate the profiles of increasing cognitive dysfunction to the heterogeneous regional distribution of neuropathological changes (MRI patterns of cortical atrophy) and based on these findings, (3) differentiate AD from other dementing diseases and follow its progression through the preclinical-prodromal-dementia continuum.

20.8 Conclusion

Dementia is a mental syndrome involving at least two different cognitive domains, with incapacity to function in common activities of daily life (ADL). A major issue is to diagnose their main cause, Alzheimer's disease (AD), in its prodromal or MCI phase. A diagnosis of "probable AD" can be established when there is progressive cognitive decline or evidence of a genetic mutation or biomarkers of AD pathological process, but the specificity of these biomarkers is controversial, since they are found in other diseases and even in normal aging. On the other hand, about 20% of patients with typical AD dementia have normal PIB-PET or CSF Aβ42 and no AD neuropathology (neurofibrillary tangles and plaques of insoluble fibrillar Aβ) but instead other conditions as TDP-43 encephalopathy (LATE).

Even more challenging is to diagnose AD in its asymptomatic preclinical phase. The recently proposed NIA-AA Research Framework is based exclusively on biological biomarkers, without considering clinical symptoms and/or functional impairment, thus carrying the risk of diagnosing AD in people who will never develop dementia, since abnormal Aβ biomarkers and AD neuropathologic changes are found in up to 40% of cognitively normal elderly, and in large long-term prospective cohort studies, almost 20% of the elderly maintain their high-level memory performance, even in their 90s. Thus, a better approach for diagnosing preclinical or prodromal AD would be to combine biological and neuropsychological biomarkers in a predictive algorithm with each putative biomarker getting a weight extracted from population-based longitudinal studies.

Another problem is the cognitive assessment of early AD using a single test (e.g., MMSE) plus global CDR scores, resulting in high rates of false-positive diagnostic errors. A more accurate diagnosis could be attained using a qualitative and actuarial neuropsychological approach by (1) evaluating at least episodic memory, executive/attentional, language, and visuospatial domains; (2) increasing sensitivity by defining impairment as below −1SD and reliability by requiring impairment in at least two tests within a domain; and (3) assessing instrumental ADL with CDR Scale Sum of Boxes scores or Pfeffer's FAQ or, especially in forensic cases, with objective evaluation of subject-performed instrumental tasks. Neuropsychological data gathered in this way has strongly been correlated to neuroimaging and CSF biomarkers, besides contributing to differentiate AD from other dementing disorders.

References

1. McKhann GM, Knopman DS, Chertkow H, Hyman BT, Jack CR Jr, Kawas CH, Klunk WE, Koroshetz WJ, Manly JJ, Mayeux R, Mohs RC, Morris JC, Rossor MN, Scheltens P, Carrillo MC, Thies B, Weintraub S, Phelps CH (2011) The diagnosis of dementia due to Alzheimer's disease: recommendations from the National Institute on Aging Alzheimer's Association workgroups on diagnostic guidelines for Alzheimer's disease. Alzheimer's Dement 7(3):263–269
2. Lehmann S, Gabelle A, Paquet C (2015) Can we rely only on ratios of cerebrospinal fluid biomarkers for AD biological diagnosis? Alzheimer's Dement 11:1125–1126
3. Michell AJ, Shiri-Feshki M (2009) Rate of progression of mild cognitive impairment to dementia – meta-analysis of 41 robust inception cohort studies. Acta Psychiatr Scand 119:252–265
4. Wahlund L-O, Pihlstrand E, Jönhagen ME (2003) Mild cognitive impairment: experience from a memory clinic. Acta Neurol Scand 107(Suppl 179):21–24
5. Albert MS, DeKosky ST, Dickson D, Dubois B, Feldman HH, Fox NC et al (2011) The diagnosis of mild cognitive impairment due to Alzheimer's disease: recommendations from the National Institute on Aging – Alzheimer's Association workgroups on diagnostic guidelines for Alzheimer's disease. Alzheimers Dement 7:270–279

6. Dubois B, Feldman HH, Jacova C, Hampel H, Molinuevo JL, Blennow K et al (2014) Advancing research diagnostic criteria for Alzheimer's disease: the IGW2 criteria. Lancet Neurol 13:614–629
7. Petersen RC, Smith GE, Waring SC, Ivnik RJ, Tangalos EG, Kokmen E (1999) Mild cognitive impairment: clinical characteristics and outcome. Arch Neurol 56:303–308
8. Petersen RC, Caracciolo B, Brayne C, Gauthier S, Jelic V, Fratiglioni L (2014) Mild cognitive impairment: a concept in evolution. J Intern Med 275:214–228
9. Petersen RC (2004) Mild cognitive impairment as a diagnostic entity. J Intern Med 256:183–194
10. Petersen RC, Morris JC (2005) Mild cognitive impairment as a clinical entity and treatment target. Arch Neurol 62:1160–1163
11. Delano-Wood L, Bondi MW, Sacco J, Abeles N, Jak AJ, Libon DJ et al (2009) Heterogeneity in mild cognitive impairment: differences in neuropsychological profile and associated white matter lesion pathology. J Int Neuropsychol Soc 15:906–914
12. Lopez OL, Jagust WJ, DeKosky ST, Becker JT, Fitzpatrick A, Dulberg C et al (2003) Prevalence and classification of mild cognitive impairment in the Cardiovascular Health Study Cognition Study. Arch Neurol 60:1385–1399
13. Ferman TJ, Smith GE, Kantarci K, Boeve BF, Pankratz VS, Dickson DW et al (2013) Nonamnestic mild cognitive impairment progresses to dementia with Lewy bodies. Neurology 81:2032–2038
14. Tröster AI (2011) A précis of recent advances in the neuropsychology of mild cognitive impairment(s) in Parkinson's disease and a proposal of preliminar research criteria. J Int Neuropsychol Soc 17:393–406
15. Gorelick PB, Scuteri A, Black SE, Decarli C, Greenberg SM, Idecola C et al (2011) Vascular contributions to cognitive impairment and dementia: a statement for healthcare professional from the American Heart Association/American Stroke Association. Stroke 42:2672–2713
16. Taragano FE, Allegri RF, Krupitzki H, Sarasola DR, Serrano CM, Loñ L, Lyketsos CG (2009) Mild behavioral impairment and risk of dementia: a prospective cohort study of 358 patients. J Clin Psychiatry 70(4):584–592
17. Risacher SL, Saykin AJ, West JD et al (2009) Baseline MRI predictors of conversion from MCI to probable AD in the ADNI cohort. Curr Alzheimer Res 6:347–361
18. Den Heijer T, van der Lijn F, Koudstaal PJ et al (2010) A 10-year follow-up of hippocampal atrophy on magnetic resonance imaging in early dementia and cognitive decline. Brain 133:1163–1172
19. Drachman DA (2014) The amyloid hypothesis, time to move on: amyloid is the downstream result, not cause, of Alzheimer's disease. Alzheimers Dement 10:372–380
20. Bondi MW, Edmonds EC, Salmon DP (2017) Alzheimer's disease: past, present, and future. J Int Neuropsychol Soc 23:818–831
21. Braak H, Zetterberg H, Del Tredici K, Blennow K (2013) Intraneuronal tau aggregation precedes diffuse plaque deposition, but amyloid-changes occur before increases of tau in cerebrospinal fluid. Acta Neuropathol 126:631–641
22. Thies W, Bleiler L (2011) Alzheimer's disease facts and figures. Alzheimers Dement 7:208–244
23. Corder EH, Saunders AM, Strittmatter WJ, Schmechel DE, Gaskell PC, Small GW, Roses AD, Haines JL, Pericak-Vance MA (1993) Gene dose of Apolipoprotein E type 4 allele and the risk of Alzheimer's disease in late onset families. Science 261(5123):921–923
24. Guerreiro R, Wojtas A, Bras J, Carrasquillo M et al (2013) TREM2 variants in Alzheimer's disease. N Engl J Med 368:117–127
25. Jonsson T, Stefansson H, Steinberg S, Jonsdottir I, Jonsson PV et al (2013) Variant of TREM2 associated with the risk of Alzheimer's disease. N Engl J Med 368(2):107–116
26. Holtzman DM, Herz J, Bu G (2012) Apolipoprotein E and apolipoprotein E receptors: normal biology and roles in Alzheimer's disease. Cold Spring Harb Perspect Med 2:a006312
27. Koistinaho M, Lin S, Wu X, Esterman M, Koger D, Hanson J, Higgs R, Liu F, Malkani S, Bales KR et al (2004) Apolipoprotein E promotes astrocyte colocalization and degradation of deposited amyloid-β peptides. Nat Med 10:719–726

28. Jiang Q, Lee CY, Mandrekar S, Wilkinson B, Cramer P, Zelcer N, Mann K, Lamb B, Willson TM, Collins JL et al (2008) ApoE promotes the proteolytic degradation of Aβ. Neuron 58:681–693
29. Takahashi K, Prinz M, Stagi M, Chechneva O, Neumann H (2007) TREM2-transduced myeloid precursors mediate nervous tissue debris clearance and facilitate recovery in an animal model of multiple sclerosis. PLoS Med 4:e124
30. Krabbe G, Halle A, Matyash V et al (2013) Functional impairment of microglia coincides with Beta-amyloid deposition in mice with Alzheimer-like pathology. PLoS One 8(4):e60921. https://doi.org/10.1371/journal.pone.0060921
31. Guerreiro R, Hardy J (2014) Genetics of Alzheimer's disease. Neurotherapeutics 11(4):732–737
32. Wang Y, Ulland TK, Ulrich JD, Song W, Tzaferis JA, Hole JT, Yuan P, Mahan TE, Shi Y, Gilfillan S, Cella M, Grutzendler J, DeMattos RB, Cirrito JR, Holtzman DM, Colonna M (2016) TREM2-mediated early microglial response limits diffusion and toxicity of amyloid plaques. J Exp Med 213(5):667–675
33. Zhong L, Wang Z, Wang D et al (2018) Amyloid-beta modulates microglial responses by binding to the triggering receptor expressed on myeloid cells 2 (TREM2). Mol Neurodegener 13:15. https://doi.org/10.1186/s13024-018-0247-7
34. Sperling RA, Aisen PS, Beckett LA, Bennett DA, Craft S, Fagan AM, Iwatsubo T, Jack JCR, Kaye J, Moantine TJ, Park DC, Reiman EM, Rowe CC, Siemers E, Stern Y, Yaffe K, Carrillo MC, Thies B, Morrison-Bogorad M, Wagster MV, Phelps CH (2011) Toward defining the preclinical stages of Alzheimer's disease: recommendations from the National Institute on Aging-Alzheimer's Association workgroups on diagnostic guidelines for Alzheimer's disease. Alzheimers Dement 7:280–292
35. De Strooper B, Karran E (2016) The cellular phase of Alzheimer's disease. Cell 164:603–615
36. Hardy J, Selkoe DJ (2002) The amyloid hypothesis of Alzheimer's disease: progress and problems on the road to therapeutics. Science 297:353–356
37. Nelson PT, Alafuzoff I, Bigio EH, Bouras C, Braak H, Caims NJ et al (2012) Correlation of Alzheimer disease neuropathologic changes with cognitive status: a review of the literature. J Neuropathol Exp Neurol 71:362–381
38. Selkoe DJ (2008) Soluble oligomers of the amyloid-beta protein impair synaptic plasticity and behavior. Behav Brain Res 192:106–113. https://doi.org/10.1016/j.bbr.2008.02.016
39. Shankar GM, Li S, Mehta TH, Garcia-Munoz A, Shepardson NE, Smith I, Brett FM, Farrell MA, Rowan MJ, Lemere CA, Regan CM, Walsh DM, Sabatini BL, Selkoe DJ (2008) Amyloid-beta protein dimers isolated directly from Alzheimer's brain impair synaptic plasticity and memory. Nat Med 14:837–842
40. Hsieh H, Boehm J, Sato C, Iwatsubo T, Tomita T, Sisodia S, Malinow R (2006) AMPAR removal underlies Ab-induced synaptic depression and dendritic spine loss. Neuron 52:831–843
41. Selkoe DJ, Hardy J (2016) The amyloid hypothesis of Alzheimer's disease at 25 years. EMBO Mol Med 8:595–608. https://doi.org/10.15252/emmm.201606210
42. Umeda T, Ramser EM, Yamashita M, Nakajima K, Mori H, Silverman MA, Tomiyama T (2015) Intracellular amyloid β oligomers impair organelle transport and induce dendritic spine loss in primary neurons. Acta Neuropathol Commun 3:51. https://doi.org/10.1186/s40478-015-0230-2
43. Ruy Y, Zheng JQ (2016) Amyloid β oligomers elicit mitochondrial transport defects and fragmentation in a time-dependent and pathway-specific manner. Mol Brain 9(1):79. https://doi.org/10.1186/s13041-016-0261-z
44. Guerrero-Muñoz MJ, Gerson J, Castillo-Carranza DL (2015) Tau oligomers: the toxic player at synapses in Alzheimer's disease. Front Cell Neurosci 9:464. https://doi.org/10.3389/fncell.2015.00464
45. Sengupta U, Guerrero-Muñoz MJ, Castillo-Carranza DL, Lasagna-Reeves CA, Gerson JE, Paulucci-Holthauzen AA et al (2015) Pathological interface between oligomeric alpha-synuclein and tau in synucleinopathies. Biol Psychiatry 78:672–683. https://doi.org/10.1016/j.biopsych.2014.12.019

46. Braak H, Braak E (1991) Neuropathological staging of Alzheimer-disease changes. Acta Neuropathol 82:239–259
47. Jucker M, Walker LC (2011) Pathogenic protein seeding in Alzheimer disease and other neurodegenerative disorders. Ann Neurol 70:532–540
48. Sengupta U, Nilson AN, Kayed R (2016) The role of amyloid-β oligomers in toxicity, propagation, and immunotherapy. EBioMedicine 6:42–49
49. Guerrero-Muñoz MJ, Castillo-Carranza DL, Krishnamurthy S, Paullucci-Holthauzen AA, Sengupta U, Lasagna-Reeves CA, Ahmad Y, Jackson GR, Kayed R (2014) Amyloid-β oligomers as a template for secondary amyloidosis in Alzheimer's disease. Neurobiol Dis 71:14–23. https://doi.org/10.1016/j.nbd.2014.08.008
50. Nelson PT, Braak H, Markesbery WR (2009) Neuropathology and cognitive impairment in Alzheimer disease: a complex but coherent relationship. J Neuropathol Exp Neurol 68(1):1–14. https://doi.org/10.1097/NEN.0b013e3181919a48
51. Resende R, Marques SC, Ferreiro E, Simões I, Oliveira CR, Pereira CM (2013) Effect of α-synuclein on amyloid β-induced toxicity: relevance to Lewy body variant of Alzheimer disease. Neurochem Res 38(4):797–806. https://doi.org/10.1007/s11064-013-0982-7
52. Nelson PT, Jicha GA, Schmitt FA et al (2007) Clinicopathologic correlations in a large Alzheimer disease center autopsy cohort: Neuritic plaques and neurofibrillary tangles "do count" when staging disease severity. J Neuropathol Exp Neurol 66:1136–1146
53. Brundel M, de Bresser J, van Dillen JJ, Kappelle LJ, Biessels GJ (2012) Cerebral microinfarcts: a systematic review of neuropathological studies. J Cereb Blood Flow Metab 32:425–436
54. Damasceno BP (2012) Relationship between cortical microinfarcts and cognitive impairment in Alzheimer's disease. Dement Neuropsychol 6(3):131–136
55. Westover MB, Bianchi MT, Yang C, Schneider JA, Greenberg SM (2013) Estimating cerebral microinfarct burden from autopsy samples. Neurology 80:1365–1369
56. Villeneuve S, Wirth M, La Joie R (2015) Are AD-typical regions the convergence point of multiple pathologies? Front Aging Neurosci. https://doi.org/10.3389/fnagi.2015.00042
57. Adamczuk K, De Weer AS, Nelissen N, Dupont P, Sunaert S, Bettens K, Sleegers K, van Broeckhoven C, van Laere K, Vandenberghe R (2016) Functional changes in the language network in response to increased amyloid β deposition in cognitively intact older adults. Cereb Cortex 26(1):358–373. https://doi.org/10.1093/cercor/bhu286
58. Dickerson BC, Bakkour A, Salat DH, Feczko E, Pacheco J, Greve DN et al (2009) The cortical signature of Alzheimer's disease: regionally specific cortical thinning relates to symptom severity in very mild to mild AD dementia and is detectable in asymptomatic amyloid-positive individuals. Cereb Cortex 19:497–510. https://doi.org/10.1093/cercor/bhn113
59. Dubois B, Hampel H, Feldman HH, Scheltens P, Aisen P, Andrieu S et al (2016) Preclinical Alzheimer's disease: definition, natural history, and diagnostic criteria. Alzheimers Dement 12(3):292–323. https://doi.org/10.1016/j.jalz.2016.02.002
60. Jack CR, Bennett DA, Blennow K, Carrillo MC, Dunn B, Haeberlein SB et al (2018) NIA-AA Research Framework: Toward a biological definition of Alzheimer's disease. Alzheimer's Dement 14:535–562. https://doi.org/10.1016/j.jalz.2018.02.018
61. Nelson PT, Dickson DW, Trojanowski JQ, Jack CR Jr, Boyle PA, Arfanakis K et al (2019) Limbic-predominant age-related TDP-43 encephalopathy (LATE): consensus working group report. Brain 142:1503–1527
62. Khachaturian ZS, Mesulam M-M, Mohs RC, Khachaturian AS (2016) Toward a consensus recommendation for defining the asymptomatic-preclinical phases of putative Alzheimer's disease? Alzheimer's Dement 12:213–215
63. Price JL, McKeel DW Jr, Buckles VD, Roe CM, Xiong C et al (2009) Neuropathology of nondemented aging: presumptive evidence for preclinical Alzheimer disease. Neurobiol Aging 30:1026–1036
64. Josefsson M, de Luna X, Pudas S, Nilsson L-G, Nyberg L (2012) Genetic and lifestyle predictors of 15-year longitudinal change in episodic memory. J Am Geriatr Soc (JAGS) 60(12):2308–2312

65. Nyberg L, Nilsson L-G, Letmark P (2016) Det Åldrande Minnet: Nycklar till att bevara hjärnans resurser. Natur & Kultur, Stockholm (in Swedish)
66. De Frias CM, Annerbrink K, Westberg L, Eriksson E, Adolfsson R, Nilsson LG (2004) COMT gene polymorphism is associated with declarative memory in adulthood and old age. Behav Genet 34(5):533–539
67. Wolk DA, Sadowski C, Safirstein B et al (2018) Use of flutemetamol F18-labeled positron emission tomography and other biomarkers to assess risk of clinical progression in patients with amnestic mild cognitive impairment. JAMA Neurol 75(9):1114–1123
68. Papp KV, Rentz DM, Mormino EC, Schultz AP, Amariglio RE, Quiroz Y, Johnson KA, Sperling RA (2017) Cued memory decline in biomarker-defined preclinical Alzheimer disease. Neurology 88:1431–1438
69. Schindler SE, Jasielec MS, Weng H, Hassenstab JJ, Grober E, McCue LM, Moris JC, Holtzman DM, Xiong C, Fagan AM (2017) Neuropsychological measures that detect early impairment and decline in preclinical Alzheimer disease. Neurobiol Aging 56:25–32
70. Landau SM, Horng A, Jagust WJ, for the Alzheimer's Disease Neuroimaging Initiative (2018) Memory declines accompanies subtreshold amyloid accumulation. Neurology 90(17):e1452–e1460. https://doi.org/10.1212/WNL.0000000000005354
71. Sheline YI, Raichle ME, Snyder AZ et al (2010) Amyloid plaques disrupt resting state default mode network connectivity in cognitively normal elderly. Biol Psychiatry 67:584–587
72. Jones DT, Knopman DS, Gunter JL et al (2016) Cascading network failure across the Alzheimer's disease spectrum. Brain 139:547–562
73. Weiler M, Northhof G, Damasceno BP, Balthazar MLF (2016) Self, cortical midline structures and the resting state: implications for Alzheimer's disease. Neurosci Biobehav Rev 68:245–255
74. Buckley RF, Scultz AP, Hedden T et al (2017) Functional network integrity presages cognitive decline in preclinical Alzheimer's disease. Neurology 89:29–37
75. Palop JJ, Mucke L (2010) Amyloid-β induced neuronal dysfunction in Alzheimer's disease: from synapses toward neural networks. Nat Neurosci 13(7):812–818
76. Busche MA, Konnerth A (2016) Impairments of neural circuit function in Alzheimer's disease. Philos Trans R Soc B 371:20150429. https://doi.org/10.1098/rstb.2015.0429
77. Donovan NJ, Hsu DC, Dagley AS, Schultz AP, Amariglio RE, Mormino EC, Okereke OI, Rentz DM, Johnson KA, Sperling RA, Marshall GA (2015) Depressive symptoms and biomarkers of Alzheimer's disease in cognitively normal older adults. J Alzheimers Dis 46(1):63–78
78. Donovan NJ, Okereke OI, Vannini P, Amariglio RE, Rentz DM, Psy D, Marshall GA, Johnson KA, Sperling RA (2016) Association of higher cortical amyloid burden with loneliness in cognitively normal older adults. JAMA Psychiat 73(12):1230–1237
79. Donovan NJ, Locascio JJ, Marshall GA, Gatchel J, Hanseeuw BJ, Rentz DM, Johnson KA, Sperling RA (2018) Harvard Aging Brain Study. Longitudinal association of amyloid beta and anxious-depressive symptoms in cognitively normal older adults. Am J Psychiatry 175(6):530–537. https://doi.org/10.1176/appi.ajp.2017.17040442
80. Zhou J, Greicius MD, Gennatas ED, Growdon ME, Jang JY, Rabinovici GD et al (2010) Divergent network connectivity changes in behavioral variant frontotemporal dementia and Alzheimer's disease. Brain 133:1352–1367
81. Balthazar ML, Pereira FR, Lopes TM, da Silva EL, Coan AC, Campos BM et al (2014) Neuropsychiatric symptoms in Alzheimer's disease are related to functional connectivity alterations in the salience network. Hum Brain Mapp 35:1237–1246
82. Fredericks CA, Sturm VE, Brown JA, Bilgel AYHM, Wong DF, Resnick SM, Seeley WW (2018) Early affective changes and increased connectivity in preclinical Alzheimer's disease. Alzheimer's Dement Diagnos Assess Dis Monit 10:471–479
83. Murray ME, Graff-Radford NR, Ross OA, Petersen RC, Duara R, Dickson DW (2011) Neuropathologically defined subtypes of Alzheimer's disease with distinct clinical characteristics: a retrospective study. Lancet Neurol 10:785–796

84. Winblad B, Palmer K, Kivipelto M, Jelic V, Fratiglioni L et al (2004) Mild cognitive impairment – beyond controversies, towards a consensus: report of the International Working Group on Mild Cognitive Impairment. J Intern Med 256:240–246
85. Libon DJ, Xie SX, Eppig J, Wicas G et al (2010) The heterogeneity of mild cognitive impairment: a neuropsychological analysis. J Int Neuropsychol Soc 16:84–93
86. Edmonds EC, Delano-Wood L, Clark LR, Jak AJ, Nation DA et al (2015) Susceptibility of the conventional criteria for MCI to false positive diagnostic errors. Alzheimers Dement 11(4):415–424
87. Edmonds EC, Eppig J, Bondi MW, Leyden KM, Goodwin B, Delano-Wood L, CR MD, for the Alzheimer's Disease Neuroimaging Initiative (2016) Heterogeneous cortical atrophy patterns in MCI not captured by conventional diagnostic criteria. Neurology 87:2108–2116
88. Bondi MW, Smith GE (2014) Mild cognitive impairment: a concept and diagnostic entity in need of input from neuropsychology. J Int Neuropsypchol Soc 20:129–134
89. Nordlund A, Rolstad S, Klang O, Lind K, Pedersen M, Blennow K, Wallin A (2008) Episodic memory and speed/ attention deficits are associated with Alzheimer-typical CSF abnormalities in MCI. J Int Neuropsychol Soc 14:582–590
90. Hantke N, Nielson KA, Woodard JL, Guidotti Breting LM, Butts A, Seidenberg M, Rao SM (2013) Comparison of semantic and episodic memory BOLD fMRI activation in predicting cognitive decline in older adults. J Int Neuropsychol Soc 19:11–21
91. Stricker NH, Salat DH, Foley JM, Zink TA, Kellison IL, McFarland CP, Leritz EC (2013) Decreased white matter integrity in neuropsychologically defined mild cognitive impairment is independent of cortical thinning. J Int Neuropsychol Soc 19:1–13
92. Heaton RK, Miller SW, Taylor MJ, Grant I (2004) Revised comprehensive norms for an expanded Halstead-Reitan Battery: demographically adjusted neuropsychological norms for African American and Caucasian adults. Lutz/Psychological Assessment Resources, Inc., Odessa
93. Jak AJ, Preis SR, Beiser AS, Seshadri S, Wolf PA, Bondi MW, Au R (2016) Neuropsychological criteria for MCI and dementia risk in the Framingham Heart Study. J Int Neuropsychol Soc 22(9):937–943
94. Chang YL, Bondi MW, McEvoy LK, Fennema-Notestine C, Salmon DP, Galasko D, Hagler DJ, Dale AM, for the Alzheimer's Disease Neuroimaging Initiative (2011) Global clinical dementia rating of 0.5 in MCI masks variability related to level of function. Neurology 76:652–659
95. O'Bryant SE, Waring SC, Cullum CM, Hall J, Lacritz L, Massman PJ, Lupo PJ, Reisch JS, Doody R, Texas Alzheimer's Research Consortium (2008) Staging dementia using Clinical Dementia Rating Scale sum of boxes scores. Arch Neurol 65(8):1091–1095
96. Jak AJ, Bondi MW, Delano-Wood L, Wierenga C, Corey-Bloom J, Salmon DP, Delis DC (2009) Quantification of five neuropsychological approaches to defining mild cognitive impairment. Am J Geriatr Psychiatry 17:368–375
97. Bondi MW, Edmonds EC, Jak AJ, Clark LR, Delano-Wood L, McDonald CR, Nation DA, Libon DJ, Au R, Galasko D, Salmon DP, for the Alzheimer's Disease Neuroimaging Initiative (2014) Neuropsychological criteria for mild cognitive impairment improves diagnostic precision, biomarker associations, and progression rates. J Alzheimers Dis 42(1):275–289

Index

B. Damasceno, *Research on Cognition Disorders*,
https://doi.org/10.1007/978-3-030-57267-9

W

Z

The manufacturer's authorised representative in the EU is Springer Nature Customer Service Centre GmbH, Europaplatz 3, 69115 Heidelberg, Germany. If you have any concerns regarding our products, please contact ProductSafety@springernature.com

Printed and bound by CPI Group (UK) Ltd, Croydon, CR0 4YY
30/09/2026
02225497-0010